Second Edition

Stuttering and Other Fluency Disorders

Franklin H. Silverman
Marquette University
Medical College of Wisconsin

Allyn and Bacon
Boston • London • Toronto • Sydney • Tokyo • Singapore

Series Editor: Kris Farnsworth
Editorial Assistant: Christine M. Shaw
Senior Marketing Manager: Kathy Hunter
Editorial-Production Administrator: Joe Sweeney
Editorial-Production Service: Walsh Associates
Composition Buyer: Linda Cox
Manufacturing Buyer: Megan Cochran
Cover Administrator: Suzanne Harbison

Library of Congress Cataloging-in-Publication Data
Silverman, Franklin H.
    Stuttering and other fluency disorders : an overview for beginning
clinicians / Franklin H. Silverman. — 2nd ed.
      p.   cm.
    Includes bibliographical references and indexes.
    ISBN 0-205-17514-7
    1. Stuttering. I. Title.
    [DNLM: 1. Stuttering. WM 475 S587s 1995]
RC424.S57   1995
616.85'54–dc20
DNLM/DLC
for Library of Congress   95-24637
                                         CIP

Printed in the United States of America
10 9 8 7 6 5 4 3 2 1   00 99 98 97 96 95

This book is dedicated to the memory of three giants on whose shoulders I have been privileged to stand who refused to allow their stuttering to keep them in chains: Wendell Johnson, Charles Van Riper, and Dean Williams.

Contents

Preface

This second edition, like the first, presents the topics that usually are addressed in stuttering and fluency disorder courses. The literature review has been updated and material on the other fluency disorders has been expanded (see Chapter 8). This book is still the only one currently in print that reviews the literature on all fluency disorders. Its purpose is to provide upper-division undergraduate and master's level graduate students as well as working clinicians with the information they need to be helpful to persons with these disorders.

I don't believe that it's possible to really understand the symptomatology and management of a disorder and the effect it can have on people's lives merely by reading about it. You have to encounter its various aspects through simulations and other types of experiences. Thus, each chapter contains assignments, simulation and experiential ones, to increase your understanding of the symptomatology of fluency disorders, their management, and the attitudes of children and adults who have them.

The abnormal behaviors exhibited by all children and adults who have a particular fluency disorder are not the same. Clinicians need a structure, therefore, for evaluating and describing behaviors that define the stuttering problems of their clients. They also need one for differentiating stuttering from normal disfluency and other fluency disorders. An approach that provides such structures is described in this book.

Also provided are a number of tasks and questionnaires for describing aspects of a client's fluency disorder and his or her reactions to it (Appendix C) and wordings and structures abstracted from evaluation reports by experienced clinicians that can be helpful when preparing such reports (Appendix A).

Clinicians also need a structure for establishing therapy goals and for developing intervention strategies to achieve them. An approach, described in this book, provides such a structure and takes into consideration why the clinician believes the client is behaving in a particular way. Considerable emphasis is placed on the principle that the approach a clinician uses to modify a behavior should be based on his or her assumption (hypothesis) about the reason(s) a client exhibits it.

Authorities do not agree about the etiology of stuttering. Some view it as completely physiological, some as completely psychological, and some (including myself) as a combination of the two. Both contemporary and historical theories concerning its etiology are discussed in this book. Like all authors of books on stuttering, I have beliefs about this that influence both the amount of space devoted to discussing individual theories (and topics related to them) and how certain studies are interpreted. To judge the credibility of my viewpoints you should know my background and experience with stuttering. I have taught courses dealing with stuttering for more than twenty years, and for more than thirty years have treated children and adults who have the disorder. I was a research associate in the Stuttering Research Program at the University of Iowa and have authored or coauthored more than fifty papers on stuttering. Most were published in the *Journal of Speech and Hearing Disorders,* the *Journal of Speech and Hearing Research,* and the *Journal of Fluency Disorders.* I have served as an editorial consultant for papers on fluency disorders for these and other journals, and for three years I was associate editor of the *Journal of Speech and Hearing Research* with responsibility for the editorial processing of all papers submitted on these disorders. And for several years I facilitated a self-help/support group that was affiliated with the National Stuttering Project for persons who stutter. Finally, I have had more than fifty years of personal experience with stuttering since I have done so since early childhood.

Franklin H. Silverman

▶ 1

Stuttering and Normal Disfluency: An Overview

My intent in this book is to provide clinicians, particularly beginning ones, with the information they need to be helpful to persons who stutter or have another fluency disorder. Almost all the information on stuttering is in the first seven chapters. Although much of the information about the other fluency disorders is in Chapter 8, there is information in the other chapters—particularly in Chapters 6 and 7—that is relevant for their management. No previous knowledge about fluency disorders is assumed.

To be helpful to a person who has a problem you have to understand the problem. You have to understand what the person is experiencing and how it affects his or her life.

The manner in which a problem affects your life can contribute to—become a part of—the problem. The amount it prevents you from doing what you want to do determines the degree to which it causes you to be handicapped. Persons who have fluency disorders can be handicapped as much or more by their reactions to their abnormal disfluency than by the disfluency itself (e.g., Attanasio, 1987b; Carlisle, 1985; Johnson, 1930; Murray & Edwards, 1980; Sugarman, 1980; Van Riper, 1984). Hence, reducing the severity of their problem may involve, in part, modifying their reactions to their hesitations.

STUTTERING AND THE STUTTERING PROBLEM

My primary objective in this section is to define stuttering and to begin acquainting you with the various dimensions of the stuttering problem. Note that the terms *stuttering* and *stuttering problem,* as used in this book, have different meanings.

1

Stuttering

There is disagreement about how the term *stuttering* should be defined (e.g., see Adams & Runyan, 1981; Alfonso, 1990; Andrews et al., 1983; Bloodstein, 1990; Conture, 1990a; Cordes & Ingham, 1995a; Culatta & Leeper, 1988; Hegde, 1978; Ingham, 1990a; Moore & Perkins, 1990; Perkins, 1983a, 1990a, 1990b; Smith, 1990a; Van Riper, 1982; Wingate, 1981a, 1984a, 1987). Almost all definitions mention repetitions of sounds and syllables and prolongations of speech sounds. And almost all mention difficulty in beginning to say words, that is, the person knows what he or she wants to say, but has to "strain" to say it. This type of abnormal speech disfluency has been referred to as *stammering*. The following extract illustrates how authorities once attempted to differentiate stammering from stuttering.

> *Formerly, authorities tried to differentiate between stuttering and stammering by saying, for example, that stuttering was a physical and stammering a psychological defect; that stuttering was a rapid repetition of one sound (c-c-c-cat) and stammering was an inability to produce voice; that stuttering was a halt on consonants and stammering was a halt on vowels; or, again, that stuttering was a disorder met with only in young children which developed into stammering if incorrectly treated. (Boome & Richardson, 1931, p. 7)*

The term stammering is now rarely used in the United States because the hesitations associated with it are thought to have the same etiology (or etiologies) as stuttering-type sound and syllable repetitions (Van Riper, 1982).

Before we examine some definitions of stuttering, we will consider several reasons why there are differences in how it is defined. One is that those who did the defining attended to (or "abstracted") different attributes of the behavior (Johnson, 1946). When you describe an event, you talk about those attributes you consider to be significant. Two people viewing an event (in this case, stuttering) are unlikely to abstract the same attributes of it and are therefore unlikely to describe it in the same way. This is illustrated by the fable of the six blind men and the elephant:

> *Six blind men who attempted to describe an elephant came up with six different descriptions. They differed in part because they had observed (felt) different parts (attributes) of the animal. However, even if they had observed (felt) the same thing, they likely would have "abstracted" (attended to) different aspects of the experience and, hence, still would have come up with different descriptions. (Johnson, 1958, p. xii)*

Since each blind man felt a different part of the elephant, he only described one attribute of it: however, all their definitions contained some "kernel of truth." Likewise, those who have tried to define stuttering have not necessarily attended to (abstracted) the same aspects (attributes) of it: hence, their definitions are different.

Another reason why definitions of stuttering differ is that some are partially or wholly based on hypotheses about its etiology. Rather then *describing* stuttering they try to *explain* it. Wendell Johnson (1958), for example, defined stuttering as an "anticipatory, apprehensive, hypertonic avoidance reaction." Coriat (1933) defined it as "a psychoneurosis caused by the persistence into later life of early pregenital oral nursing, oral sadistic, and anal sadistic components." And Brutten and Shoemaker (1967) defined it as "that form of fluency failure that results from conditioned negative emotion."

Now that we have considered a few of the reasons why definitions of stuttering tend to differ, we will attempt to glean the "kernel of truth" from several of them. This discussion is intended to lay a foundation for developing an intuitive understanding of the symptomatology and phenomenology of the disorder.

Some definitions of stuttering deal only with audible aspects of speaking behavior. The following are representative of such definitions:

> *Stuttering is a deviation in the ongoing fluency of speech, an inability to maintain the connected rhythms of speech. (Van Riper, 1982, p. 11)*

> *There is a consensus that repetitions and prolongations are necessary and sufficient for the diagnosis of stuttering to be made. (Andrews et al., 1983, p. 227)*

The "kernel of truth" in these is that the stutterer does exhibit a disturbance in the ongoing rhythm or fluency of speech. He or she repeats, prolongs, or both. However, normal speakers—both children and adults—also repeat and prolong. In fact, some persons who are regarded by themselves and others as normal speakers repeat and/ or prolong sounds more frequently than some who are regarded by themselves and others as stutterers (see Johnson, 1961; Johnson & Associates, 1959; Silverman, 1974). Such definitions are inadequate, therefore, for differentiating *moments of stuttering* from normal speech prolongations and repetitions (i.e., from *disfluencies*). They also are inadequate for determining whether a person, particularly a preschool-age child, is beginning to stutter. Normal speaking preschool-age children, for example, repeat sounds, syllables, and words (particularly single syllable ones) a great deal (see Conture, 1990a; Davis, 1939; Metraux, 1950; Johnson & Associates, 1959; Silverman & Williams, 1972a; Yairi, 1981, 1982, 1990).

Definitions that deal solely with audible aspects of speaking behavior are inadequate for a second reason. They do not allow the differentiation between stuttering and other fluency disorders.

The following are three somewhat more complex definitions of stuttering:

> *Stuttering occurs when the forward flow of speech is interrupted by a motorically disrupted sound, syllable, or word, or by the speaker's reactions thereto. (Van Riper, 1982, p. 15)*

Disorders in the rhythm of speech in which the individual knows precisely what he wishes to say, but at the time is unable to say it because of an involuntary, repetitive prolongation or cessation of a sound. (World Health Organization, 1977, p. 202)

Stuttering is the involuntary disruption of a continuing attempt to produce a spoken utterance. (Perkins, 1990a, p. 376)

The first of these definitions considers not only the audible disruptions in the forward flow of speech, but the speaker's reactions to them. Perhaps one of the most significant ways that stutterers' speech hesitations differ from those of normal speakers is that stutterers tend to react to theirs and normal speakers do not (Bloodstein, 1987). Stutterers react to their abnormal disfluencies with fear and embarrassment and *try to minimize (avoid) them.* One of the most "successful" strategies they can use for this purpose is not talking, particularly when stuttering is anticipated. When a stutterer doesn't speak, he or she doesn't stutter! While reducing verbal output minimizes stuttering, it also interferes with communication, thereby adversely affecting interpersonal relationships.

The second, which is a definition that is used internationally because it was promulgated by the World Health Organization, includes the fact that the abnormal repetitions and prolongations exhibited by stutterers are *involuntary.* This is considered by some to be the "most invariant fundamental characteristic" of the disorder (see Cooper, 1968; Manning, 1977; Perkins, 1994). The inclusion of this word is essential for differentiating the disfluencies of stuttering from normal disfluencies, for the following reason:

If the essence of clinical stuttering is in the involuntary aspect of disfluency, and not in its overt form, then the question arises whether or not a particular disfluency is stuttered or normal. If normal, the presumption seems to be that it is a manifestation of linguistic uncertainty, and therefore is a characteristic shared by all speakers. If stuttered, the disfluency presumably is a motor speech blockage, an atypical abnormal form of disfluency. (Perkins, 1983a, p. 247)

The third of these definitions, like the second, stresses the involuntary nature of stuttering, but defines the disorder from the stutterer's perspective, rather than that of the listener. According to Perkins (1990a):

... stuttering is a problem of involuntary disruption of a word the speaker is otherwise attempting to utter, rather than the resulting acoustic event, which is what the listener perceives.... Because all types of disfluency characteristic of stuttering also occur as nonstuttered disfluency, the listener can only guess which is which.... From the stutterer's vantage point,

however, the judgment is categorical: Either involuntary blockage has or has not occurred to some degree. If it has not occurred, then what sounds like stuttering to the observer would not feel like stuttering to the speaker. The reason that this distinction is categorical is because the proposed definition posits that loss of control of the ability to voluntarily continue a disrupted utterance is the essence of stuttering. If the disruption is not involuntary to some degree, then it is not a stuttered disfluency. Moreover, the stutterer would not react to it with apprehension, struggle, or avoidance as if it were stuttered. (p. 376)

For commentaries on this definition see Bloodstein (1990), Ingham (1990a), Perkins (1990b, 1991), Siegel (1991), and Smith (1990b).

We will consider next the "standard definition" proposed by Wingate (1964), which is more complex than the previous ones:

The term "stuttering" means: I. (a) disruption in the fluency of verbal expression, which is (b) characterized by involuntary, audible, or silent repetitions or prolongations in the utterance of short speech elements, namely: sounds, syllables, and words of one syllable. These disruptions (c) usually occur frequently or are marked in character and (d) are not readily controllable. II. Sometimes the disruptions are (e) accompanied by accessory activities involving the speech apparatus, related or unrelated body structures, or stereotyped speech utterances. These activities give the appearance of being speech-related struggle. III. Also, there not infrequently are (f) indications or reports of the presence of an emotional state, ranging from a general condition of "excitement" or "tension" to more specific emotions of a negative nature such as fear, embarrassment, irritation, or the like. (g) The immediate source of stuttering is some incoordination expressed in the peripheral speech mechanism; the ultimate cause is presently unknown and may be complex or compound. (p. 498)

This definition, which is among the most frequently cited ones (see Alfonso, 1990; Conture, 1990b; Martin & Haroldson, 1981), provides additional information about moments of stuttering. It can be gleaned from this definition that some moments of stuttering are partially or completely silent. They do not consist of sound prolongations or repetitions. However, there may be audible sounds associated with tension when they occur between words. Such pauses between words for this reason have been labeled *tense pauses* (Williams, Silverman, & Kools, 1968). There may also be visible signs of tensing—particularly in the facial area—during them.

It also can be gleaned from this definition that moments of stuttering may occur frequently, but not on every word. Even the most severe stutterer says some words fluently. This suggests both that the functioning of stutterers' speech mechanisms is adequate for speaking fluently at least some of the time and that they know how to do so.

A third such kernel of truth is that moments of stuttering frequently are accompanied by movements (gestures) not needed for producing the phonemes in the message. Such movements can involve the musculature of the speech mechanism, the head and neck, and/or the extremities and can also involve utterances of sounds, words, or phrases that are not a part of the message being communicated. Examples of movements involving the speech mechanism would be pressing the lips together when attempting to produce phonemes that are not bilabials and attempting to speak with inadequate breath support. Examples involving the head and neck would be closing the eyes and moving the head back. Those involving the extremities would be swinging an arm or tapping a foot. And examples of extraneous sounds, words, or phrases would be single or multiple productions of a vowel such as the schwa, a word such as "well," or a phrase such as "it is." Such utterances may be devices that the stutterer uses to keep from stuttering or has used in the past for this purpose and, although no longer working, have become a habitual part of this person's stuttering behavior. These extraneous movements sometimes are referred to as *secondary symptoms* or *secondaries.*

A final kernel that can be gleaned is that stuttering frequently is accompanied by an emotional state. Listeners may be aware of this state or it may be experienced solely by the stutterer. The emotional state may be one of fear, anxiety, tension, shame, embarrassment, or some combination of these. While speaking, a stutterer may evince both tension and embarrassment: He or she may communicate tension by voice quality and embarrassment by not maintaining normal eye contact while stuttering (Atkins, 1988; Tatchell et al., 1983). Whether these emotional states are associated with the cause of stuttering or are a result of it has not been established unequivocally.

The Stuttering Problem

The term *stuttering problem* as used here refers to abnormal speaking behaviors exhibited by persons who stutter as well as to the undesirable behaviors, attitudes, and feelings caused by their attempts to cope with (minimize) anticipated negative reactions to their stuttering (see Hulit & Wirtz, 1994). Such behaviors would include not speaking in certain situations in which it would be advantageous to do so (e.g., asking questions in class) and not pursuing a desired vocation or avocation. While persons who stutter may have "reality-based" reasons for avoiding certain vocations or avocations, most of those avoided by persons with whom I have worked were ones in which they probably could have performed competently judging, in part, by the fact that others who stutter have been successful in them. These include medicine, nursing, law, teaching, politics, sales, social work, theater, sports, business administration, writing, and speech pathology. Some persons who were very prominent in such fields in spite of the fact they stuttered were King George VI of

England, Winston Churchill, Lenin, Theodore Roosevelt, Washington Irving (author), George Washington, Charles Lamb (author), Charles Darwin, Moses, Aesop, Virgil, Aristotle, Demosthenes, and Napoleon the First. Others include Michael Ramsey (one hundredth Archbishop of Canterbury), Mel Tillis (country-western singer), Lewis Carroll (author), Marilyn Monroe (actress), Clara Barton (founder of the Red Cross), Somerset Maugham (author), Moses Mendelssohn (eighteenth-century Jewish philosopher), Annie Glenn (wife of U.S. Senator and Astronaut John Glenn), Carly Simon (composer-performer), and John Updike (author). For information about the impacts that stuttering has had on the lives of "successful" persons see Attanasio (1987b), De Keyser (1973) and Tillis & Wager (1984).

The severity of a person's stuttering problem is determined both by the amount he or she stutters and the amount of negative impact that stuttering has on the person's life. Hence, a person who stutters very little but avoids talking could have a more severe stuttering problem than one who stutters quite a bit but does not avoid talking.

Stuttering as a Component of the Stuttering Problem

Now that we have defined the terms stuttering and stuttering problem, we will consider further how the behaviors to which they refer differ. Abnormal disfluencies and other behaviors that occur during moments of stuttering are one aspect of the stuttering problem. According to Sheehan (1984):

> *Defining stuttering [solely] as a fluency problem ignores the person; it ignores his feelings about himself; it ignores the significance of stuttering in his life;... it ignores the principle that just because an individual stutters, that is not necessarily the chief problem with which a clinician need be concerned. (p. 226)*

The stuttering problem of a particular person is likely to include behaviors other than the ones we have just discussed, and its severity is not necessarily determined by their frequency or duration. For example, a person who stutters very little but usually tries to conceal the problem (e.g., by not talking unless absolutely necessary) can have a more severe stuttering problem than one who stutters quite a bit, but usually does not let it become a hinderance to communicating or otherwise doing what he or she wants to do.

The stuttering problem of a particular child or adult at any point in time can be defined by a *set of behaviors*. This set is likely to include behaviors that are not a part of the moment of stuttering. Some of these behaviors may occur while the person is not stuttering or even speaking. The severity of a person's stuttering problem is a function of the number and types of behaviors in the set that defines it. Viewed from this perspective, the goal of the evaluation process (assuming that it has been established that the person has a stuttering problem) is to identify the set of behaviors that define it. And the goal of the intervention process is either to eliminate or reduce the frequency of as many of these behaviors as possible. The intervention strategy that would be used for modifying each would depend on why the clinician believed the client was doing it. Clinicians with different beliefs about the etiology of stuttering probably would agree fairly well on the behaviors in the set that define a particular stutterer's problem, but they may not agree on intervention strategies for modifying them. Hence, clinicians are likely to find the approach to evaluation and therapy that is described in this book (which is based on viewing a particular client's problem as being defined by a set of behaviors) to be usable regardless of their beliefs about the etiology of the disorder.

The sets of behaviors that define the stuttering problems of individual clients are not identical. Also, the extents to which persons in their environment are aware of these behaviors are not identical. Some persons are likely to be more aware of them than others and, consequently, would tend to regard these behaviors as being more severe than would others. Persons with whom a stutterer has interacted for a long period of time (such as family members) are likely to pay less attention to the stuttering than they did at first if *the stutterer is not constantly signaling them that he or she is embarrassed about it* (Trotter & Kools, 1955).

The behaviors in the set that define a stutterer's problem tend to change as a function of age (see Chapter 4). While there tend to be common elements in the stuttering problems of preschool children, school-age children, and adults, new behaviors tend to be added to or substituted for existing ones as the problem develops.

HISTORICAL PERCEPTIONS OF STUTTERING

People have been aware of and have tried to explain and cope with stuttering for thousands of years. The ancient Egyptians are said to have had a hieroglyphic symbol for it (Curlee, 1993b, see Figure 1-1). Perhaps what this hieroglyph depicts is a tremor—an earthquake—being conducted from the ground to the mouth: If this is so, then the Egyptians used the earthquake as a metaphor for the moment of stuttering.

Stuttering is dealt with several times in the Bible. Moses, who is thought to have stuttered, exhibited a behavior that is frequently a component of the stuttering problem—a desire to avoid talking. Because of his "slow tongue," he wanted God to have his brother Aaron speak to the Pharaoh instead of him:

> *And Moses said unto the Lord: "Oh Lord, I am not a man of words, neither heretofore, nor since Thou has spoken unto Thy servant; for I am slow of speech, and of a slow tongue." And the Lord said unto him: "Who hath made man's mouth? and who maketh a man dumb, or deaf, or seeing, or blind? Is it not I the Lord? Now therefore go, and I will be with thy mouth, and teach thee what thou shalt speak." (Exodus 4:10-12)*

FIGURE 1-1 **Egyptian hieroglyphic symbol for stuttering. From Curlee, 1993b.**

The cause of Moses' stuttering, according to the Talmud, was physiological—abnormal functioning of his oral speech mechanism (Goldberg, 1989):

> *While Moses was still an infant the Pharaoh was advised to kill him, for one day, it was predicted, Moses would rise up against him. The Pharaoh at first shrugged, then decided to put Moses to the test. He placed two bowls before Moses, one filled with gold, the other, with hot coals. If Moses chose the gold, he would be slain. Of course Moses reached for the gleaming gold, but an angel intervened and struck his hand. So he grabbed a hot coal and put it in his mouth. And thereafter stuttered. (p. 71)*

During this century, some authorities have expressed the belief that stuttering is caused, at least in part, by an abnormality in the functioning of the peripheral speech mechanism. Some of the abnormalities to which they have attributed it are discussed elsewhere in this section and in Chapter 5.

The Bible also refers to stuttering in Isaiah (32:4): "And the tongue of the stam-merers shall be ready to speak plainly."

In this section we will consider how stuttering has been viewed historically—the reader needs to understand where we came from to understand where we are now. Our present views on both the etiology and management of stuttering are built upon the experience of the past. Clinicians who are unaware of how stuttering has been treated in the past are more likely to use intervention strategies that have been shown again and again to be of little or no long-term value than are those who have this knowledge. These strategies may produce a rapid reduction in stuttering sever-ity, but the vast majority of clients on whom they are used are likely to relapse within five years following termination of therapy (Boberg, 1981; Boberg, Howie, & Woods, 1979).

People have attempted to explain stuttering (and stammering) in various ways during the past 5,000 years. Their explanations have usually reflected what physi-cians, psychologists, psychiatrists, theologians, and philosophers thought at the time to be the cause of misfortune or abnormal behavior. Almost all such explanations (theories) have one of the following themes:

1. Punishment for sin
2. Physiological factors other than those directly related to the speech mechanism
3. Defects in the structure and/or function of the speech mechanism
4. Symptom of psychopathology
5. Learned behavior

Representative explanations having each theme are discussed in the following sec-tions. For further information about how stuttering has been viewed historically, see Appelt (1911), Clark (1964), Eldridge (1968), Freund (1966), Hunt (1861), Kling-beil (1939), Moeller (1975), Murray & Edwards (1980), Paden (1970), Rieber (1977), Shames & Rubin (1986), Van Riper (1970, 1973, 1982), and Wingate (1976).

Punishment for Sin

These explanations, which have been around for thousands of years, imply that stut-tering is a punishment for sin—either that of the person who stutters or that of some-body in his or her family. Battus (the son of Polymnestros, a notable Theraean of the 5th century B. C.) went to Delphi to inquire of the prophetess how to cure his stam-mering. She indicated that his disability resulted from angering Apollo and that he must follow her instructions to placate the god and, hopefully, doing so would cause him to be merciful (Herodotus, 1821).

Though this explanation, to my knowledge, has not been advocated by any con-temporary authorities on stuttering, one occasionally encounters a stutterer or par-ents of a stutterer who appears to believe it. They may say they believe that this is the cause of their or their child's stuttering or they may indicate such a belief indirectly by praying for a cure or participating in healing services. There appears to be a fairly generally held belief in our society that "bad things happen to bad people" judging, for example, by the popularity of such books as *Why Bad Things Happen to Good People* (Kushner, 1981).

Physiological Factors Other Than Those Directly Related to the Speech Mechanism

Stuttering has been attributed for thousands of years to physiological processes that are not directly related to the mechanisms of respiration, phonation, and/or articulation. Hippocrates, the father of medicine (the author of the Hippocratic oath), stated in the fifth century B. C. that speech disorders, including stuttering, were caused by a disturbance in the harmonious mingling of the four "humours," which are referred to as either heat, cold, moisture, and dryness or blood, bile, phlegm, and a "watery humour" (Hippocrates, 1923a, 1923b, 1923c). Mercurialis, a 16th century physician, felt that the cause of chronic stuttering was a disturbance in the humidity of the brain (Appelt, 1911). Twentieth-century theories of this type have attributed stuttering to abnormalities in (1) the structure and/or function of the hearing mechanism, (2) the bones of the head, (3) the endocrine system, (4) the autonomic nervous system, and (5) the central nervous system (see Chapter 5).

Defects in the Structure or Function of the Speech Mechanism

These theories attribute stuttering to some abnormality in the structure or function of the mechanisms of respiration, phonation, and/or articulation. Demosthenes, in the fourth century B. C., is reported to have overcome stuttering by practicing speaking with pebbles under his tongue: A generally accepted theory of the time cited the tongue as being responsible for all abnormalities of speech (Cicero, 1942). Aristotle (who had been born in the same year as Demosthenes) also blamed the tongue for causing stuttering:

> *When people stammer it is due, not to an affection of the veins, but to the movement of the tongue; for they find a difficulty in changing the position of the tongue when they have to utter a second sound. (Cited in Eldridge, 1968, pp. 15–16)*

The belief that an abnormality in the structure and/or function of the tongue causes stuttering appears to have been the most widely held one between the time of Aristotle and the Renaissance (about A. D. 1500).

Between the Renaissance and the beginning of the twentieth century the tongue continued to be blamed for stuttering. Other abnormalities of the structure and/or function of the speech mechanism also were regarded as the cause of stuttering. Several scholars during the seventeenth century blamed the hyoid bone for stuttering. A seventeenth-century Italian anatomist believed that two holes of abnormal size, somewhere in the middle region of the palate, were responsible for stuttering. An eighteenth-century scholar attributed stuttering to a weakness of the soft palate, uvula, and root of the tongue.

During the nineteenth century there was considerable speculation about the cause of stuttering, much of which focused on a defect in the structure or function of the speech mechanism. Itard, a French physician, in a book published in 1817, speculated that stuttering was caused by a general debility of the nerves that stimulated the movements of the tongue and larynx (Hunt, 1967). This was one of the first times that the etiology of stuttering was attributed to the larynx, a topic on which there was considerable research during the 1970s and 1980s. Itard recommended exercises for improving tongue strength that involved placing a fork beneath the tongue.

In early nineteenth century America a physician named Yates developed what became known as the "American Method" for treating stuttering. This method apparently regarded the etiology of stuttering as involving, at least in part, the functioning of the tongue, because it instructed the stutterer to keep the tip of the tongue resting continually on the alveolar ridge (Appelt, 1911). At night a small roll of wet linen was placed under the tongue to help the person maintain this position. Between 1825 and 1830 more than one hundred cases were reported to have been cured by this method.

Colombat de l'Isère in 1831 classified moments of stuttering into two groups: (1) those in which the blockings resulted from spasms of the lips and tongue and (2) those in which the spasms occurred in the larynx, pharynx, and/or the respiratory muscles (Eldridge, 1968). He recommended various types of exercises for improving the functioning of the mechanisms of respiration, phonation, and articulation. He also developed a small metronome-type device—known as the muthonome—with which stutterers were encouraged to pace their speech (Wingate, 1976, p. 155). More than one hundred years later (late 1960s) there was again considerable interest in the use of miniature metronomes for stutterers (see Chapter 7).

A German surgeon, Johann Frederick Dieffenbach, who believed that stuttering was caused by a spasm of the glottis, early in 1841 began treating it by surgery (Lebrun & Bayle, 1973). His operation to cure this spasm consisted of making a horizontal incision at the root of the tongue and excising a triangular wedge across it. More than 250 stutterers in France and Germany were reported to have undergone this operation in 1841 (incidentally, without anesthesia). Though Dieffenbach claimed successful results, some stutterers who underwent the procedure died, and other surgeons who experimented with it did not substantiate his results. Consequently, by the end of the year 1841 the procedure was apparently abandoned (Hunt, 1861).

Dieffenbach's approach was not the only medical-surgical one to be tried and abandoned during this period. According to Eldridge (1968), others included severing the hypoglossal nerve, piercing the tongue with hot needles, blistering the tongue with embrocations, encouraging smoking as a sedative for the vocal folds, and administering tincture of peppermint oil and chloroform to allay diaphragmatic spasms. The use of surgical approaches unfortunately did not cease after the nineteenth century. People underwent operations at the beginning of this century under the impression that such measures would cure their stuttering. According to Blanton & Blanton (1936):

> The commonest was tonsillectomy and the removal of adenoids. The clipping of the frenum and uvula were quite common. A method popular around 1922 and 1923 was the widening of the dental arch. Occasionally a patient was seen whose tongue has been nicked, and, very rarely, cases were recorded of trepanning, or cutting a hole in the skull. (p. 119)

During the second half of the nineteenth century theories continued to be advanced that attributed stuttering to a defect in the structure and function of the speech mechanism, though the primary emphasis during this period appeared to be on psychological mechanisms. A number of devices were introduced, presumably, to help overcome the effect of such defects on speech and, thereby, to cure stuttering (Katz, 1977). One of these, which was invented by an American named Bates, consisted of a narrow flattened tube of silver, seven-eighths of an inch in length and three-eighths of an inch in diameter, which was held in close proximity to the hard palate by a piece of wire that was fastened to the anterior teeth (Rieber, 1977). The tube was positioned so that the anterior end was lodged just behind the teeth and the posterior opened into the mouth, looking upward and backward toward the fauces. The tube was intended to overcome spasms when producing lingua-palatal sounds by preserving a continuous flow of air. The Committee of Science and Arts of the Franklin Institute in Philadelphia (which was one of the most respected U.S. institutions supporting science and technology during this period) in 1854 presented Bates with one of their most prestigious awards for "his ingenious and useful invention."

Another such instrument invented during this period consisted of a collar that was secured around the neck under a "stock or a cravat" (Rieber, 1977). It was fitted with a metal plate designed to rest upon the thyroid cartilage. A screw, resting in a spring, regulated the pressure of the plate on the cartilage. When the pressure was strong enough "to approximate the thyroid and arytenoid cartilages," muscular spasms of the glottis were claimed to be overcome.

There were also attempts during this period to overcome the defect in the structure or function of the speech mechanism by encouraging the stutterer to speak in a nonhabitual manner. One authority recommended that stutterers open the glottis when beginning to block by pronouncing or droning the schwa vowel. He also recommended the substitution of a "soft drawl" for a stutter (Eldridge, 1968). Encouraging stutterers to speak in nonhabitual manners continued throughout the twentieth century, even though it was demonstrated repeatedly through both clinical experience and systematic research that the reduction in stuttering severity resulting from the use of such strategies was almost always temporary.

During the twentieth century many persons who treated stuttering stated a belief, or demonstrated one indirectly by the strategies they used for treating stuttering, that the condition was caused by a defect in the structure or function of some part of the speech mechanism. Breathing exercises and various types of vocal gymnastics were advocated. Persons who treated stuttering in this manner included those both with and without medical training. Those without medical training included speech (elocution) instructors and public school teachers who had little or no formal training in the treatment of speech disorders as well as those who had received significant amounts of such training, persons who had been trained to be speech therapists (pathologists), and persons without formal training in speech disorders but who felt they had been successful in overcoming their own stuttering and offered to share their "secret" for doing so (for a price) with others. Some persons in this latter group in the early part of the twentieth century began what are known as *commercial stuttering schools* (Wingate, 1976). One of the most infamous of these was the Bogue Institute in Indianapolis. Such schools, most of which used "secret methods" and were residential, offered a "guaranteed cure" for a fairly high tuition that was usually payable in advance. The following is an example of the type of guarantee that was offered by commercial stuttering schools:

> *No matter what caused your stammering, no matter how old you are, how long you have stammered, how many times you have tried to be cured—no matter what you think about your case or whether you believe it is curable—if I have diagnosed your trouble and pronounced it curable, then I can cure YOU.... I not only claim to be able to do this for you, I back it up with a past record of success in treating hundreds of cases similar to your own. Like cures like. What has cured others like you, will cure YOU. But I don't ask you to risk a single penny upon even that evidence and proof. The moment you enroll in the Bogue Institute, I will issue to you and place in your hands, a written Guarantee Certificate, over my own signature, binding me to cure you of stammering or refund every cent of the money which you have paid me for tuition fee, and asking you only to follow the easy instructions given under the Bogue Unit Method. (Bogue, 1926, pp. 236–237)*

Some, like the above, offered to refund the tuition if the stutterer was not cured. In most cases, when a stutterer relapsed after leaving the school and asked for a refund, he or she was held at fault for the relapse—that is to say, the stutterer was told that if he or she had followed instructions precisely, the problem would have been cured.

There have been a number of attempts since the end of World War II to attribute stuttering (at least in part) to a defect in the functioning of some aspect of the speech mechanism. Many speech pathologists now believe that such a defect does contribute to the etiology of stuttering. Both these theories and the research that supports them are dealt with in Chapters 4 and 5.

Symptom of Psychopathology

Explanations of this type, which are based on the *medical* model, regard stuttering as a symptom of some type of psychopathology. By classifying it as a symptom, the implication is that it indicates the presence of a psychological pathological process in much the same way as a fever indicates the presence of a physiological pathological process (an infection). Just as a physician usually would not treat a fever (symptom) but the infection causing it, a clinician who believes that stuttering is a symptom of psychopathology usually would not treat the stuttering (symptom) but the psychological pathological process believed to cause it. Theoretically, if the physician were successful in treating the infection, the fever would go down; and if the clinician were successful in treating the psychopathology, the client would stutter less severely. We will consider in this section how a psychological pathological process underlying stuttering has been conceptualized historically—that is, up to the end of World War II.

There appear to have been few attempts prior to the nineteenth century to attribute stuttering to psychopathology. One of the earliest attempts to do so was by the eighteenth-century philosopher Moses Mendelssohn, who attributed stuttering to "a collision between many ideas, flowing simultaneously from the brain" (Eldridge, 1968, p. 36). The belief that persons stutter because "they think faster than they can talk" or because "they do not think of what they are going to say before they say it," incidentally, still is held by many stutterers and others. It is not unusual, for example, for a preschooler whom parents believe is beginning to stutter to be told to think of what he or she is going to say before saying it. Unfortunately, such a suggestion may be more likely to increase stuttering than to reduce it (see Chapter 5).

During the first half of the nineteenth century there were several attempts to attribute stuttering to psychopathology—specifically, a lack of harmony between thought and speech. Rullier, for example, stated that stuttering "was caused by a disproportion between the rate at which the brain can produce thoughts and that at which it can transfer them to the different stages of innervation" (Appelt, 1911). And Blume held that it was caused by "a lack of harmony between thinking and speaking" (Appelt, 1911).

Interest in theories that view stuttering as a symptom of psychopathology increased considerably during the latter half of the nineteenth century. Klencke (1860) published an influential book in which he indicated that stammering reflected the stammerer's need of psychological help—his whole personality needed treatment; further, Klencke advocated attention to environmental influences, and opened a sanatorium as a place of retreat and treatment for stammerers. He was one of the first clinicians to view stuttering as a symptom of an environmentally induced personality disturbance and to stress the importance of treating the whole person—not just the mouth.

During the first two decades of the twentieth century there continued to be considerable interest in theories that viewed stuttering as a symptom of psychopathology. This was due, in large part, to the influence of Freudian psychology and psychoanalysis: There was a marked tendency during this period to view these as a panacea for many ills. A paper was published in Germany in 1908 entitled "Nervous disorders and their treatment," in which stuttering was discussed as an anxiety neurosis from the psychoanalytic point of view. Another published in Germany in 1909 was entitled "A new treatment for stuttering" and discussed the application of psychoanalytic techniques to the treatment of stuttering. And in 1911 Appelt published the book *Stuttering and Its Permanent Cure,* which strongly advocated the use of psychoanalytic techniques for the treatment of stuttering.

Considerable enthusiasm was generated by these publications and a number of psychoanalytically trained clinicians attempted to use these methods for treating stuttering. Isidor Coriat (1931) held that every stutterer should have psychoanalysis. However, he expressed doubts about whether a complete cure could be expected because he had seen many examples of relapse. Another psychoanalyst, Abraham Brill (1923), after eleven years of treating a total of sixty-nine stutterers through psychoanalysis claimed only five cures, of which one was reported to have relapsed.

Among the persons who were reported to be skeptical about the value of psychoanalysis in treating stuttering was Sigmund Freud himself. According to a personal communication by Esti Freud (Freund, 1966, p. 174), he was of the opinion that psychoanalysts did not understand the mechanism of stuttering and that psychoanalytic techniques had been valueless in treating it.

Edward Scripture, an American physician who had cooperated with Brill in applying psychoanalysis to stuttering, advocated a modified Freudian approach to the treatment of stuttering. He felt that even after psychoanalytic techniques had resolved the emotional problem causing stuttering, the stutterer would still be likely to have some bad speech habits that he or she would have to be taught to eliminate (Scripture, 1931). This was one of the first attempts to combine psychotherapy and speech therapy in the treatment of stuttering. Such a combination of therapies has also been recommended by some contemporary psychotherapists who are psychoanalytically oriented (see Barbara, 1982; Freund, 1966; Glauber, 1982).

During and immediately following World War I many soldiers on both sides who developed stuttering as a symptom of war neurosis ("shell shock") were treated at military hospitals. Since their condition was assumed to be psychological in origin (a neurosis), psychotherapy often was used. Some of the physicians who were treating them felt that psychotherapy alone could not eliminate all the abnormal behaviors that occurred during their moments of stuttering because they were habits (learned responses) and thus advocated treating moments of stuttering directly.

There was an awakening of interest during the 1920s in training clinicians who were not physicians to treat communicatively handicapped persons, including stutterers. These persons offered speech correction services in such settings as university speech clinics and public schools. Many of them had been specialists in speech training and belonged to the National Association of Teachers of Speech. In 1925 some members of this organization who were primarily interested in therapeutic aspects of speech training formed the American Academy of Speech Correction—now, the American Speech-Language-Hearing Association (Paden, 1970). Since most of the clinicians who viewed stuttering as a symptom of psychopathology were physicians, and since after the 1920s most of the clinicians in the United States who were treating stutterers were not physicians, it is not particularly surprising that there was less interest after this period in treating stuttering through psychotherapy alone.

Learned Behavior

These theories, which view stuttering as a bad habit or learned behavior, have been around for at least three centuries. Amman (1700/1965) was perhaps the first to state in print that stuttering is a bad habit. He attempted to help stutterers break the habit by, among other things, encouraging them to practice speaking loudly and slowly. Approximately one hundred years later Erasmus Darwin (1800), who was the grandfather of Charles Darwin and was a stutterer, attributed the disorder to emotionally conditioned interruptions of motoric speech. His recommendations included encouraging stutterers to begin plosive sounds with loose contacts. Madame Leith, who believed that the disorder resulted from an abnormal tongue thrust habit, in 1825 trained patients to speak with the tonguetip up against the palate (Hunt, 1861). Arnott (1828), who believed that stuttering resulted from a learned "spasm of the glottis," sought to prevent it by teaching stutterers to prefix each word with an "e" vowel. There were also others during the first half of the nineteenth century who viewed the etiology of stuttering in this way (Hunt, 1861).

The belief that stuttering was a bad habit (learned response) attained widespread acceptance, particularly in the United States and Britain, during the middle of the nineteenth century (Van Riper, 1982). One of the persons responsible for bringing this about was Alexander Melville Bell, the grandfather of Alexander Graham Bell (inventor of the telephone). Bell wrote several books promoting the view that stuttering was a habit and recommending that it be treated as such. He stated that "The impediment has been shown to be a habit; it is therefore beyond the province either of medical or surgical treatment, and within that, exclusively, of the educator" (Bell, 1853, p. 47). This view was also accepted by many practitioners during the last third of the nineteenth century (Van Riper, 1982).

During the first third of the twentieth century some persons continued to view stuttering as learned behavior, though the prevailing view (due to the influence of Freudian psychoanalysis) was that stuttering was a symptom of psychopathology—a neurosis. One of the most influential persons during this period who viewed it in this way was Knight Dunlap (1932). He believed that the habit of stuttering could be weakened by voluntarily practicing stuttering. Based on this theory (which Dunlap termed the *beta hypothesis*) the stutterer was told that "when the critic [clinician] commands 'again' he is to say the word over (or to say the initial syllable again if stopped on a syllable) in the same way as that in which he said it before, or in a way as near as possible to the erroneous one" (Dunlap, 1932). After the stutterer did so several times the clinician would say "right" and the stutterer would attempt to say it without stuttering.

The number of persons who viewed stuttering as learned behavior increased considerably during the middle third of the twentieth century. This was due, in part, to the fact that a number of persons who entered the field of speech pathology with strong interests in stuttering during the thirties, forties, and fifties received at least some of their graduate training in departments of psychology. The University of Iowa was the institution from which many of these persons received their Ph.D. degree (Moeller, 1975). Two of the most influential of them were Wendell Johnson and Charles Van Riper. There was considerable interest during this period in departments of psychology (particularly at Iowa) in the possibility that at least some abnormal behaviors that were viewed as symptoms of psychopathology were learned. Hence, during this period a number of theories were formulated and intervention strategies were developed that looked upon stuttering as being learned behavior (see the section dealing with "The Iowa Development" in Bloodstein, 1987). The impact of this view on stuttering theory and management during the final third of this century is discussed in Chapter 5.

HOW DOES STUTTERING DIFFER FROM NORMAL SPEECH HESITATION?

The findings of a large number of studies indicate that most, if not all, children and adults hesitate some while they speak (Starkweather, 1987). They *repeat* sounds, syllables, words, and phrases; they *interject* syllables, words, and phrases (such as "um" and "well"); they *revise* (correct) what they said; they *pause* at places where pauses usually do not occur; they produce *incomplete phrases;* and they *prolong* sounds. These phenomena tend to occur relatively frequently in the speech of children—particularly preschool ones.

If all speakers—both stutterers and nonstutterers—are disfluent, how does stuttering differ from normal disfluency? Are they points on the same continuum (they just differ qualitatively) or are they different phenomena (they differ categorically)? Considerable research was published during the past fifty years that provided data relevant to these questions (Bloodstein, 1987; Starkweather, 1987; Van Riper, 1982). Unfortunately, authorities do not agree on how they should be interpreted. Some have interpreted them as supporting the view that stuttering and normal disfluency are probably on the same continuum (see Andrews et al., 1983; Bloodstein, 1987; Conture, 1990b; Cordes & Ingham, 1995b; Johnson & Associates, 1959; Perkins, 1983a; Yairi & Clifton, 1972). And there are others who have interpreted them as supporting the opposite view (see Adams & Runyan, 1981; Wingate, 1984a, 1987).

Regardless of whether normal disfluency and stuttering differ categorically or are points on a continuum, it is necessary to be able to differentiate between them for several reasons. First, it is necessary to be able to do so to determine whether a person (particularly a preschool-age child) is beginning to stutter. And second, it is necessary to be able to do so for planning and evaluating therapy. Reducing the severity of stuttering may involve encouraging clients to be disfluent in ways that listeners are likely to regard as being more normal (Van Riper, 1973). To assist them in doing so, it is necessary to know how normal disfluencies differ from those that occur during moments of stuttering.

Many studies have been reported in which disfluency behaviors of stutterers were compared to those of their nonstuttering peers (Starkweather, 1987). The subjects studied ranged in age from less than two years to more than seventy years. A number of attributes of their disfluency behaviors were compared including type, duration, and degree of accompanying tension Some of the major findings of this research are summarized in this section. Additional information on this topic is presented in Chapter 2.

Types of Disfluency Behaviors

Disfluency behaviors (hesitation phenomena) in the speech of stutterers and nonstutterers have been categorized in several ways by linguists (see Blankenship & Kay, 1964; Goldman-Eisler, 1968; Levin & Silverman, 1965; Maclay & Osgood, 1959) and by speech pathologists (Starkweather, 1987). The scheme that has been used most often for comparing the disfluencies of stutterers and nonstutterers is one that was developed by Wendell Johnson and his associates at the University of Iowa (Johnson, 1961; Johnson & Associates, 1959; Williams et al., 1968). It includes the following types of disfluency behaviors:

1. *Part-word repetitions.* These are sound and syllable repetitions. They occur most often at the beginnings of words and almost never at the ends of words. Though the number of times a particular sound or syllable is repeated can be relatively high, it is usually only once or twice. The repetitions may be accompanied by audible and/ or visible signs of tensing. Level of awareness of their occurrence can be relatively high or relatively low. The repetitions may be voluntary though they usually are involuntary.

2. *Word repetitions.* These are repetitions of an entire word. In most cases it is a single-syllable word. While a word may be repeated a relatively large number of times, it is usually repeated only once or twice. These repetitions, like part-word ones, may be accompanied by audible and/or visible signs of tensing, may be voluntary or involuntary, and may vary with how aware the speaker is of their occurrence.

3. *Phrase repetitions.* These are repetitions of units consisting of two or more words. Such units usually are repeated only once or twice. They may be accompanied by audible and/or visible signs of tensing, may be voluntary or involuntary, and may vary with how aware the speaker is of their occurrence.

4. *Interjections of sounds, syllables, words, and phrases.* These sound units, which occur between words, usually do not perform a linguistic function in messages—that is to say, the denotative meanings of messages usually are not affected by their presence. Examples are "um" and "you know." They may be accompanied by audible and/or visible signs of tensing, they may be voluntary or involuntary, and the speaker may or may not be aware of their occurrence.

5. *Revisions—incomplete phrases.* These include instances in which the speaker becomes aware of making an error and corrects it. The error may be in how a word was pronounced or it may be related to the meaning of the word(s) that were said. Also included are instances in which the speaker begins a utterance, but obviously does not complete it.

6. *Disrhythmic phonations.* These are disturbances in the normal rhythm of words. The disturbance may be attributable to a prolonged sound, an accent or timing that is notably unusual, an improper stress, a break (usually between syllables), or any other speaking behavior not compatible with fluent speech. Included here are phenomena that some investigators have referred to as "broken" words (e.g., "I am g--oing to the store"). Disrhythmic phonations may be accompanied by audible and/or visible signs of tensing, may be voluntary or involuntary, and may vary with how aware the speaker is of their occurrence.

7. *Tense pauses.* These are phenomena that occur between words, part words, and interjections. They consist of pauses in which there are barely audible manifestations of heavy breathing or muscle tightening. The same phenomena within a word would place the word in the category of disrhythmic phonation. Tense pauses vary with how aware the speaker is of their occurrence.

To what extent do the frequencies of these disfluency (hesitation) types allow persons who stutter to be distinguished from normal speakers? Representative data on the frequency of occurrence of these behaviors in the spontaneous speech of preschool, elementary school, and adult male stutterers and nonstutterers are presented in Tables 1-1, 1-2, and 1-3. The same types of data are reported in all three tables. The only differences are the age levels of the subjects from whom speech samples were elicited and whether data were reported for tense pause. For a particular type for a particular group, the *lowest index* is the frequency of disfluencies per hundred words spoken by the subject who had the fewest occurrences; the *highest index* is the frequency found in the subject who had the most occurrences; Q_2 (the median) is the frequency exceeded by 50 percent of the subjects; Q_1 is the frequency exceeded by 75 percent of the subjects; and Q_3 is the frequency exceeded by 25 percent of the subjects.

These data indicate that among preschoolers (Table 1-1), elementary schoolers (Table 1-2), and adults (Table 1-3), the "typical" person (the one designated by Q_2) who stutters is disfluent more often than his or her "typical" nonstuttering peer. For all three age groups, the median disfluency frequency in "all categories" for the stutterers exceeded that for the nonstutterers. This finding should not be particularly sur-

TABLE 1-1   **Range and quartile distribution of the frequency indices of disfluency (number of disfluencies per 100 words) for each of the six disfluency (hesitation) types and for all types combined for 68 young male stutterers (MS) and 68 matched young male nonstutterers (MN). The majority of the subjects in both groups were preschoolers. The values for Q_1 and Q_3 are interpolations from the decile distribution in which the data are reported.**

Disfluency Category and Group	Lowest Index	Quartiles			Highest Index
		Q_1	Q_2	Q_3	
Interjections					
MS	0.0	1.6	2.9	4.9	15.2
MN	0.0	1.0	2.0	4.6	12.7
Part-word repetitions					
MS	0.0	1.2	3.1	6.8	36.6
MN	0.0	0.1	0.6	0.8	2.4
Word repetitions					
MS	0.0	2.2	3.2	5.8	14.8
MN	0.0	0.4	1.0	1.6	4.6
Phrase repetitions					
MS	0.0	0.4	1.0	1.7	7.1
MN	0.0	0.1	0.5	0.9	2.5
Revisions—incomplete phrases					
MS	0.0	0.5	1.1	2.5	6.9
MN	0.0	0.6	1.1	2.3	8.8
Disrhythmic phonations					
MS	0.0	0.1	0.6	1.9	20.0
MN	0.0	0.0	0.0	0.2	2.0
All categories					
MS	3.3	9.5	13.6	24.5	46.5
MN	0.6	3.8	7.1	10.2	18.3

From Johnson & Associates, 1959, p. 206.

prising since excessive disfluency is almost universally considered to be a defining characteristic of stuttering (Alfonso, 1990; Conture, 1990a).

Although the typical stutterer is disfluent more often than the typical nonstutterer, there is considerable overlap between the groups. That is, there are persons

TABLE 1-2　**Range and quartile distribution of the frequency indices of disfluency (number of disfluencies per 100 words) for each of the seven disfluency (hesitation) types and for all types combined for 56 elementary school male stutterers (MS) and 56 matched elementary school male nonstutterers (MN).**

Disfluency Category and Group	Lowest Index	Quartiles			Highest Index
		Q_1	Q_2	Q_3	
Interjections					
MS	0.0	0.0	0.0	0.2	3.2
MN	0.0	0.0	0.0	0.1	2.2
Part-word repetitions					
MS	0.0	1.0	1.9	5.3	21.2
MN	0.0	0.4	0.9	1.7	4.7
Word repetitions					
MS	0.0	0.0	1.0	3.1	12.5
MN	0.0	0.0	0.4	0.9	1.8
Phrase repetitions					
MS	0.0	0.0	0.0	1.0	3.2
MN	0.0	0.0	0.0	0.9	2.3
Revisions—incomplete phrases					
MS	0.0	0.0	1.0	2.1	4.2
MN	0.0	0.9	1.5	3.0	6.1
Disrhythmic phonations					
MS	0.0	0.0	0.5	1.5	40.0
MN	0.0	0.0	0.0	0.6	3.0
Tense pauses					
MS	0.0	0.0	0.0	0.0	5.6
MN	0.0	0.0	0.0	0.0	0.6
All categories					
MS	0.0	4.2	7.3	13.7	80.0
MN	0.0	2.6	3.5	6.1	16.7

From Silverman, 1974.

who are not regarded by themselves or others as stutterers, yet who hesitate more often than persons who are regarded by themselves and others as being stutterers. Twenty-five percent of the elementary school nonstutterers, for example, hesitated more often than 25 percent of the elementary school stutterers (see Table 1-2), that

TABLE 1-3   **Range and quartile distribution of the frequency indices of disfluency (number of disfluencies per 100 words) for each of the six disfluency (hesitation) types and for all types combined for 50 adult male stutterers (MS) and 50 matched adult male nonstutterers (MN). The values for Q_1 and Q_3 are interpolations from the decile distribution in which the data are reported.**

Disfluency Category and Group	Lowest Index	Quartiles			Highest Index
		Q_1	Q_2	Q_3	
Interjections					
MS	0.0	3.0	7.2	15.0	71.6
MN	0.0	1.4	2.6	6.8	15.3
Part-word repetitions					
MS	0.0	1.9	4.2	9.5	52.2
MN	0.0	0.0	0.2	0.4	1.2
Word repetitions					
MS	0.0	1.3	3.1	5.3	13.5
MN	0.0	0.3	0.6	1.2	2.5
Phrase repetitions					
MS	0.0	0.3	0.9	1.9	5.5
MN	0.0	0.0	0.2	0.6	1.3
Revisions—incomplete phrases					
MS	0.0	0.9	1.2	2.1	32.0
MN	0.3	0.7	1.2	2.1	5.6
Disrhythmic phonations					
MS	0.0	0.0	0.7	4.0	37.4
MN	0.0	0.0	0.0	0.0	1.0
All categories					
MS	4.6	12.6	22.6	40.3	135.8
MN	0.7	3.4	6.6	9.3	19.9

From Johnson, 1961, p. 10, 14.

is, the frequency exceeded by 25 percent of the nonstutterers (6.1) was greater than that for 25 percent of the stutterers (4.2). This same trend also was evinced by the preschoolers and adults.

We will now consider the disfluency types individually (see Tables 1-1, 1-2, and 1-3). There is considerable overlap between the groups of stutterers and of nonstutterers for four of the types: word repetitions, phrase repetitions, revisions-incomplete phrases, and interjections. For part-word repetitions and disrhythmic phonations there is much less overlap between the groups: These are the types, incidentally, that most persons tend to regard as stuttering (Wingate, 1964). The type that seems to differentiate stutterers from nonstutterers most sharply is tense pause (see Table 1-2). It is almost never observed in the speech of normal speakers. Most stutterers do not exhibit it either. Therefore, while its presence suggests that the person is a stutterer, its absence does not indicate that he or she is a normal speaker.

In conclusion, the available data indicate that there is no disfluency type (with the possible exception of tense pause) that stutterers produce and normal speakers do not. Hence, attempting to differentiate persons who stutter from those who do not solely on the basis of whether a particular type of disfluency occurs in their speech would tend to be risky. Since labeling a normal speaker as a stutterer may precipitate the disorder (see Chapter 5), the consequences of such an error could be serious.

Duration of Individual Moments of Disfluency

Speakers not only differ in how often they are disfluent, they also differ in how long their moments of disfluency tend to last. That is, speakers differ in the maximum number of times they tend to repeat words and part words and in the maximum number of seconds their disrhythmic phonations tend to last. In this section we will compare stutterers and nonstutterers on the basis of the duration of their instances of disfluency.

The "typical" (median) stutterer's moments of disfluency tend to last longer than those of the "typical" (median) nonstutterer (Johnson, 1961; Johnson & Associates, 1959). However, there appears to be some overlap between stutterers and nonstutterers in how long their longest moments of disfluency tend to last. Some nonstutterers, particularly preschoolers, occasionally repeat sounds, syllables, and single syllable words more than four times (Silverman, 1972b). And some stutterers rarely, if ever, make such repetitions more than once or twice. Similar overlap exists between groups for the duration of sound prolongations and inappropriate pauses within words. It would then appear that the presence of occasional words and part words that are repeated a relatively large number of times and/or occasional disrhythmic phonations that are relatively long, by themselves, would not allow persons who stutter to be differentiated reliably from their normal-speaking peers.

Degree of Tension While Being Disfluent

A speaker may appear relatively relaxed while being disfluent or may produce audible and/or visible signs of tensing during at least some of his or her disfluencies. Such tensing can be manifested in a number of ways (singly or in combination) including tense pauses, audible tension (strain) evinced in the voice while speaking, abnormally rapid rates of syllable repetition, audible manifestations of irregularities in breathing, and visible manifestations of excessive tensing of muscle groups in the speech mechanism and elsewhere. The presence of a significant degree of tension while being disfluent does appear to differentiate persons who stutter (or who are at risk of developing stuttering) from their normal-speaking peers (Bloodstein, 1987; Starkweather, 1987; Van Riper, 1973).

ASSIGNMENTS

Stuttering Simulation

This chapter has introduced you to stuttering. To develop a deeper understanding of the impact that having this disorder can have on a person, I recommend that you simulate stuttering in at least three situations and observe the effect it has on communication, how other people react to you, and how you feel about their reactions.

How typical are the experiences of persons who simulate stuttering of those of persons who have the disorder? Judging by feedback I have received from hundreds of students who have done this assignment and others (see Ham, 1990a, Hulit, 1989; Leahy, 1994), they tend to be quite representative. This conclusion is based both on my experiences as a stutterer and on those of persons with fluency disorders whom I have treated.

Identification of Moments of Stuttering

Watch a videotape of a stutterer reading a passage and on a copy of it mark each word on which a moment of stuttering occurred. Have a fellow student (or some other person) also do this task. How well do your judgments agree? Why are their disagreements? Is your identification of moments of stuttering reliable enough for clinical purposes?

Delayed Auditory Feedback

While the simulation assignment described above provides insight into how people react to persons who have fluency disorders and how those who have them are likely to react to their reactions, it does not provide insight into what it is like to be unable to speak fluently. One way that you can gain this insight is to speak while your auditory feedback is being delayed. The instrumentation used for this purpose is a special audiotape recorder that plays back through headphones what a person says a fraction of a second (usually approximately 0.2 seconds) after he or she says it. Most normal speakers experience some disruption in their speech fluency when they attempt to speak under this condition. As well as you can describe them in words, what are your reactions to not being able to control your fluency, that is, speak fluently?

Autobiography

Another way that you can gain some insight into how stuttering and other fluency disorders can affect a person's life is by reading autobiographical books and articles. Such books include ones by Johnson (1930) and Tillis & Wager (1984). Most issues of the National Stuttering Project's (NSP) newsletter *Letting Go* contain at least one article of this type. The NSP also publishes other autobiographical material, including a book, *To Say What Is Ours,* and a videotape "Voices in Exile."

Depiction of Stutterers in the Arts and Literature

One way to gain a little insight into how stutterers are viewed in a particular culture is to observe how they are portrayed in the arts and literature of that culture. Characters who stutter appear in novels, children's books, movies, dramas, and operas (Anderson, 1994; Benecken, 1994; Silverman & Trotter, 1976). For a listing of some of the novels in which they appear, see Silverman & Trotter (1976). How are stutterers depicted in the arts and literature of your culture? Has the manner in which they are depicted changed during the course of this century? If you feel that it has changed, how has it done so?

2

Symptomatology and Phenomenology of Stuttering

A description of the abnormal disfluency behavior associated with stuttering (i.e., the "moment of stuttering") in children and adults is presented in this chapter. Few of the behaviors and phenomena discussed here are exhibited by all persons who have the disorder and some are far more likely to be exhibited by adults than by children, particularly preschoolers (see Chapter 4). Behaviors that occur during moments of stuttering are described from four perspectives: auditory, visual, physiological, and introspective. Conditions under which they tend to increase or decrease in frequency (the phenomenology of these behaviors) are also described.

Few, if any, stutterers stutter on all the words they say (see Johnson, 1961; Johnson & Associates, 1959; Silverman, 1974). While speech-language pathologists agree that almost all stutterers appear at times to be saying some words and utterances fluently, they often disagree on the percentages of words on which stuttering occurs in particular speech samples (see Cordes & Ingham, 1994, for a review of the literature on the identification and measurement of moments of stuttering). Those who attempt to determine these percentages from audiotape recordings may identify fewer moments of stuttering than those who derive them from videotapes, introspective reports, and various types of physiological recordings.

We will refer in this section to periods of time during which stuttering appears to be occurring as *moments of stuttering*. These periods have also been referred to as stutterings, instances of stuttering, stuttering events, and stuttering blocks. They are regarded by stutterers as being involuntary (Kelly & Conture, 1988). Their duration can range from slightly less than one second to several minutes (Sheehan, 1974). It is sometimes difficult to specify their exact duration because of uncertainty about when they begin and end (Ingham, Cordes, Ingham, & Gow, 1995). There is wide variability from stutterer to stutterer with regard to the behaviors that occur during these moments (Starkweather, 1987). While one could argue that the moment of stuttering continues to be an accepted entity (judging by the frequency with which it has been referred to in recent papers published in the *Journal of Fluency Disorders* and other professional and research journals), there are data that suggest that for some stutterers periods of speech between moments of stuttering may contain perceptible or physiological abnormalities (Adams, 1981; Colcord & Gregory, 1987; Conture, Colton, & Gleason, 1988; Healey & Gutkin, 1984; Healey & Ramig, 1986; McClean, 1990; Prosek, Montgomery, Walden, & Hawkins, 1987; Prosek, Montgomery, & Walden, 1988; van Lieshout, Peters, Starkweather, & Hulstijn, 1993; Williams, 1957; Wingate, 1986; Winkler & Ramig, 1986). The degree of abnormality that was observed in most of these studies was relatively small (McClean, 1990).

The section begins with descriptions of those behaviors that occur during moments of stuttering that can be seen and/or heard by a listener. Next, conditions that have been reported to influence the location (loci) and frequency of moments of stuttering are described. Finally, the moment of stuttering is described from two other perspectives—physiological and introspective.

Why is it necessary to view the moment of stuttering from several perspectives in order to understand it? Because by doing so one can obtain a more complete description. As the fable of the six blind men and the elephant demonstrates (see Chapter 1), the description of a phenomenon (such as the moment of stuttering) is determined in large part by the perspectives from which it is viewed.

OBSERVABLE BEHAVIORS DURING MOMENTS OF STUTTERING

There are a number of types of behavior that occur during moments of stuttering that can be seen and/or heard (Costello & Hurst, 1981). Some of these also occur in the speech of normal speakers (see Chapter 1), though they may differ qualitatively from those present during moments of stuttering (Onslow, 1992b; Wingate, 1987). Those that tend to occur most often are described in this section.

Sound, Syllable, and Word Repetitions

One of the behaviors that can occur during moments of stuttering of which listeners are likely to be aware is repetition of sounds, syllables, and words (particularly single-syllable ones). These are observable in the speech of young children who are beginning to stutter as well as in that of persons in their seventies who have stuttered all their lives (Johnson, 1961; Johnson & Associates, 1959). Most repetitions occur on the initial syllables of words and almost never occur on their final syllables (Lebrun & Van Borsel, 1990; Stansfield, 1995). The sound or syllable repeated may be the next one in the word the person is trying to say or it may be some other one. The number of times a sound, syllable, or word is repeated (the number of units of repetition) by most stutterers is usually five or fewer (Van Riper, 1982). The person may appear relatively relaxed while repeating or relatively tense. Children are more likely than adults to appear relaxed while repeating (Bloodstein, 1987). If the person is tense while repeating, one or more of the sounds during each repetition may be prolonged or otherwise spoken disrhythmically (Van Riper, 1982).

Disrhythmic Phonations

These, as mentioned in Chapter 1, include any disturbances in the normal rhythm or timing of elements in words other than sound and syllable repetitions (Williams et al., 1968). Hence, this is a within-word rather than a between-word phenomenon. It is also a "wastebasket" category because it includes all the abnormalities in timing and rhythm that occur during production of words that are not repetitions. The two most frequently occurring behaviors in this category are prolongations and "broken" words (pauses within words that usually occur between syllables).

Prolongations usually occur on the initial sounds of words and almost never on the final sounds (Bloodstein, 1987). While they can last almost any length of time, most are less than five seconds (Sheehan, 1974). They may begin with a complete, or almost complete, blockage of airflow though the articulators (Van Riper, 1982). (Because of this blockage, moments of stuttering containing them sometimes are referred to as "blocks.") Such blockages are particularly likely to occur during the production of plosive sounds and often are accompanied by visible tensing in muscle groups that are not directly involved with respiration, phonation, or articulation. While such tensing can occur in almost any muscle group, it usually involves the musculature of the face and neck. For example, a stutterer may tightly close his or her eyes during such a blockage.

Abnormal pauses within words—usually between syllables—are referred to as *broken* words (Johnson, 1961). Most tend to be shorter than five seconds. They may be silent or the person may produce some sound during them. If they are not silent, the sounds produced may or may not be the ones in the next syllable of the word. During such pauses, there is often observable tensing of muscle groups (particularly in the facial area) that are not directly involved with respiration, phonation, or articulation.

Tense Pauses

Tense pauses are abnormally long pauses between words during which sound, caused by tensing of muscles in the speech mechanism, particularly the larynx, is evident (Williams et al., 1968). They usually occur before words that the person appears to be having difficulty saying (initiating breath flow for) the initial sound. The duration of these pauses is usually less than five seconds, and the tensing associated with them may be evident visually as well as auditorily. It may, in fact, be more evident visually than auditorily.

The mechanism underlying these pauses appears to be the same as that underlying broken words. With both, pauses tend to occur because the person is having difficulty saying (initiating breath flow for) the next sound.

Incomplete Phrases

These are utterances that a person begins, but does not complete. An example would be the statement "I want a . . . ." (Johnson, 1961). They occur in the speech of both normal speakers and stutterers (Johnson, 1961). However, they sometimes occur in the speech of stutterers for a reason they would not do so in the speech of normal speakers—the avoidance of stuttering (Van Riper, 1982). If a stutterer feels himself or herself, in an utterance, beginning to block or anticipates blocking, he or she may decide not to complete the utterance. While doing so may avoid the stuttering, it could confuse the listeners.

Interjections of Sounds, Syllables, Words, or Phrases

All speakers occasionally interject into their utterances sounds, syllables, words, and phrases that do not appear to affect the meaning (Johnson, 1961). Examples would be "um," "er," and "you know." Some types of interjection are referred to as *filled pauses* (Wingate, 1984b). Interjecting these can be a strategy for holding a listener's attention while deciding what to say next. Some stutterers also use interjections as a device to avoid stuttering (Van Riper, 1982). By interjecting a sound, syllable, word, or phrase before attempting to say a word on which they expect to stutter, they believe they can reduce the severity of their stuttering upon that word. Such interjections have been referred to as *starters* (Van Riper, 1982).

Revisions

When speakers realize that they have made an error, they are likely to correct it, particularly if they believe that not doing so could cause their message to be misunderstood (Johnson, 1961). Some stutterers tend to avoid revising errors if they believe that they are likely to stutter while doing so (Silverman & Williams, 1973). In addition, some of them use revision as a device to reduce the severity of the stuttering. When they begin to stutter on a word they do not complete it, but instead substitute a synonym they think they can say more fluently (Van Riper, 1982).

Abnormal Speaking Rate

There are several reasons why stutterers may have relatively slow speaking rates. One is the act of stuttering itself. Since stuttering blocks consume time, their presence obviously reduces speaking rate. Another reason why they may speak relatively slowly is to reduce the severity of their stuttering. Some stutterers tend to stutter less severely when they do so (Bloodstein, 1987).

Some stutterers use an abnormally rapid speaking rate as a device to avoid stuttering. They appear to believe that if they pause they are likely to stutter more severely (Van Riper, 1982).

Abnormal Loudness or Pitch Level

One occasionally encounters a stutterer whose speech is usually abnormally loud or soft or whose voice is abnormally high- or low-pitched for his or her age and sex. While these behaviors may not be related to the person's stuttering, they may be devices that he or she is purposefully using to reduce stuttering severity (Van Riper, 1982).

Tensing of Muscle Groups That Are Not Involved with Speech Production

Tensing of muscle groups that are not involved with respiration, phonation, or articulation may occur during moments of stuttering (Van Riper, 1982). Such tensing may be visually obvious or not. Visually observable movements (i.e., gestures) associated with such tensing include closing the eyes and moving the head backward. An example that would not be visually obvious (without special instrumentation) would be tensing of the musculature of the ear, particularly that of the tympanic membrane.

While authorities agree that such tensing occurs, they do not agree on the reasons for it. One hypothesis is that the person is either currently using it as a device to reduce stuttering severity or has used it in the past for this purpose and although it no longer works, it has become an habitual component of the person's moments of stuttering (Wingate, 1964; Brutten & Shoemaker, 1967).

Use of Gestures

Some evidence exists that adult stutterers tend to gesture less and include less detail in their gestures during moments of stuttering than they would otherwise (Shenker, Mayberry, Scobble, Grothe, & White, 1994).

DISTRIBUTION OF MOMENTS OF STUTTERING IN THE SPEECH SEQUENCE

Moments of stuttering are not distributed randomly in the speech sequence. They are more likely to occur at some locations (loci) than at others (Brown, 1945). A location in this context can be a word or a syllable within a word.

Why is it important that moments of stuttering are more likely to occur on words possessing certain attributes than on others and on some syllables of words than on others? The main reason is that this phenomenon tends to make some explanations (theories) for the etiology of stuttering more plausible than others. Those who propose theories for the etiology of stuttering must explain how they would account for what is known about the phenomenology of the disorder, if they want their theories to be taken seriously. Since the approaches clinicians use for managing stuttering should be influenced by their beliefs about its etiology (Williams, 1968), the presence of such phenomena could have clinical as well as theoretical implications.

While stuttering tends to occur on certain words and at certain locations within words more often than would be expected by chance, it is important to remember that it can occur on any word and at any location within a word. Some of the characteristics (attributes) of words and syllables that have been shown to influence the loci of moments of stuttering are described below. For further information about them see Bloodstein (1987), Brown (1945), Starkweather (1987), Van Riper (1982), and Wingate (1982, 1986a, 1986b).

The Position of a Word in an Utterance

Moments of stuttering are considerably more likely to occur at some word positions in utterances (sentences) than at others (Jayaram, 1984). They occur more often on the first, second, or third words of utterances than would be expected by chance—that is, than if their distribution based on this attribute were random (Brown, 1938, 1945; Logan & Conture, 1995; Wingate, 1982). This is true for school-age children and adult stutterers during both oral reading and spontaneous speech (Wingate, 1982). Word position, incidentally, is the only attribute discussed in this section that does not appear to influence the distribution of hesitations in the speech of normal speakers in the same way as it does the speech of stutterers (Chaney, 1969; Silverman & Williams, 1967; Williams, Silverman, & Kools, 1969b; Wingate, 1982). Hence, the tendency to be considerably more disfluent at the beginning of an utterance than at other positions in the utterance appears to be a characteristic of stuttering rather than of disfluency in general.

Do the sentences on which stuttering tends to occur on the first three words differ from others? There is some evidence (Gaines, Runyan, & Meyers, 1991) that they tend to be ones that are both relatively long and grammatically complex.

The Grammatical Function of a Word

Moments of stuttering during both oral reading and spontaneous speech are more likely to occur on *lexical* words (nouns, verbs, adverbs, and adjectives) than on *function* words (articles, prepositions, conjunctions, and pronouns) when the relative frequencies of occurrence of these two types of words are taken into consideration (Brown, 1945; Williams et al., 1969b). This is true for both school-age children and adults who stutter (Brown, 1945; Williams et al.). It also is true for hesitations (disfluencies) in the spontaneous speech and oral reading of school-age children and adults who do not stutter (Chaney, 1969; Silverman & Williams, 1967; Williams et al., 1969b). This phenomenon, therefore, appears to be a characteristic of speech disfluency in general rather than of stuttering.

The Length of a Word

Moments of stuttering during both oral reading and spontaneous speech are more likely to occur on relatively *long* words than on relatively *short* ones, when the relative frequency with which these two types of words occur is taken into consideration (Brown, 1945). This is true for both school-age children and adults (Brown, 1945; Williams et al., 1969b). It also is true for hesitations (disfluencies) in the spontaneous speech and oral reading of school-age children and adults who do not stutter (Chaney, 1969; Silverman & Williams, 1967; Williams et al., 1969b). Thus, this phenomenon, like grammatical function, appears to be a characteristic of speech disfluency rather than just of stuttering.

The Initial Phoneme of a Word

Moments of stuttering during both oral reading and spontaneous speech are more likely to occur on words beginning with *consonants* than with *vowels*, when, again, the relative frequency with which words beginning with consonants and vowels occur is taken into consideration (Brown, 1945; Wells, 1983). This is true for both school-age children and adults (Brown, 1945; Williams et al., 1969b). It also is true for hesitations (disfluencies) in the spontaneous speech and oral reading of school-age children who do not stutter (Chaney, 1969; Silverman & Williams, 1967; Williams et al., 1969b). The cause does not appear to be phonological difficulty, at least for young children who stutter (Throneburg, Yairi, & Paden, 1994). This phenomenon, like grammatical function and word length, appears to be a characteristic of speech disfluency in general rather than of stuttering.

The Speaker's Degree of Familiarity with a Word

There is a little evidence suggesting that both stutterers and nonstutterers are less likely to be disfluent on words with which they are familiar than on those with which they are not familiar, particularly during oral reading (Hubbard & Prins, 1994). This finding, if replicated, would suggest that difficulties with word retrieval and/or phonological encoding can precipitate moments of stuttering (Hubbard & Prins, 1994).

Syllable Stress

Moments of stuttering on polysyllabic words appear more likely to occur on stressed syllables than on unstressed ones (Prins, Hubbard, & Krause, 1991). Perhaps this is why moments of stuttering rarely occur on the final syllable of polysyllabic English words.

The Consistency Effect

Moments of stuttering, during both oral reading and spontaneous speech, occur on words on which they occurred previously more often than would be expected by chance (Johnson & Knott, 1937b; Cullinan, 1988; Wingate, 1986a, 1986b). This phenomenon, which is referred to as the *consistency effect,* is present in the speech of both school-age children and adults (Johnson & Knott, 1937b; Williams, Silverman, & Kools, 1969a). This also appears to be true for hesitations (disfluencies) in the spontaneous speech and oral reading of persons who do not stutter (Williams, Silverman, & Kools, 1969a). Consequently, this phenomenon—like grammatical function, word length, and initial phoneme—appears to be a characteristic of speech disfluency rather than just of stuttering.

The Location within a Word

Moments of stuttering during both oral reading and spontaneous speech are more likely to occur on the *initial syllables* of multisyllable words than on any of their other syllables (Starkweather, 1987). They almost never occur on final syllables (Lebrun & Van Borsel, 1990).

Distance from Previously Stuttered Words

For some stutterers, moments of stuttering tend to occur in clusters more often than would be expected by chance (Hubbard & Yairi, 1988; Still & Griggs, 1979). This phenomenon, which has been observed in the speech of children as well as that of adults (Hubbard & Yairi, 1988), is referred to as the *adjacency effect.*

THE EXPECTANCY (ANTICIPATION) PHENOMENON

The tendency for moments of stuttering not to be distributed randomly may be at least partially due to the *expectancy (anticipation) phenomenon.* This is the ability exhibited by some stutterers to predict the words on which they are going to stutter *with greater than chance accuracy* (Johnson & Sinn, 1937; Johnson & Solomon, 1937; Knott, Johnson, & Webster, 1937; Van Riper, 1936). The words "greater than chance accuracy" were italicized because few, if any, stutterers appear able to predict *all* of their moments of stuttering (Johnson & Sinn, 1937; Johnson & Solomon, 1937; Knott et al., 1937; Van Riper, 1936). This ability is not observed as frequently in children as in adults (Silverman & Williams, 1972a). Anticipatory physiological changes prior to stuttering that are correlated with such predictions have been observed in some stutterers (e.g., Baumgartner & Brutten, 1983). Some authorities believe that this phenomenon contributes to the precipitation of stuttering (see Chapter 5).

CONDITIONS THAT AFFECT STUTTERING SEVERITY

Stutterers tend to stutter more severely under some conditions than under others (Andrews et al., 1983). While there are individual variations with respect to how specific conditions influence stuttering severity, there are some conditions that appear to affect the majority of stutterers similarly—that is, to increase or reduce their stuttering severity.

Why is it important that stuttering severity varies in a predictable manner under certain conditions? One reason is that such phenomena (like those associated with the distribution of moments of stuttering) tend to make some explanations (theories) for the etiology of stuttering more plausible than others. Another is that they have been incorporated into intervention strategies to reduce stuttering severity. These phenomena, therefore, have clinical as well as theoretical implications.

Some conditions that have been reported to reduce stuttering severity are described in the next section, and some that have been reported to increase it, in the section that follows. The order in which conditions are considered in each section is not intended to imply anything about their relative importance.

Conditions That Reduce Stuttering Severity

There are a number of conditions under which stuttering severity tends to be reduced, including the following:

Speaking in a Nonhabitual (Novel) Manner
If stutterers modify their speaking behavior in any way, the result is likely to be a temporary reduction in stuttering severity (Bloodstein, 1987). Such a reduction can last as long as several years (see Silverman, 1976b).

In what ways have stutterers modified their habitual speaking behavior that have resulted in increased fluency? They have changed their speaking rate, in most cases reducing it (Andrews, Howie, Dozsa, & Guitar, 1982; Johnson & Rosen, 1937); changed their pitch (Johnson & Rosen, 1937); whispered (Cherry & Sayers, 1956); simulated accents (Andrews et al, 1982; Mowrer, 1987); changed the intonational pattern of their speech—as in speaking in a monotone (Adams, Sears, & Ramig, 1982) or in a singsong manner (Bloodstein, 1950); and prolonged vowel sounds (Andrews et al., 1982). They have also interjected sounds, syllables, words, and/or phrases before words on which they expected to stutter (Van Riper, 1982) and have accompanied speech with movements such as arm swinging (Andrews et al., 1982).

Reading in Chorus

Few, if any, stutterers will stutter while reading aloud in chorus (unison) with someone (Adams & Ramig, 1980; Andrews et al., 1982; Barber, 1939; Ingham & Packman, 1979; Johnson & Rosen, 1937). The person with whom they read can be a normal speaker or another stutterer. Even if the person is a stutterer, neither of them is likely to stutter. When the person stops reading with the stutterer, he or she will usually begin stuttering again almost immediately. Choral reading differs from most of the other conditions described in this section because its ability to facilitate fluency does not seem to wear off.

"Shadowing"

Some stutterers become more fluent while shadowing, or concurrently repeating, another person's speech (Andrews et al., 1982; Cherry & Sayers, 1956; Wingate, 1981c). Shadowing is the spontaneous speech equivalent of reading in chorus. A variation of shadowing is speaking in chorus with ones echo: This phenomenon, incidentally, is widely used in Poland as a component of treatment programs for stuttering (Adamczyk, 1994).

Singing

Few, if any, stutterers stutter while singing (Andrews et al., 1982; Healey, Mallard, & Adams, 1976; Wingate, 1976; Witt, 1925). I have worked with two extremely severe stutterers who sang semiprofessionally and neither stuttered while doing so. Also, Mel Tillis, a contemporary country-western singer who is a moderately severe stutterer, apparently never stutters while singing.

Some clinicians who treated stuttering during the first half of the twentieth century utilized this phenomenon in their therapy programs. They encouraged stutterers to speak in a singsong manner (Eldridge, 1968; Van Riper, 1973). While this strategy may have reduced stuttering severity (at least temporarily), it probably caused more adverse attention to be called to these people then did their stuttering.

Using a Metronome

Many stutterers stutter less frequently (at least initially) when they pace their speech with a metronome—one word or syllable per beat (Andrews et al., 1982; Johnson & Rosen, 1937; Martin & Haroldson, 1979; Martin, Johnson, Siegel, & Haroldson, 1985). The metronome beat can be delivered auditorily, visually, tactilely, or by some combination of these senses. The effect for some stutterers, however, wears off after a period of time (Silverman, 1976b). Some normal speakers also tend to be disfluent less frequently while speaking under this condition (Silverman, 1971).

Since the early part of the nineteenth century stutterers periodically have been encouraged to pace their speech with the beats of a miniature metronome (Wingate,

1976). There was considerable interest in this approach during the late 1960s and early 1970s (Brady, 1968, 1969, 1971; Silverman & Trotter, 1973a, 1973b, 1974, 1975). Miniature electronic metronomes intended for this purpose were built into hearing-aid housings (see Figure 2-1).

Speaking in the Presence of Loud Masking Noise
Many stutterers tend to stutter less severely (at least temporarily) while speaking in the presence of masking ("white") noise that presumably is loud enough to keep them from hearing their own speech (Cherry & Sayers, 1956; Garber & Martin, 1977; Martin et al., 1985; Martin, Haroldson, & Triden, 1984). The masking noise may be generated either by an audiometer or a device specifically designed for this purpose. It is presented to the stutterer binaurally, using either standard-size head-phones or the miniature type used with hearing aids. Some normal speakers also tend to be disfluent less frequently while speaking under this condition (Silverman & Goodban, 1972).

There have been attempts to utilize this phenomenon in stuttering therapy (Moore & Adams, 1985; Silverman & Trotter, 1973a, 1973b, 1974, 1975; Walle, 1980). Beginning in the mid-1960s, miniature masking-noise generators built into body-type hearing-aid housings were made available to stutterers. Some used manual switches to turn the sound on and off (Trotter & Lesch, 1967; Trotter & Silverman, 1973) and others used voice-actuated ones (Ingham, Southwood, & Horsburgh,

FIGURE 2-1   **Behind-the-ear hearing-aid housing
containing a metronome intended for stutterers.**

1981). With the latter, a small disk-shaped microphone is attached to the neck (usually using tape disks that are sticky on both sides) over the thyroid cartilage of the larynx. When the stutterer begins to phonate, the microphone detects the vibration and turns on the masking noise, and when he or she stops phonating, the noise is turned off. Some stutterers feel that they have benefited from using such a device (see Carlisle, 1985).

Experiencing Delayed Auditory Feedback
Some stutterers stutter less severely when they experience delayed auditory feedback while they speak (Andrews et al., 1982; Fukawa, Yoshioka, Ozawa, & Yoshida, 1988; Goldiamond, 1965; Kalinowski et al., 1993; Martin, Siegel, Johnson, & Haroldson, 1984). Ordinarily we hear what we say almost immediately after we say it. With delayed auditory feedback we hear what we say a short period of time (usually 0.2 seconds) after we say it. The experience is somewhat similar to that of speaking in an environment in which there is an echo. The electronic device used for creating delayed auditory feedback functions like an audiotape recorder in all but one significant way: It can "record" and "play back" at the same time. The stutterer talks into a microphone and his or her speech is recorded and played back through headphones a fraction of a second later. The recording may be stored on magnetic tape or in a computer's memory. These devices have been made small enough to be used by stutterers outside of the therapy room (Craven & Ryan, 1984; Muellerleile, 1981).

Reducing Speaking Rate
Some stutterers stutter less severely than usual if they speak slowly (Andrews et al., 1982; Johnson & Rosen, 1937; Kalinowksi, Armson, Roland-Mieszkowski, Stuart, & Gracco, 1993). It has been hypothesized that some of the conditions mentioned in this section (such as pacing speech with a metronome) reduce stuttering severity because they cause stutterers to speak slower than usual (Bloodstein, 1987).

Speaking While Alone and to Animals and Young Children
Stutterers have been reported to stutter less severely when they speak or read aloud in an environment where no one can hear them (Porter, 1939; Quinn, 1971). They also have been reported to do so when they speak to animals (Andrews et al., 1982) and very young children (Andrews et al., 1982; Ramig, Krieger, & Adams, 1982).

Articulating without Phonating (Lipped Speech)
Some stutterers have been reported to stutter less severely if they do not phonate while producing the articulatory gestures required for speech (Commodore & Cooper, 1978; Perkins, Rudas, Johnson, & Bell, 1976).

Speaking in a Monotone
Some stutterers have been reported to stutter less severely if they speak or read in a monotone (Adams et al., 1982; Bloodstein, 1950). A monotone is a type of speech

pattern in which each syllable is produced at approximately the same pitch and loudness level (Adams et al., 1982).

Speaking a Language in which the Person Tends to Be Relatively Fluent

Many stutterers who are bilingual report that they stutter less severely in one language than the other. This has been confirmed in some cases (Bernstein-Ratner & Benitez, 1985; Nwokah, 1988).

Response-Contingent Stimulation of Stuttering

The operant model of B. F. Skinner indicates that behavior that is learned in a particular way—that which is an operant response—can be manipulated in frequency through response-contingent punishment and reinforcement (James, 1981; Luper, 1968; Mowrer, 1968a). Shames and Sherrick published a theoretical paper in 1963 in which they suggested that both normal disfluency and moments of stuttering may be operant responses (Curlee, 1993a). Their hypothesis was based in part on a study by Flanagan, Goldiamond, & Azrin (1958) in which the frequency of moments of stuttering was temporarily reduced by contingent presentations of a 105 dB tone. Following publication of the Shames & Sherrick (1963) paper, there was a great deal of research dealing with the effect of response-contingent presentation of stimuli assumed to be "punishing" on the frequency of various behaviors that occurred during moments of stuttering. A number of types of stimuli were used in this research including electric shock (Martin & Siegel, 1966a, 1966b), blue light (Martin & Siegel, 1966a, 1966b), verbal punishment, such as saying the word "wrong" (Christensen & Lingwall, 1983; Martin & Siegel, 1966b), loud noise (Reed & Lingwall, 1976), intervals of delayed auditory feedback (Goldiamond, 1965), and removal of money (Halvorson, 1971). There also was research in which stimuli assumed to be neutral (e.g., the word "tree") or positive (the word "right") were presented in the same response-contingent manner (Cooper, Cady, & Robbins, 1970). The findings of these and other studies indicate that response-contingent stimulation of behaviors associated with moments of stuttering, *regardless of the nature of the stimulation,* reduces the frequency at which they occur (Andrews et al., 1983; Ingham & Andrews, 1973; James, 1981; Martin & Haroldson, 1982; Prins & Hubbard, 1988; Shames, 1975; Shames & Egolf, 1976; Shames & Rubin, 1986; Shames & Sherrick Jr., 1963; Siegel, 1970). Authorities do not agree about the reason (Bloodstein, 1987). Identical noncontingent stimulation, incidentally, in experimentally naive subjects produces no such effect (Andrews et al., 1983; Ingham & Andrews, 1973; Lanyon & Barocas, 1975).

Utilizing Electromyographic (EMG) Biofeedback from Speech Muscles

Some stutterers have been reported to stutter less severely while monitoring the degree of tension in parts of their speech musculature utilizing electromyography (EMG) biofeedback instrumentation (Craig & Cleary, 1982; Guitar, 1975; Lanyon,

1977). EMG biofeedback, as it is used with stutterers, is a procedure for monitoring muscle tension to produce relaxation. Electrodes are attached to the skin over the muscle being monitored and the amount of tension in the muscle is communicated to the client in some concrete manner, such as by the pitch of a tone: for example, the more tense the muscle, the higher the pitch. The client is told to change the feed-back stimulus in some way. If it were a tone, he or she would be told to lower its frequency. Doing so would result in the muscle becoming more relaxed.

Not Desiring to Conceal (Avoid) Stuttering

The less important many stutterers feel it is to conceal or avoid stuttering, the less severely they tend to stutter (Van Riper, 1982). In fact, when they want to stutter, they may not be able to do so. I once offered a severe stutterer money for each time he stuttered "for real" during a specified time period. He did not stutter even once during it, but began doing so again immediately after it ended. The following case report (Frankl, 1985) also illustrates this phenomenon:

> A similar case ... was related to me by a colleague. ... It was the most severe case of stuttering he had met in his many years of practice. Never in his life, as far as the stutterer could remember, had he been free from his speech trouble, even for a moment, except once. This happened when he was twelve years old and had hooked a ride on a streetcar. When caught by the conductor, he thought that the only way to escape would be to elicit his sympathy, and so he tried to demonstrate that he was just a poor stut-tering boy. At that moment, in which he tried to stutter, he was unable to do so. (p. 127)

Perhaps one reason why some stutterers tend to be more fluent while speaking to animals and young children and while alone is that they do not attempt to conceal their stuttering.

Not Thinking about or Attending to Speech

Anecdotal reports from stutterers indicate that there is a decrease in stuttering sever-ity when they are not thinking about or attending to speech (Bloodstein, 1987; Kamhi & McOsker, 1982). There is some evidence that stutterers tend to devote more attention to speech than do nonstutterers—for example, they perform more poorly than the latter on attention-demanding tasks that accompany speech (Kamhi & McOsker, 1982).

Playing a "Role"

Stutterers who function as actors or actresses may not stutter while doing so. Among the actors and actresses who had a stuttering problem are Marilyn Monroe and Peter Bonerz (the actor who played Pete the dentist on the Bob Newhart television show in the 1970s). Stutterers who attempt to project an image that they feel is not really them may stutter less severely while doing so. This is particularly likely to be true if the image they are trying to project is more forceful than their usual one (Fransella, 1972).

Suggestion

If stutterers believe that they will stutter less severely than usual under certain conditions, there is likely to be a *temporary* reduction in their stuttering severity under these conditions (Hulit & Haasler, 1989). The message that causes them to develop this belief could be self-generated or communicated to them while they were in a "waking" or "hypnotic" state (Bloodstein, 1987). Some therapies, incidentally, that use relaxation techniques (see Jacobson, 1938; Wolpe, 1958) tend to produce a state that is similar to, or perhaps identical to, a hypnotic one.

Performing an Adaptation Task

Most stutterers become progressively more fluent if they repeat a speaking task a number of times, one after the other. An example of such a task would be reading aloud a passage five times without pausing more than a few seconds between readings (Horii & Ramig, 1987; Johnson & Knott, 1937b; Prins & Hubbard, 1992; Wingate, 1986a, 1986b; Zimmermann & Hanley, 1983). Most stutterers would have fewer moments of stuttering during their second reading than during their first and fewer during their third, fourth, and fifth readings than during either their first or second (see Figure 2-2). This phenomenon, which is referred to as the *adaptation*

FIGURE 2-2 **Performance of a typical stutterer on an oral reading adaptation task.**

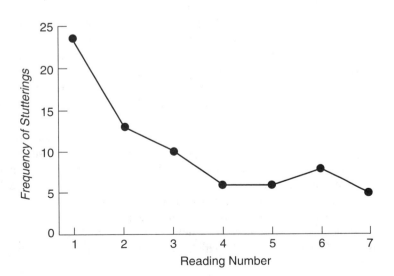

effect, also has been studied using repetitions of a spontaneous speech task (Bloom & Silverman, 1973; Kroll & Hood, 1974). The tasks that have been used for this purpose include consecutive repetitions of a single word on which stuttering initially occurs (Silverman & Williams, 1972b) and repeated descriptions (one after the other) of an object or event (Bloom & Silverman, 1973). The latter task differs from the others in this paragraph in that the word(s) said each time is (are) not exactly the same. Most stutterers do not become as fluent while performing spontaneous speech adaptation tasks as they do while performing oral reading ones. Some normal speakers also tend to exhibit the adaptation effect (Silverman, 1970a, 1970c, 1970d; Williams et al., 1968).

Conditions That Increase Stuttering Severity

A number of conditions that are reported to reduce stuttering severity for many stutterers were discussed in the preceding section. There also are conditions that have been reported to increase the severity of many stutterers' stuttering, at least temporarily (Young, 1985). Some of them are described in this section.

Speaking on the Telephone

Many stutterers tend to stutter more severely than usual while talking on the telephone (Georgieva, 1994; Leith & Timmons, 1983). In fact, some stutter so severely that they avoid using the telephone whenever possible. To cope with this problem, they have someone (such as their spouse) make calls for them. Or they talk to people face-to-face when it would be sensible to do so on the phone. For example, they may travel to stores, rather than phone, to find out if certain items are available.

One explanation that has been offered for this phenomenon is that, at least in part, it is due to the desire to make a good impression (Van Riper, 1982). When stutterers talk to people face-to-face, the listeners' impressions of them are based on both visual and auditory information. Although their speech may not communicate that they are mature, intelligent persons, their visual appearance (such as the way they are dressed) may do so. The impressions people form over the telephone are based solely on auditory data. Hence, stutterers probably have a stronger desire to avoid stuttering while talking on the telephone than they would in other situations. This would tend to increase their stuttering severity on the telephone.

Another explanation that has been offered for this phenomenon is that stutterers fear that people will hang up the telephone if they are unable to initiate speech (Van Riper, 1982). They may have difficulty saying "hello" when they answer the telephone or they may have difficulty beginning to speak after a person they are calling answers. The person being phoned may assume that the call is a "crank" one (particularly if he or she hears sounds associated with heavy breathing) and hang up. Obviously, a stutterer who had such a fear would not want to stutter on the telephone, particularly at the beginning of a call, which would tend to increase his or her stuttering severity.

A third possible explanation is that stutterers feel under pressure to communicate quickly while speaking on the telephone. Consequently, they wouldn't want to stutter because doing so makes it take longer to communicate. This desire to avoid stuttering tends to increase their stuttering severity.

Saying One's Name

Many stutterers stutter relatively severely when they say their name (Bloodstein, 1987). This occurs both when they are asked their name and when they voluntarily say it (as when introducing themselves). They also may do so when they say their address and telephone number. A strong desire to avoid stuttering and knowing that they cannot do so by substituting or circumlocuting may be the reason for this.

Telling Jokes

Some stutterers stutter relatively severely when they tell jokes (Van Riper, 1982). They are particularly likely to do so on their punch lines. Stuttering on a punch line can ruin a joke. The reason for increased stuttering under this condition is probably a strong desire to avoid doing it.

Repeating a Misunderstood Message

When asked to repeat a message some stutterers tend to stutter more severely than when they say it the first time (Bloodstein, 1987). They may even stutter when repeating a message that they said fluently. Perhaps this increased stuttering results from their desire to transmit the message successfully when they repeat it and a belief that stuttering could keep them from doing so.

Waiting to Speak

For some stutterers, the longer they have to wait to say something, the more severely they are likely to stutter while doing so (Young, 1985). If they are a member of a group in which people are taking turns introducing themselves, they are likely to stutter more severely if they are one of the last persons to do so than if they are one of the first. Some stutterers report experiencing an increase in their anxiety level as the time when they will have to introduce themselves gets closer and closer. The increase in stuttering severity that occurs under this condition probably is a function of both the desire to not stutter when introducing oneself and the longer time available to anticipate and fear stuttering while waiting to speak.

An increase in anxiety while waiting to respond may not be unique to stutterers. There is some evidence that nonstutterers experience it also (Miller & Watson, 1992).

Speaking to Authority Figures

Many stutterers tend to stutter more severely when they speak to people whom they regard as authority figures (Bloodstein, 1987). Such persons could include their parents, employers, and teachers (Georgieva, 1994). Actually, it could include anyone on whom they want to make a good impression.

Speaking to a Relatively Large Audience

Some stutterers tend to stutter more severely while speaking to a relatively large audience than to a relatively small one (Porter, 1939; Martin & Haroldson, 1988; Siegel & Haugen, 1964; Young, 1985). Perhaps this is true, in part, because they have a stronger desire than usual to be fluent while speaking to a such an audience. Others, at times, tend to be relatively fluent while speaking to large audiences. This seems particularly likely to occur if they believe that they are viewed by their listeners as an authority figure and they are willing to bring their stuttering out into the open (Johnson, 1946, 1961).

Failing to Bring Their Stuttering Out into the Open

Not acknowledging to their listeners verbally or otherwise—as through a message printed on a T-shirt (Silverman, 1988; Silverman, Gazzolo, & Peterson, 1989)—that they have a stuttering problem tends to cause many stutterers to stutter more severely (Johnson, 1946, 1961). For this reason, clinicians usually encourage stutterers to bring their stuttering out into the open.

Desiring to Avoid Stuttering

Stutterers tend to stutter most when they want to stutter least (Williams, 1982). This may partially explain why some of the other conditions mentioned in this section result in increased stuttering.

Spontaneous Recovery

The tendency for stutterers to become progressively more fluent during a series of readings of a passage in which there is no more than a few seconds pause between readings (referred to as the "adaptation effect") has been described in this chapter. If a stutterer pauses for a period of time after reading a passage repeatedly in this manner and then begins to read the passage yet again, he or she probably will stutter more severely during the first reading of the second series than during the final reading of the first series (see Figure 2-3). This phenomenon, which is referred to as *spontaneous recovery* (Johnson & Knott, 1937a), does not appear to be exhibited by nonstutterers (Silverman & Bloom, 1973). Hence, it seems to be one that does differentiate stuttering from normal speech disfluency (Silverman & Bloom, 1973).

Experiencing Positive Emotional Arousal (Excitement)

The conditions that have been discussed in this section thus far are associated with negative emotional arousal (e.g., anxiety). There have been reports of children's stuttering increasing in severity under conditions that are thought by their parents to generate positive emotional arousal—for example, being excited about their birthday (Adams, 1992). Whether such an increase in severity results from positive emotional arousal or from the conditions actually producing a negative emotional state is uncertain (Adams, 1992).

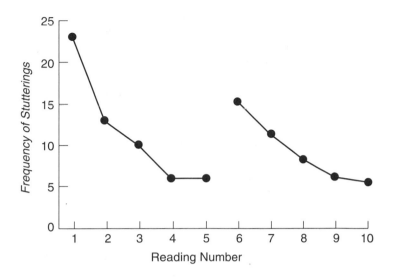

FIGURE 2-3   **Spontaneous recovery following adaptation on an oral reading adaptation task. Note that the frequency of stuttering is higher on the sixth reading than on the fifth.**

SECONDARY BEHAVIORS (SYMPTOMS) THAT ACCOMPANY MOMENTS OF STUTTERING

There are some behaviors other than disfluencies that may occur during moments of stuttering. These behaviors—which are referred to in the stuttering literature as *secondary symptoms* or *secondaries*—are more common in the speech of adult stutterers than in that of preschool-age and primary-school-age ones (Van Riper, 1982). Some investigators have questioned whether the difference between children and adults with regard to the presence of secondaries is as large as has been previously assumed (see Yairi, Ambrose, & Niermann, 1993).

Observations concerning the presence or absence of secondaries can be helpful when deciding whether a young child is beginning to stutter. Their presence in the disfluent speech of a preschooler would suggest that he or she is doing so (see Conture & Kelly, 1991).

What types of behaviors have been classified as secondaries? Among those that tend to occur most often are the following:

1. Looking away from the listener while stuttering, that is, maintaining poor eye contact with the listener (Atkins, 1988)
2. Jerking or other movements of the head

3. Blinking (closing) the eyes and/or wrinkling the forehead
4. Distortions of the mouth (such as pressing the lips tightly together)
5. Quivering of the nostrils
6. Interjections of sounds, syllables, words, and phrases that do not contribute to communicating the person's message and that are being used as "starters"
7. Abnormal variations in the loudness and/or pitch of the voice
8. Abnormal variations in speaking rate

Such behaviors may occur by themselves or in various combinations (Prins & Lohr, 1972).

Why do these behaviors accompany moments of stuttering? The most widely accepted explanation is that they began as devices for avoiding these moments or at least reducing their severity (Bloodstein, 1987). If a stutterer anticipates stuttering on a word, he or she may attempt to avoid it by doing something prior to saying the word. Or if the person begins to stutter on a word, he or she may attempt to do something to reduce the duration of the block. A stutterer is likely to continue using the device until he or she no longer believes that doing so will reduce the duration of blocks. By this time, the behavior has become an habitual (learned) component of the blocks. Thus, as mentioned in a previous section, such behaviors may accompany moments of stuttering either because they are being used as devices for coping with moments of stuttering or they are ones that were used for this purpose in the past that no longer work but have become habitual components of them.

Assuming that these devices represent current or past attempts to cope with stuttering, why do they work and why do they stop working? There are several reasons why they may do so. First, they cause stutterers to speak in nonhabitual manners. As was noted previously, many stutterers tend to become more fluent when they do so. However, once such a device becomes a habitual part of a stutterer's speaking behavior, it no longer facilitates fluency.

A second reason why such devices may work and eventually stop working has to do with the stutterers' beliefs regarding their efficacy. So long as they believe that a device will in some "magical" way facilitate fluency it is likely to do so. According to Barbara (1982):

> *The various bodily movements and contortions used by a person when he stutters . . . carry with them a sense of implied magic ritual. The pressing of both hands against the sides of the body, the pinching of himself to get started, the blinking of his eyelids, the placing of the palm of his hand over his mouth, etc., are just some of the many bodily magic gestures used in a particular difficult speaking situation. (p. 50)*

However, if a stutterer loses confidence in a device's ability to facilitate fluency, it is likely to do so. *Anticipation of fluency tends to lead to fluency in the same manner that anticipation of stuttering tends to lead to stuttering.*

A third reason why such devices may work and eventually stop working is a combination of the previous two reasons. Devices initially work because they cause stutterers to speak in a nonhabitual manner. The fluency that they experience while using them causes stutterers to anticipate further fluency. The initial fluency-enhancing effect, therefore, is a function of *both* speaking in a nonhabitual manner and anticipating fluency. Once the nonhabitual manner of speaking begins to become habitual, such devices tend to work less well. This tends to result in a loss of confidence in their ability to facilitate fluency which, in turn, tends to make them less effective at doing so.

A stutterer may continue consciously to use a device beyond the point that it is effective in reducing his or her stuttering severity. This person may believe that using the device tends to make his or her blocks shorter. Obviously, there is no objective way of determining how long a block would have lasted if a device had not been used. He or she may also believe that using the device sometimes prevents stuttering on a particular word. Of course, he or she might have been fluent while saying that word without the device. We know that the ability of stutterers to predict their moments of stuttering is far from perfect (Johnson & Sinn, 1937; Johnson & Solomon, 1937; Knott et al., 1937, Van Riper, 1936). The belief that a device sometimes "works" causes its use to be reinforced on a *partial reinforcement schedule* (Brutten & Shoemaker, 1967). The findings of a large number of studies conducted by experimental psychologists suggests that behaviors that are learned on such a schedule are extremely difficult to extinguish (Brutten & Shoemaker, 1967).

PHYSIOLOGICAL EVENTS THAT ACCOMPANY MOMENTS OF STUTTERING

Thus far, we have considered moments of stuttering from the perspective of their observable, or rather, acoustic and visual characteristics. There are several other perspectives from which they can be viewed. One of these is physiological. Moments of stuttering are accompanied by abnormal physiological events that intermittently influence the processes of respiration, phonation, and/or articulation (Caruso, Conture, & Colton, 1988; Denny & Smith, 1992; McClean, Goldsmith, & Cerf, 1984).

Because abnormal physiological events occur during moments of stuttering does not necessarily mean that they are at least partially responsible for them. Physiological *consequences* of a psychological process may be the cause of their occurrence. If, for example, moments of stuttering were at least partially caused by anxiety, there would be an increase in the level of activity of the sympathetic division of the autonomic nervous system (Brutten & Shoemaker, 1967). A number of abnormal physiological events tend to occur whenever there is such an increase (Brutten & Shoemaker, 1967).

Some abnormal physiological events associated with respiration, phonation, and articulation that have been reported to occur during moments of stuttering are described in this section. Other aspects of physiological functioning that have been reported to differentiate persons who stutter from their peers are described in Chapter 3.

Respiration

Abnormalities in respiratory functioning sometimes occur during moments of stuttering (Baken, McManus, & Cavallo, 1983; Murdoch, Killin, & McCaul, 1989; Watson & Guitar, 1986). There were efforts during the first half of this century to partially explain stuttering on this basis (see Fletcher, 1914; Fossler, 1932). The types of abnormalities that have been reported include "antagonisms between abdominal and thoracic breathing, irregularities of consecutive respiratory cycles, prolonged expirations or inspirations, complete cessation of breathing, interruptions of expiration by inspiration, and attempts to speak on intake of air" (Bloodstein, 1987, p. 11). Most stutterers tend not to exhibit these abnormalities when they are silent or speaking fluently (Bloodstein, 1987).

Phonation

A number of abnormalities in the functioning of the laryngeal mechanism during moments of stuttering have been reported (Borden, Baer, & Kenney, 1985; Conture, Schwartz, & Brewer, 1985; Freeman, 1979; Mallard, Hicks, & Riggs, 1982; Newman, Harris, & Hilton, 1989). In fact, there were a number of attempts during the 1970s and 1980s to explain stuttering on the basis of such abnormalities. Among those that are commonly observed clinically are breath-holding and glottal fry. Many stutterers have reported to their clinicians that their "throat closes tightly" during moments of stuttering.

A number of studies on laryngeal functioning during moments of stuttering have utilized instrumentation-based measurement approaches such as electroglottography and electromyography (Borden et al., 1985). Among the reported abnormalities in laryngeal functioning during moments of stuttering are the following:

> Breaks in the rhythm of vocal fold vibration and a clonic fluttering of the folds (Borden et al., 1985)
>
> Vocal folds fixed in either an open or closed position (Conture, McCall, & Brewer, 1977)
>
> A more gradual buildup in voicing than in fluent utterances (Bakker & Brutten, 1990; Borden et al., 1985; Hayden, Adams, & Jordahl, 1982; Hayden, Jordahl, & Adams, 1982; Healey & Gutkin, 1984)
>
> Excessive muscular activity (Freeman & Ushijima, 1978)
>
> Simultaneous contractions of antagonistic (abductor and adductor) laryngeal muscles (Freeman & Ushijima, 1978)

Articulation

The functioning of the articulators during moments of stuttering has been studied extensively through the use of such techniques as electromyography, x-ray motion pictures, and measures of intraoral air pressure and rate of airflow. Among the abnormalities that have been reported are the following:

> Defective synchronization of the action potentials of the paired musculature—such as the masseter muscles (Williams, 1955)
>
> A buildup of muscular tension, reaching a peak near the termination of a block (Sheehan & Voas, 1954)
>
> Excessive muscular activity (Shapiro, 1980; Thurmer, Thumfart, & Kittel, 1983)
>
> Tremors (Platt & Basili, 1973; Van Riper, 1982)
>
> Prolonged articulatory postures on stop consonants (Hutchinson, 1975)
>
> Lack of coordination between articulatory movements and onset of phonation (Hutchinson & Watkin, 1976)
>
> Abnormally rapid articulatory movements at the moment of release from a block (Hutchinson & Watkin, 1976)

STUTTERERS' PERCEPTIONS OF MOMENTS OF STUTTERING

Thus far, we have examined the moment of stuttering from the perspective of listeners and physiologists. One important perspective we have not yet considered is that of persons who stutter. What they experience prior to and during moments of stuttering and how they react to it not only can influence their attitude toward their stuttering, but their stuttering behavior itself.

Stutterers ordinarily experience their moments of stuttering auditorily and through feelings they report to be associated with muscle tension and anxiety (Brutten & Shoemaker, 1967; Craig, 1990; Perkins, 1990a; Peters & Hulstijn, 1984). These feelings may occur before moments of stuttering as well as during them. In fact, they may partially explain the ability of many stutterers to predict their moments of stuttering with greater-than-chance accuracy (Johnson & Sinn, 1937; Johnson & Solomon, 1937; Knott et al., 1937; Van Riper, 1936).

Stutterers' Auditory Perception of Their Moments of Stuttering

Stutterers probably do not experience their moments of stuttering auditorily in exactly the same manner as do their listeners. Some seem surprised when they hear audiotape recordings of their speech. There could be several reasons for this difference. One is that while they are speaking stutterers are attempting to cope with, or reduce, the severity of their stuttering, which would tend to divert their attention from monitoring their speech auditorily (Van Riper, 1982). Another is that during at least some of their moments of stuttering they experience "a kind of momentary loss of 'contact'" (Bloodstein, 1987, p. 24).

Stutterers' Tactile-Kinesthetic Perception of Their Moments of Stuttering

Stutterers experience their moments of stuttering tactile-kinesthetically as well as auditorily. They experience them as feelings of abnormal muscle tensing (Snidecor, 1955) and as feelings resulting from the articulators touching (contacting) each other with excessive force. If, for example, stutterers were blocking on /f/, they probably would be aware of their upper teeth pressing against their lower lip. If a block is a particularly "hard" one, the stutterer may experience pain. This is particularly likely if a stutterer blocks and bites his or her tongue while producing a voiced or voiceless *th*.

Stutterers may judge the severity of their stuttering in a particular situation as much, if not more, on the basis of how it "felt" than how it "sounded." If they didn't perceive much abnormal muscle tension or many "hard contacts" while they spoke, stutterers may conclude that their stuttering was not very severe. On the other hand, if they were aware of a great deal of abnormal muscle tensing or a number of hard contacts (particularly of those accompanied by pain) while they spoke, they are likely to conclude that their stuttering was relatively severe.

We have considered elsewhere in this chapter how a stutterer's desire to avoid stuttering can result in increased stuttering. One reason why a stutterer may desire to avoid stuttering is to avoid the discomfort—the abnormal muscle tensing and hard contacts associated with it. Few people enjoy biting their tongue or lip!

Listeners may not be aware of all a stutterer's stuttering and for this reason will experience it differently than the stutterer does. Some moments of stuttering that are unlikely to be detected by a listener visually or auditorily can be detected by a stutterer who experiences them as they occur as abnormal feelings of muscle tensing or abnormally hard contacts between articulators. For some stutterers, the majority of their moments of stuttering tend to be of this type. These have been referred to as *internal stutterers* (Freund, 1966).

Stutterers' Perceptions of Anxiety prior to Moments of Stuttering

We dealt in the preceding section with feelings associated with the muscle tensing that occurs during moments of stuttering. Similar feelings can occur before moments of stuttering. Such feelings have been reported to be associated with increases in anxiety level. According to Bloodstein (1987):

> *Prior to the block there is often an apprehension of impending difficulty, varying in severity from mild uneasiness to extreme panic.... (p. 24)*

Whether such apprehension causes stutterers to anticipate stuttering or whether their stuttering is caused by their doing so has not been unequivocally established.

ASSIGNMENTS

Stuttering Checklist

From a videotape of a stutterer reading a passage or doing a spontaneous speech task, select six words on which moments of stuttering occur. Use the Checklist of Stuttering Behaviors (see Appendix C) to catalogue the behaviors that occur during each of these moments. The behaviors you will be cataloging have been described in this chapter. Have a fellow student (or some other person) also do the checklist for these words. How well do your judgments agree? Why are their disagreements? Is your use of the checklist reliable enough for clinical purposes?

Stuttering Severity Rating

Watch a videotape of a stutterer reading a passage or doing a spontaneous speaking task and rate the severity of the stuttering on the Iowa Scale of Severity of Stuttering (see Appendix C). Have a fellow student (or some other person) also perform this task. How well do your severity ratings agree? If they are different, how do you explain the difference? Is your use of this scale reliable enough for clinical purposes?

▶ 3

The Person
Who Stutters

Do persons who stutter *as a group* have anything in common other than the fact they stutter? That is, do they share any attributes? This chapter focuses on the literature that addresses these questions.

While there is some overlap between the literature reviewed in this chapter and the preceding one, the orientation is different. In this chapter the focus is on the person who stutters rather than on stuttering behavior or the moment of stuttering per se. Characteristics of persons who stutter were discussed in Chapter 2 to help explain the symptomatology and phenomenology of stuttering. Relevant data are used in this chapter to help explain how persons who stutter function physiologically, how they feel about and react to themselves and others, and how they communicate aside from their moments of stuttering.

Caution is necessary when interpreting the information presented in this chapter. Even if the majority of persons who stutter appear to differ in some way from their normal-speaking peers, it is not safe to assume that the difference is related somehow to the etiology of their stuttering. It may be the result, for example, of living with the disorder rather than a cause of it.

A second reason why caution should be exercised is that "mind" and "body" are not independent entities. Physiological differences between groups can result from psychological differences between them and vice versa (Kent, 1983). A difference in anxiety level, for example, can produce a difference between groups in physiological events that occur when the level of activity of the sympathetic division of the autonomic nervous system is increased—for example, an increase in the amount of perspiration on the skin (Brutten & Shoemaker, 1967).

It is important for clinicians to be aware of how persons who stutter have been reported to differ from their normal-speaking peers in ways other than speech fluency. There are several reasons. First, it provides them with information they need to formulate hypotheses about the etiology of behaviors they want to modify. Before an intervention strategy for modifying a behavior can be formulated, it is necessary to make an assumption, or formulate an hypothesis, about why it occurs. If the strategies clinicians develop are consistent with their hypotheses and their hypotheses are valid, they are more likely to be successful in modifying the behavior (Williams, 1979).

Second, this awareness can help them understand their clients' attitudes, feelings, and reactions. If they do not understand these, they will tend to be less effective regardless of the therapy approaches they are using (Van Riper, 1979).

Third, it provides them with information they need to identify the set of behaviors that defines a client's stuttering problem. This set is likely to include behaviors other than those directly related to the moment of stuttering (Silverman, 1980a, 1980b). While no client is likely to exhibit all the behaviors referred to in this chapter, those mentioned occur often enough that they are worth checking for during an evaluation.

Fourth, the awareness can influence the prognosis for improvement. The presence or absence of certain attitudes, feelings, and reactions can influence (reduce or increase) the likelihood that a client will benefit from therapy (Van Riper, 1979).

PHYSIOLOGICAL CHARACTERISTICS

There has been considerable research during the past one hundred years on the physiological functioning of persons who stutter. Most of the subjects in these studies have been beyond elementary school age. Some findings that pertain to the following questions are summarized here:

- What physiological processes of persons who stutter have been investigated?
- How do persons who stutter, as a group, differ from normal-speaking peers in physiological functioning?
- Are there subgroups of stutterers who function in physiologically abnormal ways that may contribute to the onset or maintenance of their stuttering?

What Physiological Processes Have Been Investigated?

Many physiological processes have been investigated (directly or indirectly) in an attempt to identify an organic cause for stuttering. Those to which the most attention has been directed during the past one hundred years are discussed in this section, and the findings of studies pertaining to them are summarized in the next section.

Many of the processes discussed in this section and in a following one on psychological processes are interrelated. This has several implications. First, it suggests that when an investigator studies one process, he or she is likely to be indirectly studying others. For example, when an investigator studies respiration, he or she also *indirectly* studies biochemical, central nervous system, and autonomic nervous system functioning. Second, it suggests that an investigator has to be cautious when interpreting the results of his or her studies. If a difference is found between persons who stutter and their normal speaking peers, the cause may not be the process being investigated, but one related to it. For example, if an investigator found an anomaly in the functioning of their respiratory system, the cause may be an anomaly in the functioning of their central or autonomic nervous systems. Or it could even arise from an anomaly in psychological functioning or from learning!

Respiration
The respiratory functioning of persons who stutter has been compared both to that of normal speakers and to their own while silent or while they appear to be speaking fluently (Baken et al., 1983; Beech & Fransella, 1968).

Cardiovascular Functioning
Investigators have attempted to determine whether the cardiovascular functioning of persons who stutter differs from that of their normal-speaking peers (Beech & Fransella, 1968).

Biochemical Functioning
Three research approaches have been used to determine whether the biochemical functioning of stutterers differ from that of their normal-speaking peers. First, studies have compared the levels of specific biochemicals in the bodies of stutterers to those in nonstutterers (Hill, 1944a; Rastatter & Harr, 1988; Schleier, Schelhorn, & Groh, 1991). Second, there have been studies in which biochemical abnormalities were inferred by observing the effect of certain drugs (such as haloperidol) on their speech fluency (Rosenberger, 1980). And third, there have been studies on the incidence of stuttering among persons who have particular disturbances in biochemical functioning, such as diabetes (Van Riper, 1982).

Central Nervous System Functioning
Movements of the speech musculature are controlled, in part, by the central nervous system (CNS). Since stuttering blocks consist of abnormal movements of this musculature, it is not particularly surprising that there has been a great deal of research on the functioning of this system in stutterers. Among the investigated phenomena mediated by this system are the following: action potentials from the bilaterally paired musculatures of the speech mechanism (Travis, 1934; Williams, 1955), motor control (McClean, 1990), brain waves (Moore, 1984, 1986), hemispheric asymmetries for language processing (Hand & Haynes, 1983; Johannsen & Victor, 1986; Kent, 1983; Moore, 1976, 1990; Rastatter & Dell, 1987b; Rastatter, Loren, & Colcord, 1987), involuntary movements including tremors (Hill, 1944b), manual motor performance (e.g., Starkweather, Franklin, & Smigo, 1984; Till, Reich, Dickey, &

Seiber, 1983; Webster, 1989), muscular tension (Brown & Shulman, 1940), reflex activity (Smith & Luschei, 1983), oral motor coordination (Caruso et al., 1988; Perkins et al., 1976; Riley & Riley, 1986), performance on neuropsychological tests (Cox, 1982), and performance on self-paced rhythmic tasks (Brown, Zimmerman, Linville, & Hegmann, 1990).

Autonomic Nervous System Functioning

The *positive* relationship between the level of activity of the sympathetic division of the autonomic nervous system and anxiety is well established: Increases in anxiety tend to be associated with increases in level of activity (Brutten & Shoemaker, 1967). It also is well established that there is a *negative* relationship between its level of activity and relaxation—that is, increases in relaxation tend to be associated with decreases in its level of activity (Brutten & Shoemaker, 1967). In addition, it is generally accepted that anxiety level can affect motor performance, including that associated with respiration, phonation, and articulation (Brutten & Shoemaker, 1967). Investigators have attempted to determine whether stutterers differ from their normal-speaking peers in the functioning of their autonomic nervous system, particularly as it pertains to anxiety (Craig, 1990; Kraaimaat, Janssen, & Brutten, 1988).

Sensori-Perceptual Functioning

Investigators have attempted to determine whether the auditory, tactile-kinesthetic, and visual systems of persons who stutter differ from their normal-speaking peers. They have studied the prevalence of stuttering among persons with pathology in these systems—for example, those who are hearing-impaired (Montgomery & Fitch, 1988)—as well as the functioning of these systems in persons who stutter but who have not been diagnosed as having such pathology. One reason is that a disturbance in such functioning can affect speech fluency. For example, speaking in the presence of delayed auditory feedback or masking ("white") noise can reduce stuttering severity (see Chapter 2).

How Does the Physiological Functioning of Persons Who Stutter, as a Group, Differ from Their Normal-Speaking Peers?

While no differences in physiological functioning, other than those that occur during the moment of stuttering, have been demonstrated unequivocally to differentiate persons who stutter from their normal-speaking peers (Bloodstein, 1987; Van Riper, 1982), some investigators believe that there may be such differences. This belief, in part, is based on the findings of a number of studies that report such differences. Also, some believe that investigators may have failed to find them because they searched in the wrong place and/or used methodologies that were not sufficiently sensitive.

If there are physiological differences between persons who stutter and those who don't other than those occurring during moments of stuttering, where would they be most likely to be found? Since such differences probably would be most likely to be found where previous research suggests they exist, a summary of the findings of studies in the various areas mentioned in the preceding section is presented here.

Respiration

Because of the obvious anomalies in breathing movements that occur during moments of stuttering, it is not particularly surprising that this was one of the first areas in which investigators searched for a physiological cause for stuttering. Systematic research on the breathing movements of persons who stutter started at the beginning of this century (Beech & Fransella, 1968). Most research findings support the following conclusions:

- Various kinds of abnormalities in breathing movements may occur during moments of stuttering (Travis, 1927; Blackburn, 1931; Starbuck & Steer, 1954).
- Breathing patterns of stutterers during fluent speech may be abnormal (Johnston, Watkin, & Macklem, 1993; Williams & Brutten, 1994).
- The same types of breathing abnormalities tend to occur during both moments of stuttering and expectancy of stuttering (Van Riper, 1936).
- Patterns of chest wall posturing for phonation exhibited by stutterers are qualitatively identical to those exhibited by nonstutterers (Baken et al., 1983).
- Abnormalities observed in the breathing movements of persons who stutter during moments of stuttering usually are not present during silence (Bloodstein, 1987).
- During silence, the breathing movements of persons who stutter do not differ from those of their normal-speaking peers (Moore, 1938; Kurshev, 1968).

Cardiovascular Functioning

Systematic research on the cardiovascular functioning of persons who stutter has been ongoing for more than seventy-five years. The impetus for much of this research was the finding that the pulse rate of persons who stutter tends to increase (accelerate) before and during moments of stuttering (Fletcher, 1914). Those phenomena investigated that are associated with cardiovascular functioning include pulse rate, heart rate, sinus arrhythmia, blood pressure, and basal metabolic rate (Bloodstein, 1987). Research findings on cardiovascular functioning while stutterers are silent (and presumably not contemplating speaking) are mixed. While those of some studies (Brunner & Frank, 1976; Palmer & Gillette, 1938, 1939; Ritzman, 1943) indicate that phenomena associated with it differ in some way(s) from that of their normal-speaking peers, those of others (McCroskey, 1957; McDowell, 1928; Ritzman, 1943; Walker & Walker, 1973) do not.

Biochemical Functioning

Research on the chemical makeup of persons who stutter has been ongoing for more than sixty years. Among the biochemical phenomena that have been studied directly or indirectly are alveolar carbon dioxide level (Hill, 1944a; Johnson, Young, Sachs, & Bedell, 1959; Starr, 1928), salivary pH (Hafford, 1941; Kelly, 1932; Starr, 1928), chemical composition of the blood (Karlin & Sobel, 1940; Kopp, 1934; Podolskaya & Shklovsky, 1973), and plasma levels of adrenergic neurotransmitters and primary amino acids (Rosenberger, 1980; Rastatter & Harr, 1988). While some of these studies (such as Kelly, 1932; Kopp, 1934; Podolskaya & Shklovsky, 1973; Rastatter & Harr, 1988; Starr, 1928) report differences between stutterers and nonstutterers, others (such as Hafford, 1941; Hill, 1944a; Johnson et al., 1959; Karlin & Sobel, 1940) do not.

Central Nervous System Functioning

Research on the central nervous system (CNS) functioning of persons who stutter has been going on for more than fifty years. There were times during this period when differences between stutterers and nonstutterers appeared to have been found. During the 1930s, for example, a number of studies suggested that persons who stutter are less likely than normal speakers to have established unilateral cerebral dominance (Fitzgerald, Cooke, & Greiner, 1984).

Much of the recent physiological research on stuttering has dealt with central nervous system functioning. A number of investigators have reported finding differences between persons who stutter and their peers (Watson, Freeman, Devous, Chapman, Finitzo, & Pool, 1994). Some of those reported are considered in the following paragraphs.

A number of studies of the *cortical potentials* (brain waves) of persons who stutter suggest they may differ from those of their normal-speaking peers during silence, auditory presentation of words, visual presentation of words, anticipation of speaking, and speaking (see Table 9 in Bloodstein, 1987, pp. 136–140). However, in most studies there were stutterers whose brain waves (cortical potentials) did not differ from those of normal speakers. Also, the areas of the cerebral cortex in which irregularities were detected were not the same in all studies.

The prevalence of stuttering among persons with known brain damage has been reported to be higher than in the general population (approximately 1 percent). This conclusion is based on the findings of a number of studies. The populations surveyed included person with epilepsy (Gens, 1950; Harrison, 1947), cerebral palsy (Heltman & Peacher, 1943; Rutherford, 1938), and/or mental deficiency (Boberg, Ewart, Mason, Lindsay, & Wynn, 1978; Schlanger & Gottsleben, 1957). The prevalence of stuttering in these studies ranged from 1.5 to more than 20 percent.

An aspect of central nervous system functioning in stutterers on which there has been considerable research is *cerebral lateralization of function* (Penfield & Roberts, 1959). Investigators have used several strategies for determining (directly or indirectly) whether stutterers differ from their normal-speaking peers in the lateralization of certain functions within their cerebral cortex. Aspects of their sensory, motor, and language functioning that are thought to be mediated by either the right or left side of this structure have been studied. These strategies will now be discussed along with the major findings obtained when using them.

One of the first strategies that was used to investigate cerebral lateralization of function in persons who stutter was to assess their handedness and other manifestations of cerebral sidedness, such as eyedness and footedness (Spadino, 1941). They were required to complete questionnaires and do tasks (such as writing or catching a ball) designed to assess whether they consistently performed them with the hand, foot, and eye on the same side of the body (right or left) or whether they were ambidextrous and lacked a dominant, hand, foot, and eye. Since the cerebral cortex is responsible, in part, for the performance of such tasks, inferences can be made about the roles of the right and left halves of the cerebral cortex in carrying them out by observing how they are executed. Consistent use of the left side of the body for doing the tasks would indicate that the right side of the cerebral cortex is dominant for hand, foot, and eye functions and vice versa. However, use of both the right and left extremities and eyes for doing tasks would indicate lack of dominance of one side of the cerebral cortex over the other for mediating hand, foot, and eye functions.

Many of the early studies of peripheral sidedness (such as Van Riper, 1935) suggested that persons who stutter, as a group, are less likely than their normal-speaking peers to have established unilateral cerebral dominance: They are more likely than them to be ambidexterous. This lack of unilateral cerebral dominance was thought to be a cause of stuttering (see Chapter 5). It was hypothesized, for example, that left-handed persons who are forced to write with their right hand begin to stutter because becoming skillful with their right hand causes them to become ambidexterous and as a consequence they lose unilateral cerebral dominance (Fagan, 1931; Travis, 1931). After 1940, interest in the peripheral sidedness of persons who stutter lessened because of research suggesting that the methodology used in these studies was faulty (Williams, 1955). When these studies were replicated using methodologies regarded as appropriate, stutterers no longer seemed more likely then their peers to lack unilateral cerebral dominance.

Interest in the cerebral lateralization of persons who stutter lay dormant for several decades. There was renewed interest during the 1960s, in part, because of research indicating that cerebral lateralization for speech and language does not necessarily correspond to that for handedness and other aspects of peripheral sidedness (Penfield & Roberts, 1959). Earlier investigators of cerebral lateralization in persons who stutter appeared to have implicitly or explicitly assumed that they could infer lateralization for speech and language from that for handedness, footedness, and eyedness.

The *Wada test* was one of the first methodologies used during this period to study stutterers' cerebral lateralization for speech and language. This test is used by neurosurgeons preoperatively to determine which half of the cerebral cortex is dominant for these functions (Penfield & Roberts, 1959). Sodium amytal is injected into the right and the left carotid arteries, one at a time. The right carotid artery provides the blood supply to the right half of the cerebral cortex and left carotid artery provides it to the left half. If a person temporarily loses the ability to speak when sodium amytal is injected into a carotid artery, it is assumed that a center for mediating speech and language is located in the hemisphere of the cerebral cortex to which the artery supplies blood. By injecting sodium amytal into the carotid arteries one at a time it can be determined whether control for speech and language functions is located in the right half of the cerebral cortex, the left half of the cerebral cortex, or both. For most persons it appears to be located in one-half of the cerebral cortex, almost always the left (Penfield & Roberts, 1959).

A report was published by a neurosurgeon on four of his patients who stuttered in which he indicated that Wada tests administered before surgery demonstrated a lack of lateralization—that is, all four appeared to have a center for language processing in both hemispheres (Jones, 1966). Investigators who attempted to replicate this finding (such as Rosenfield, Jones, & Liljestrand, 1981) did not detect such a lack of lateralization in any of their stuttering subjects.

A second methodology that was used during this period to study cerebral lateralization in persons who stutter was *dichotic listening* (Blood & Blood, 1989a, 1989b; Blood, Blood, & Hood, 1987; Curry & Gregory, 1969). This task, like the Wada test, was used to infer cerebral lateralization for speech and language processing. It is administered by having the subject listen simultaneously to pairs of different words, one with the right and one with the left ear. Most persons report the words they hear through their right ear more accurately than those they hear through their left ear. Since words heard with the right ear are sent to the left half of the cerebral cortex for processing, the fact that most persons understand more of what they hear with their right than with their left ear provides additional support for the hypothesis that the left hemisphere of the cerebral cortex is usually dominant for speech and language processing.

If, on dichotic listening tasks, persons who stutter do not do as much better with their right ear as do normal speakers, this would suggest that the left hemisphere of their cerebral cortex was less dominant than is normal for language processing. In other words, it might indicate that their right hemisphere had a greater than normal role in mediating language functioning. It is not surprising, therefore, that a number of investigators have used dichotic listening to test the hypothesis that at least some persons who stutter lack unilateral cerebral dominance for speech and language processing. While the findings of some studies are consistent with this hypothesis (such as Curry & Gregory, 1969), those of others (such as Quinn, 1972; Cerf & Prins, 1974) are not. In studies that could be interpreted as supporting the hypothesis, persons who stuttered, as a group, did less well than normal speakers in comprehending words heard through their right ear.

A third methodology that has been used to study cerebral lateralization for speech and language in persons who stutter is *electroencephalography.* Changes in brain waves (usually the alpha ones) that occur in the right hemisphere are compared to those that occur in the left during tasks requiring linguistic processing (Boberg, Yeudall, Schopflocher, & Bo-Lassen, 1983; Moore, 1984). Normal speakers tend to evince a larger change in the left than in the right hemisphere while performing such tasks. Some persons who stutter, on the other hand, have been reported to evince a larger change in the right hemisphere than in the left while doing so (Moore, 1986).

One reason why some stutterers may differ from normal speakers in level of right hemisphere activity is that the tasks used may produce more stress (anxiety) in those who stutter than in those who don't. There is some evidence that stress results in greater activation of the right hemisphere (Boberg et al., 1983). Hence, the increase in right hemisphere brain wave activity evinced by some persons who stutter may have resulted from conditioned anxiety to the receptive/expressive aspects of the speech act rather than from the use of the right hemisphere for language processing (Boberg et al., 1983).

Several other methodologies have been used to study cerebral lateralization for speech and language in persons who stutter. These include auditory tracking (Neilson, Quinn, & Neilson, 1976; Sussman & MacNeilage, 1975), the presentation of words in different halves of the visual field using a tachistoscopic viewing procedure (Hardin, Pindzola, & Haynes, 1992; Johannsen & Victor, 1986; Rastatter & Dell, 1987b; Rastatter & Loren, 1988; Rastatter, McGuire, & Loren, 1988; Szelag et al., 1993), and finger tapping with right and left hands while performing speech tasks (Brutten & Trotter, 1985). The findings of studies that used these methodologies are mixed. Some findings (Johannsen & Victor, 1986; Rastatter & Dell, 1987b; Rastatter & Loren, 1988; Rastatter et al., 1988; Sussman & MacNeilage, 1975) suggest that at least some persons who stutter use their right hemisphere more than normal speakers do to process speech and language. However, those of others (Brutten & Trotter, 1985; Hardin et al., 1992; Johannsen & Victor, 1986; Rastatter & Dell, 1987b; Neilson, Quinn, & Neilson, 1976) did not indicate any differences between groups in this regard. The findings of studies using these methodologies, therefore, are the same as those using the others discussed in this section—that is, although some persons who stutter seem to evince higher levels of right hemisphere activity on some tasks involving language processing than their normal-speaking peers, the available evidence does not indicate that this is true for all persons who stutter.

The motor capabilities of the speech mechanism are determined, in large part, by the functioning of the central nervous system. Since the musculature of this mechanism functions abnormally during moments of stuttering, it is not particularly surprising that investigators have researched the possibility that persons who stutter have less than normal ability to control the movements of at least some parts of this musculature. Most of the early studies on the motor capabilities of persons who stutter dealt with general bodily coordination (Finkelstein & Weisberger, 1954; Kopp, 1946) and manual skills (Bloodstein, 1987; Finkelstein & Weisberger, 1954; Starkweather, Franklin, & Smigo, 1984; Till, Reich, Dickey, & Seiber, 1983; R. L. Webster, 1986; W. G. Webster, 1985, 1989). Investigators reasoned that if persons who stutter had a neuromuscular disorder or apraxia that affected their speech mechanism, it would be likely to affect other parts of their musculature, including that of the upper extremities. While differences were reported in some of these studies between persons who stutter and their peers (Kopp, 1946; Starkweather, Franklin, & Smigo, 1984; Webster, 1986, 1989), they were not reported in others (Bloodstein, 1987; Finkelstein & Weisberger, 1954; Till, Reich, Dickey, & Seiber, 1983; Webster, 1985). The findings of these studies, therefore, suggest that the general motor capabilities of some persons who stutter tend to be inferior to those of their normal-speaking peers, but do not establish this unequivocally for the majority of them.

During the past twenty years much of the research on the motor performance of persons who stutter has focused on the musculature of the speech mechanism. Subtle oral-motor coordination differences between them and their normal-speaking peers have been reported, particularly involving the functioning of the larynx (Perkins et al., 1976; Riley & Riley, 1986). The phrase "oral-motor discoordination" has been used to refer to these differences (Perkins et al., 1976; Riley & Riley, 1986). Many stutterers have been reported to exhibit such abnormalities in laryngeal functioning during moments of stuttering. From time to time hypotheses have been advanced suggesting that stuttering results from some disturbance in the functioning of the laryngeal mechanism. A relatively large number of studies have been published during the past twenty years (Adams, 1981, 1984, 1988; Adams & Hayden, 1976; Bakker & Brutten, 1990; Borden et al., 1985; Conture et al., 1985; Cross & Luper, 1979, 1983; Dembowski & Watson, 1991; De Nil & Brutten, 1991b; Ferrand, Gilbert, & Blood, 1991; Freeman, 1979; Hall & Yairi, 1992; Hayden, Jordahl, & Adams, 1982; Healey & Gutkin, 1984; Jäncke, 1994; Lees, 1988; Mallard et al., 1982; McFarlane & Shipley, 1981; Nudelman, Herbrich, Hess, Hoyt, & Rosenfield, 1992; Rastatter & Dell, 1987a, 1987b; Rastatter et al., 1987; Reich, Till, & Goldsmith, 1981; Starkweather, 1982; Starkweather, Franklin, & Smigo, 1984; Starkweather, Hirshman, & Tannenbaum, 1976; Till, Reich, Dickey, & Seiber, 1983; Williams & Brutten, 1994) that were designed, at least in part, to determine whether stutterers differ from nonstutterers with regard to phonatory reaction time—the time it takes a person to initiate or terminate phonation after being given a signal to do so. While the findings of most of these studies indicate that the typical (mean or median) stutterer tends to be slower than the typical normal speaker, they also indicate that some overlap exists between groups. That is, some stutterers have faster phonatory reaction times than some normal speakers. There is also some evidence, incidentally, that stutterers who tend to have relatively slow phonatory reaction times also tend to have relatively slow reaction times for nonspeech movements (Cross & Luper, 1983).

Autonomic Nervous System Functioning

For more than fifty years investigators have been interested in the possibility that abnormalities in the functioning of the autonomic nervous system contribute to the etiology of stuttering. Interest in this possibility is not particularly surprising considering that the level of activity of its sympathetic division is positively related to anxiety (Brutten & Shoemaker, 1967) and that some explanations for the moment of stuttering attribute it, at least in part, to anxiety (see Chapter 5).

Seeman (1934) was one of the first to look into the possibility that an abnormality in the functioning of the autonomic nervous system could contribute to the etiology of stuttering. He believed that such an abnormality could do so by causing the sympathetic division to become hyperactive, or more irritable than normal. His hypothesis received some support from the findings of several studies of stutterers' sympathetic reactivity during silence (Sedlacek, 1947–48). Unfortunately, the numbers of stutterers evincing particular abnormalities in these studies were not compared to those in matched control groups of normal speakers. While there is a paucity of studies designed to determine whether stutterers differ from nonstutterers in sympathetic division reactivity, it is possible that some stutterers have a tendency toward higher than normal levels of such reactivity, resulting in lower thresholds for autonomic response to stress. It should be noted, however, that in the two studies cited above not all stutterers exhibited abnormalities in autonomic nervous system functioning. It appears, therefore, that such an abnormality is *not* a necessary condition for the development of stuttering.

Auditory Functioning
Even though the prevalence of stuttering in the hearing-impaired population appears to be lower than that in the general population (Andrews et al., 1983; Montgomery & Fitch, 1988), a number of investigators have looked into the possibility that persons who stutter have an anomaly in their auditory system that somehow contributes to the etiology of their disorder. Aspects of their auditory functioning that have been investigated include the following: threshold for pure tones (St. Louis & Hinzman, 1988), relative phase angle of air- and bone-conducted sounds (Stromsta, 1957, 1972); right ear versus left ear presentation of stimuli—as in dichotic listening (Curry & Gregory, 1969; Liebetrau & Daly, 1981; McFarlane & Shipley, 1981), effect of delayed auditory feedback on oral activity not involving speech (Stark & Pierce, 1970), central auditory functioning at the level of the brain stem (Anderson, Hood, & Sellers, 1988; Bonin, Ramig, & Prescott, 1985; Decker, Healey, & Howe, 1982; Dietrich, Barry, & Parker, 1995; Hageman & Greene, 1989; Hall & Jerger, 1978; Kent, 1983; McLean-Muse, Larson, & Gregory, 1988; Stager, 1990), and reflex response of the middle ear muscles to sound (Hannley & Dorman, 1982; Horovitz, Johnson, Pearlman, Schaffer, & Hedin, 1978). The findings of these studies, like those for all aspects of the physiological functioning of persons who stutter, are mixed. While some investigators who have researched a particular aspect of auditory functioning report differences between persons who stutter and their peers (Bonin et al., 1985; Hall & Jerger, 1978; Toscher & Rupp, 1978), others do not (McLean-Muse et al., 1988). Incidentally, in many of the studies in which a group difference was reported, the author(s) concluded that the subjects who stuttered behaved more like their normal-speaking peers then they did like persons who were known to have auditory system lesions. Perhaps, as some investigators have specu-

lated, the reported differences in auditory functioning between persons who stutter and those who do not result, in part, from differences in their anxiety levels (Horovitz, Johnson, Pearlman, Schaffer, & Hedin, 1978).

Tactile-Kinesthetic Functioning

A disturbance in tactile-kinesthetic feedback can have a detrimental effect on the performance of motor acts. While such acts are occurring, information is continuously being sent to the brain from receptors in the muscles and the skin about the state of contraction of the various muscles and the location in space of the various structures involved in performing the acts. Could a disturbance in tactile-kinesthetic feedback disrupt movements of the articulators and vocal folds in a way that would cause a breakdown in speech fluency? A few investigators have attempted to answer this question. The aspects of tactile-kinesthetic functioning that they studied included threshold for vibratory sensation (Fucci, Petrosino, Gorman, & Harris, 1985), intra-oral two-point discrimination (Jensen, Sheehan, Williams, & LaPointe, 1975), and oral recognition of forms (Jensen et al., 1975; Martin, Lawrence, Haroldson, & Gunderson, 1981; Stewart, Evans, & Fitch, 1985). The findings of their studies (like those of the other aspects of physiological functioning discussed in this chapter) are mixed. While the available evidence does not rule out the possibility that a disturbance in tactile-kinesthetic feedback contributes to the etiology of stuttering, neither does it provide strong support for the existence of such an etiologic factor.

Visual Functioning

A number of investigators have studied the visual performance of persons who stutter. While the functioning of the eyes and central visual nervous system is only indirectly related to that of the speech mechanism, differences between persons who stutter and those who do not during the performance of visual tasks could point to differences between them in central nervous system functioning for speech (Hand & Haynes, 1983; Rastatter & Dell, 1988).

The aspects of visual functioning that have been studied in persons who stutter include the following: visual acuity, phoria, binocular perception, color vision, visual perseveration, and perception of visual symbols. In addition, there has been research on the prevalence of stuttering among persons who are blind and partially sighted. The findings of these studies suggest that the prevalence of stuttering among blind and partially sighted persons is the same as that in the general population (Weinberg, 1964) and that the visual acuity, phoria, binocular perception, and color vision of persons who stutter are within normal limits (Hamilton, 1940; Schindler, 1955). It is uncertain, however, whether the performance of persons who stutter is within normal limits on visual perseveration and visual symbol perception tasks. While some studies suggest that they perform differently than normal speakers on the tasks (Goldsand, 1944; Kelly, 1932), those of others do not (Hamilton, 1940; King, 1961). Consequently, these findings are the same as for most other aspects of physiological functioning discussed in this chapter—mixed.

Is There a Subgroup of Persons in the Stuttering Population Who Function Abnormally Physiologically in Ways That May Contribute to the Onset and/or Maintenance of Their Stuttering?

Does the fact that only some persons who stutter appear to evince physiological anomalies indicate that the etiology of stuttering is not the same for all persons? That is, does it indicate that there are subgroups within the stuttering population? Some of those who have written about stuttering (such as Bloodstein, 1987; Liebetrau & Daly, 1981; Sheehan, 1970; St. Onge, 1963; St. Onge & Calvert, 1964; Van Riper, 1982) suggest that there may be such subgroups. Their existence could partially explain why differences were found between stutterers and nonstutterers in some investigations of a particular physiological phenomenon, but not in others. That is, whether anomalies were found in a particular study would be at least partially a function of the proportion of stuttering subjects in it who were from the organic type. The higher this proportion, the higher the probability that a difference would be found between the groups.

PSYCHOLOGICAL CHARACTERISTICS

There is considerable information available about the psychological characteristics of persons who stutter. Some comes from research and some from anecdotal reports by clinicians, stutterers, and others. Some is applicable to most, if not all, persons who stutter and some to only a relatively small segment of the stuttering population—such as older stutterers (Manning, Dailey, & Wallace, 1984). Much of this information is summarized here, particularly that pertaining to the following questions:

- What psychological attributes of persons who stutter have been investigated?
- How do persons who stutter, as a group, tend to differ psychologically from their normal-speaking peers?

What Psychological Attributes of Persons Who Stutter Have Been Investigated?

There are few, if any, psychological attributes that have not been dealt with some-where in the stuttering literature. Many are discussed in autobiographies of persons who stutter (see Carlisle, 1985; Johnson, 1930; Murray, 1980; Wedberg, 1956). Many are also discussed in the writings of clinicians who have treated persons who stutter, including those of psychiatrists (see Barbara, 1982; Freund, 1966; Glauber, 1982; Wolpe, 1958), psychologists (see Fransella, 1972; Murphy & Fitzsimons, 1960; Sheehan, 1968, 1970), and speech pathologists (see Johnson, 1932, 1946, 1958, 1961; Van

Riper, 1958, 1973, 1979, 1982). In addition, a great deal of information about such attributes has been published in research journals, particularly those in the fields of speech pathology, psychology, and psychiatry (Goodstein, 1958; Sermas & Cox, 1982). This section makes use of information from all these sources.

Intelligence

The intelligence of persons who stutter has been investigated in several ways including determining whether their performance on intelligence tests differs from that of the general population (Andrews & Harris, 1964; Okasha, Bishry, Kamel, & Hassan, 1974; Schindler, 1955) and assessing the prevalence of the disorder among persons with mental deficiency (Bloodstein, 1987, Table 20; Keane, 1972).

Emotional Adjustment

There has been considerable research on the emotional adjustment of persons who stutter (Sermas & Cox, 1982). Most tests and other procedures that psychologists and psychiatrists have developed for evaluating emotional adjustment have been administered to them.

Personality Traits

There has also been considerable research on the personality of those who stutter (Manning et al., 1984; Sermas & Cox, 1982). A number of traits have been studied, including levels of anxiety (Fitzgerald, Djurdjic, & Maguin, 1992; Miller & Watson, 1992; Craig, 1990), depression (Miller & Watson, 1992; Richardson, 1944; Shames, 1951), obsessive-compulsiveness (Bloodstein & Schreiber, 1957), self-reliance (Perkins, 1947), capacity for abstract thinking (Meltzer, 1944), drive toward achievement (Goodstein, 1958; Sheehan & Zussman, 1951), oral and anal eroticism (Carp, 1962), passive-dependency (Katz, 1966), hostility (Bloch & Goodstein, 1971), aggression (Bloch & Goodstein, 1971), guilt (Lowinger, 1952), and locus of control orientation (McDonough & Quesal, 1988).

Self-Concept

Aspects of self-concept that have been studied include level of aspiration (Sheehan, 1979b), body image (Devore, Nandur, & Manning, 1984), thinking of yourself as a stutterer (Perkins, 1993), and sex-role identification (Broida, 1963).

How Do Persons Who Stutter, as a Group, Tend to Differ Psychologically From Their Normal-Speaking Peers?

Intelligence

While most estimates of the average IQ of stutterers that have been reported (those by Andrews & Harris, 1964; Okasha et al., 1974; Schindler, 1955) fall in the general region of 100 (the theoretical average for the population at large), in studies in which they have been compared to nonstutterers (Andrews & Harris, 1964; Okasha et al., 1974; Schindler, 1955) their IQs tended to be slightly lower, approximately half a standard deviation. This deficit is evident in both verbal and nonverbal intelligence tests (Andrews et al., 1983), and it may explain, in part, why they tend to lag approximately six months behind their peers educationally (Andrews et al., 1983; Williams, Melrose, & Woods, 1969). The prevalence of stuttering among the mentally retarded that has been reported in some studies (see Bloodstein, 1987, Table 20) is approximately 3 percent. This exceeds that in the general population, which is approximately 1 percent. While there is a little evidence that suggests the symptomatology of their stuttering can be similar to that of other persons who have the disorder (e.g., Chapman & Cooper, 1973; Lerman, Powers, & Rigrodsky, 1965; Preus, 1972; Shearer & Baud, 1970), it is uncertain for how many of them this is true.

Do college students who stutter tend to differ in IQ from their normal-speaking peers? There is a little evidence (Fruewald, 1936) that suggests that they tend, on the average, to have higher IQs than their peers. This could explain why professors generally don't expect students who stutter to be unintelligent and incompetent (Silverman, 1991).

Emotional Adjustment
While the available data (both clinical and research) do not provide strong support for the conclusion that stuttering is usually a symptom of a neurosis or other type of emotional disorder (Andrews et al., 1983; Miller & Watson, 1992; Sermas & Cox, 1982), they do not rule out the possibility that it is a symptom of such a disorder for some persons who stutter. These data come from two sources. The first is from studies in which persons who stutter were evaluated for the presence of psychopathology by means of psychological tests. And the second is from studies and case reports in which the impact of psychotherapy on stuttering was reported.

The following are some of the psychological tests that have been administered to persons who stutter by investigators who wanted to determine whether they have a type of psychopathology of which stuttering could be a symptom:

- Bell Adjustment Inventory (Duncan, 1949)
- Bernrueter Personality Inventory (Bender, 1939)
- Blacky Test (Carp, 1962)
- California Test of Personality (Prins, 1972)
- Children's Apperception Test (CAT) (Porterfield, 1969)
- Eysenck Personality Inventory (Hegde, 1972)
- Guilford Inventory of Factors (Shames, 1951)
- Junior Eysenck Personality Inventory (Okasha et al., 1974)
- Kessler PD Scale (Shopwin, 1959)
- Maslow Test of Insecurity (Brutten, 1951)

- Minnesota Multiphasic Personality Inventory (MMPI) (Horlick & Miller, 1960; Lanyon, Goldsworthy, & Lanyon, 1978; Sermas & Cox, 1982)
- Minnesota Personality Scale (Brown & Hull, 1942)
- Rathus Assertiveness Schedule (Cohen, Thompson, Ruppel, & Flaherty, 1975)
- Revised Hopkins Symptom Checklist (Sermas & Cox, 1982)
- Revised Willoughby Personality Schedule (Greiner, Fitzgerald, Cooke, & Djurdjik, 1985)
- Rogers Test of Personality Adjustment (Darley, 1955)
- Rorschach Test (e.g., Goodstein, 1958; Sermas & Cox, 1982)
- Rosenzweig P-F Study (Quarrington, 1953)
- Sarason General Anxiety Scale for Children (Andrews & Harris, 1964)
- Structured Doll Play Test (Katz, 1966)
- Thematic Apperception Test (TAT) (e.g., Sermas & Cox, 1982)
- Woodsworth-House Mental Hygiene Inventory (Johnson, 1932)

The findings of most of the studies in which these tests were used did not indicate that persons who stutter, as a group, are less well adjusted than their peers, but rather that they are more similar to them than to persons who are known to be emotionally disturbed (see Bloodstein, 1987; Cox, 1982; Sermas & Cox, 1982; Van Riper, 1982).

There are several factors that could have contributed to stutterers appearing less well adjusted than their peers on some of these tests. One was the inclusion of items that relate to attitudes toward speaking (such as "Do you find it difficult to speak in public?"). Most older children and adults who stutter are aware that, in at least some situations, they tend to have poorer speech skills than nonstutterers (Watson, 1988). They, therefore, are likely to respond "inappropriately" to such items for different reasons than do normal speakers who are emotionally disturbed. A second was their being less well adjusted than nonstutterers as a consequence of living with stuttering (Andrews et al., 1983). Living with almost any disability can adversely affect a person's emotional adjustment (Miller & Watson, 1992).

A second type of evidence that supports the conclusion that stuttering usually is not a symptom of some type of emotional disorder are reports addressing the impact of psychotherapy on stuttering. If stuttering were a symptom of an emotional disorder, we would expect it to be reduced considerably in severity or eliminated by "successful" psychotherapy, particularly successful psychoanalysis. Reports in the literature about the impact of psychoanalysis and other forms of psychotherapy on stuttering do not indicate that it is often successful by itself in eliminating it or dramatically reducing its severity (Barbara, 1982; Bloodstein, 1987; Eldridge, 1968; Freund, 1966; Van Riper, 1973; Webster, 1977). *This should not be interpreted to mean that persons who stutter are unlikely to benefit from psychotherapy.* Many have benefited from it. However, the ways in which they are likely to do so are unlikely to include the amelioration of their stuttering.

While the available evidence does not support the conclusion that stuttering is a symptom of psychopathology for the majority of persons who stutter, it does not disprove that it may be such for some persons. There are case reports suggesting that it can be such a symptom (see Luchsinger & Arnold, 1965; Van Riper, 1979). Also, the available evidence does not disprove that there are stutterers who are severely emotionally disturbed (Cox, 1986). The prevalence of severe emotional disturbance in the stuttering population is at least as great as that in the general population (Cox, 1986). Finally, the available evidence does not disprove that the emotional adjustment of persons who stutter influences the severity of their stuttering. It undoubtedly does do so for at least some persons who stutter.

Personality Traits
While there has been considerable speculation (particularly in the psychiatric literature) about personality traits common to persons who stutter, their presence has not been established empirically. There is no personality trait that almost all persons who stutter have been shown unequivocally to possess (Bloodstein, 1987).

While there do not appear to be any personality traits common to all persons who stutter, there are some that many of them appear to possess. The reason may be, in part, that they have been reacted to negatively in a similar manner by their normal-speaking peers—for example, they have often been teased, mocked, laughed at, patronized, and treated as intellectually inferior by them.

Many persons who stutter are not as outgoing as they probably would be if they did not have the disorder. This is not particularly surprising, considering how they are perceived and consequently reacted to by some people with whom they interact (Turnbaugh, Guitar, & Hoffman, 1981). They tend to avoid social situations in which they expect people to react negatively to them because they stutter. And when they do enter such situations, they tend to talk less than they would if they did not stutter. They are particularly likely to avoid social interactions that involve talking on the telephone—a situation in which most stutterers tend to stutter relatively severely (see Chapter 2). There is a little evidence, however, that at least some tend to become less concerned about their stuttering—and, consequently, less likely to avoid talking because of it—after they are fifty years old (Manning et al., 1984).

Is it an abnormal tendency on the part of many stutterers to avoid situations in which they would have to do a lot of talking? While it increases the extent to which they are handicapped by their stuttering problem, it does not appear, in most cases, to indicate the presence of psychopathology. It is normal to try to avoid pain—both physical and psychological! Since persons who stutter are likely to experience negative reactions to their stuttering as pain and since most of them probably are not masochists, their attempts to reduce the pain in their life by avoiding talking (and, hence, stuttering) whenever possible are understandable. The problem is that the price they pay for avoiding this source of pain may be too high. It can, for example, cause them to choose an occupation in which they will not have to do much talking, particularly on the telephone. Since most relatively high-paying jobs in our society do entail a great deal of talking (including on the telephone), their choice of one that does not require this can adversely affect them economically.

A second way that persons who stutter may pay too high a price for avoiding this source of pain is restricting their social relationships—including romantic relationships. Many teenage (and older) males who stutter, for example, avoid dating because of concern about how their date will react to their stuttering, particularly if they have to make the date by telephone (Carlisle, 1985). One way that a speech-language pathologist can be helpful to such persons is to increase their awareness of the price they are paying for avoiding this source of pain.

While many persons who stutter are not very outgoing, there are some who are so in spite of reactions to their stuttering. They sometimes choose occupations in which the ability to communicate well is important. Such occupations include teaching, law, medicine, sales, speech pathology (Murray & Edwards, 1980; Johnson, 1930; Van Riper, 1979), psychology, social work, entertainment (Tillis & Wager, 1984), accounting, politics, and the ministry. They may also choose avocations that cause them to be actively involved with various groups in their community.

A second personality trait that is shared by many persons who stutter is unwillingness to express anger openly when doing so would be appropriate (Barbara, 1982). This trait, which appears to result from living with stuttering, can influence its severity. The more anger they feel and the less willing they are to express it openly, the more severely they are likely to stutter. The effect of openly expressing anger on fluency can be dramatic—very few people tend to stutter while they are swearing!

Why might many persons who stutter sometimes be unwilling to express anger openly when doing so would be appropriate? One reason may be they believe that people will not like them as well if they do so. That is, they believe that openly expressing anger will cause them to be rejected (Rubin, 1969).

A third personality trait that is shared by many persons who stutter is depression related to coping with stuttering (Johnson, 1946; Miller & Watson, 1992). All depression they evince, of course, is not from this source. They can be depressed for the same reasons as their normal-speaking peers—both psychological and biochemical.

Why might stuttering cause clients to be depressed? There are several possible reasons. First, they may be depressed as a consequence of the grieving process (Tanner, 1980). This is a normal, predictable, healing process that people go through when they experience a loss. The first stage is denial, the second is anger, the third is bargaining, the fourth is depression, and the fifth is acceptance. The loss that the stutterer has sustained is the ability to speak normally and all that this implies for interpersonal relationships. While the length of time people normally spend at each stage of this process can vary considerably, depending on the nature of the loss and their ability to cope, some persons remain at a particular stage so long that it is likely that they have become *fixated* (Tanner, 1980). Some persons who stutter appear to have become fixated at the depression stage (Johnson, 1946). They have not reached the acceptance stage at which they would accept the fact that they stutter, then do what they can to reduce its severity, and get on with their lives.

A second reason why stuttering may cause clients (particularly adult ones) to become depressed is that they believe their failure to overcome stuttering is their fault. That is, they believe it is possible to overcome stuttering and their failure to do so means that they have not tried hard enough or are too weak-willed. The belief that it should be possible to cure their stuttering could have been based on information from any of several sources, including books about the disorder (such as Schwartz, 1976; Schwartz & Carter, 1986) and statements made to them by speech pathologists and other clinicians. Their belief may not be accurate (Cooper, 1987).

A third reason why clients may experience depression because of stuttering is that they are overreacting to their disfluency, possibly because they are perfectionistic (Amster, 1994). That is, they are reacting more negatively to it than others are likely to. Some persons who have become quite fluent as a result of therapy experience depression from this very source. Rather than comparing their present fluency level to what it was before therapy and feeling good about what they have accomplished, these persons compare it to an idealized one of perfect fluency. As a result, they perceive themselves as having failed and become depressed. Such persons have what Johnson (1946) referred to as the "IFD disease." That is, they go from idealism to frustration to demoralization. Their internal standard for acceptable fluency is vague and/or unrealistically high. Either would result in their judging their fluency as unacceptable, which, in turn, would lead to frustration and finally demoralization (depression). Even a few mild moments of stuttering a month could cause a person with this orientation to become depressed! Some extremely mild stutterers may become depressed for this reason.

Being a stutterer can lead to frustration for other reasons also. These include lack of emotional contact with people. Teens who stutter, for example, tend to date less often than their peers.

A fourth personality trait that is shared by many persons who stutter is guilt about stuttering (Van Riper, 1982). This guilt could have arisen from several sources. One is the belief that they are somehow responsible for beginning to stutter because they did not do what was necessary to talk correctly. This belief could have had its origin in advice they received as children from their parents and others to talk slower, or to take a deep breath before beginning to talk, or to think of what they are going to say before they say it, and it may have been reinforced by one or more of the following reactions to their stuttering:

- Being rejected, punished, or mocked because of it
- Having people (particularly their parents) look away or sometimes have a pained expression on their face while they were doing it
- Having people, particularly their parents, participate in a conspiracy of silence about it. This may communicate to them that what they are doing is so bad that it cannot even be mentioned.

All of these could be interpreted to imply that they stutter because they did not try hard enough to stop.

This belief could also have been reinforced by speech pathologists. They may, for example, have made comments to their clients suggesting that they stutter "because they do things that interfere with talking." While this may be true, and it may be necessary to make such comments to motivate clients to work on their speech, it is important to recognize that these remarks can reinforce their guilt.

A second belief that can result in such guilt is that stutterers are somehow responsible for their continuing to stutter. This belief can be reinforced by information they receive from the media and from professionals (including speech pathologists), which suggests that it is possible for them to be cured or learn to speak with considerably less abnormality. This may not be true for some persons who stutter (Cooper, 1987). Their guilt can also be reinforced by their certainty that they should be able to change any aspect of their behavior.

A third belief from which guilt can arise is that people who stutter are somehow responsible if they relapse following termination of therapy, that is, if they fail to maintain the fluency they gained while in therapy. This belief may result, in part, from comments made by their clinician suggesting that if they had been doing what they should have been doing to maintain their fluency, they would not have relapsed. This may or may not be true.

A fourth belief that may contribute to guilt is that when people stutter, they take too much of other people's time. Having this belief is likely to both put them under time pressure to speak fluently, which tends to increase stuttering severity, and motivate them to avoid words on which they expect to stutter. Stutterers, for example, may order something in a restaurant they do not want believing that if they order what they really do want, they will stutter and take too much of the server's time.

Feelings of guilt about stuttering can lead to feelings of shame or embarrassment (Van Riper, 1982). Many persons who stutter report feeling ashamed or embarrassed about doing so. This accounts, at least in part, for the poor eye contact that many of them evince during moments of stuttering. Psychologists have found that looking away is one of the main behavioral changes associated with feeling ashamed about something (Atkins, 1988). Hence, one strategy that could be used for improving the eye contact of persons who stutter would be to reduce their feelings of shame or embarrassment about stuttering.

A fifth personality trait that is shared by many persons who stutter is anxiety about speaking (Miller & Watson, 1992; Craig, 1990). Such anxiety can result from anticipating stuttering in a speaking situation and desiring to avoid it (Miller & Watson, 1992; Watson, 1988). Some authorities have speculated that it contributes to precipitating moments of stuttering (see Chapter 5).

Some persons whose stuttering is relatively mild tend to experience a higher level of such anxiety than some of those whose stuttering is relatively severe, particularly if they try to conceal the fact that they stutter. They can be successful in concealing their stuttering by using such strategies as word substitution and reduced verbal output. Anticipating stuttering while with persons from whom they have tried to conceal the disorder can cause them to experience anxiety because they are afraid that if these persons find out about it, they will no longer accept them. The longer stutterers try to conceal their stuttering and the more they value a personal relationship, the more intense this anxiety is likely to be. Persons who stutter relatively severely may experience less anxiety then they do about the effect of stuttering on their relationships because they are unable to conceal it completely. Hence, they usually find out fairly quickly whether they will be accepted.

A sixth personality trait that many be shared by many persons who stutter is an external locus of control orientation for speech (McDonough & Quesal, 1988). The construct of locus of control (Rotter, 1966) implies a continuum, the ends of which represent two different general expectancies about reinforcement: internal and external. According to McDonough & Quesal (1988):

> *An individual with an internal locus of control believes that his/her own behaviors, abilities, or attributes determine "reinforcements." Those individuals with an external locus of control believe that reinforcements are under the control of "luck," "chance," "good days," "bad days," "powerful others," etc., rather than under their personal control. (p. 98)*

While stutterers do not appear to differ from nonstutterers in their expectancies on overall locus of control, there is a little evidence that they tend to differ from them in their expectancies concerning speech-specific locus of control—they are more likely than them to believe that it is controlled by external factors (McDonough & Quesal, 1988). Since the presence of such a belief would be likely to interfere with many approaches to therapy, it should be evaluated for and, if present, addressed. Strategies for doing so are described in Chapters 7 and 8.

Self-Concept

Considerable data exists to indicate that the self-concepts of many persons who stutter are adversely affected by their stuttering (Cooper & Cooper, 1985a; Cooper & Rustin, 1985; Perkins, 1994; Van Riper, 1982). Aspects of their self-perception that have been studied include how they perceive their body, personality, and social status and how they believe others perceive them (Kalinowski, Lerman, & Watt, 1987). Some of the ways in which these aspects of self-concept are likely to be affected by stuttering are described in this section.

Persons who stutter are likely to have a conflicting body image—normal one moment and deviant the next (Van Riper, 1982). A conflicting body image can be more difficult to cope with than one by which you are always likely to be regarded by yourself and others as being abnormal in some way. One young woman who stutters stated that:

> *I'd rather be blind or deaf, or have a huge birthmark on my face, or be bald than stutter. Then I would always have the trouble and could get used to it. I'll never be able to accept a face that only sometimes suddenly jumps*

around and makes horrible sounds. How can you learn to bear something that comes and goes so erratically? (Van Riper, 1982, p. 227)

Hence, stress from living with a conflicting body image can add to the severity of a client's stuttering problem.

There are several strategies that persons who stutter may use alone or in combination to lessen the stress that results from living with a conflicting body image. The first (which has already been dealt with in several contexts) is avoiding or concealing stuttering. The less frequently a person stutters, the less often he or she experiences stress from this source.

A second strategy stutterers may use for this purpose is to secure therapy. However, even if it is successful and they become much more fluent than they were previously, they may continue to experience stress from this source. Some of them are so highly aware of their stuttering that even occasionally having a few mild blocks (ones of which most listeners probably would not be aware) can adversely affect their body image (Van Riper, 1982). Hence, reducing the severity of their stuttering, by itself, may not "normalize" their body image. Their reaction to their stuttering (or the meaning it has for them) must also change (Johnson, 1946).

A third strategy they may use is *denial*—not abstracting (paying attention to) at least some of the abnormality that occurs during their moments of stuttering (Burley & Morley, 1987). The less attention they pay to their stuttering, the less they tend to react to it and, consequently, the less likely they are to experience this source of anxiety. The use of this strategy, however, can interfere with some approaches to therapy (intervention), particularly ones that attempt to teach clients to modify or control their moments of stuttering in some way. If they are unaware of what they are doing while they are stuttering, they probably will find it difficult to learn to modify it (Van Riper, 1973).

Thus far, our discussion of aspects of self-concept that may be adversely affected by stuttering has focused on body image. This is not the only one that is likely to be so affected by it. Another is how persons who stutter view their social status.

Social status in our culture is determined primarily by one's occupation, education, and evidence of success as measured by wealth and possessions and by the number of people on whom one has claims. You acquire claims on people by putting them in your debt (such as by doing favors for them) and/or by viewing them as inferior (e.g., having the ability to hire or fire them). Persons who stutter tend to be more comfortable and, consequently, more fluent when they speak to persons on whom they have claims. In this regard, a successful businessman said:

If I know that I can hire or buy them, I don't mind stuttering so much and I don't stutter so hard. I'm on top and they're down under. I don't give a damn what they think. It's my equals who bother me. (Van Riper, 1982, p. 231)

Some stutterers who regard themselves as having relatively high status tend to stutter more severely than otherwise when talking to persons whom they believe are not aware of their status. A university professor who stutters, for example, may do so when ordering food from a waiter or waitress who is not aware of "who he is." This increase in stuttering may result, at least in part, from the belief—which is supported by research (e.g., Beech & Fransella, 1968; Burley & Rinaldi, 1986; Kalinowski et al., 1987)—that such persons are likely to regard those who stutter as "inferior" unless they have information to the contrary. Hence, they would want to be fluent while speaking to them, which would tend to increase the severity of their stuttering. Stutterers tend to stutter most when they want to stutter least!

Some persons who stutter blame the disorder for causing them to have a lower social status than they would have had otherwise. They tend to view themselves as being "a giant in chains" ("If only I hadn't stuttered, I would have achieved...."). There is evidence, incidentally, that stutterers do tend to face high levels of discrimination in the area of employment (Rice & Kroll, 1994). Others do not view themselves as having a lower social status because of stuttering (see Black, 1987; Tillis & Wager, 1984).

Persons who stutter, of course, are not the only ones who view themselves as being "a giant in chains." Many persons in our society feel that they have been kept from achieving a higher social status by some sort of chain (as in not being able to go to college). Viewing yourself in this manner can have both positive and negative consequences. Positively, it can keep your perceived lack of achievement from adversely affecting your self-concept ("I'm good, but circumstances beyond my control kept me from achieving."). Negatively, it can keep you from trying to achieve until the chains are removed. Some persons who stutter tend to assume, for this reason, that they can't achieve their goals until their stuttering is cured. Though it certainly is desirable for them through therapy to reduce the severity of their stuttering, it may not be necessary for them to wait until they have done so to get on with their lives (Black, 1987; Tillis & Wager, 1984)!

This discussion of those aspects of self-concept that are likely to be adversely affected by stuttering has focused thus far on how persons who stutter tend to view themselves, particularly with regard to body image and social status. Another aspect that is likely to be affected is how they feel others view them. How we believe others view us affects how we view ourselves. According to Van Riper (1982):

> *We construct our personal identities by internalizing the reactions and evaluations of the people who play important parts in our lives—parents, siblings, mates, friends, employers, and fellow workers. What we think we see in the eyes of others often determines what and whom we think we are. (pp. 229–230)*

The impact on self-concept of how persons who stutter believe others view them is likely to be felt early in the development of the disorder. Parents tend to look upon stuttering as undesirable behavior and respond negatively to it (Johnson & Associates, 1959). Also, teasing, mockery, and rejection from peers are common experiences for children of all ages who stutter.

In adulthood, persons who stutter may feel the force of negative evaluation from peers of both sexes. This can adversely affect their self-concept and, thereby, their behavior in a number of ways. For example, it can affect their choice of a lover or spouse (Boberg & Boberg, 1990; Carlisle, 1985). According to Van Riper (1982, p. 233), a man who stutters may seek a person who evaluates his speech with unusual tolerance and is willing to protect him against communicative trauma and stress. Such a companion probably would be willing to make some phone calls for him. He may also seek one whom he feels others would not regard as very desirable. The reason is that he believes a person whom others would regard as desirable probably would not find him attractive because of his stuttering. There is a little evidence, incidentally, that women do not tend to react as unfavorably to stuttering as do men (Burley & Rinaldi, 1986).

How stutterers *expect* others to view them can influence their perceptions concerning how others view them. People "filter" the reactions of others to support their expectations (Johnson, 1946). According to Fransella (1972):

> *It cannot be reiterated too often that how we construe an act, person, place, or thing determines how we behave in relation to that act, person, place, or thing. No situation is intrinsically dangerous, anxiety-provoking or beautiful, it is only so if we construe in that way. (p. 69)*

This impact of expectation on perception has several clinical implications. First, it has to be taken into consideration when evaluating clients' reports of how people react to their stuttering. The reactions they report may or may not be accurate. And second, knowledge about it can be used as a "tool" (in combination with others) for desensitizing clients to their stuttering. The more aware they are of how their perceptions of peoples' reactions to their stuttering can be distorted by how they expect them to react to it, the less certain they should be (in at least some situations) that people really are reacting negatively to their stuttering and, hence, the weaker should be their desire to avoid it. Also, the less certain they are that listeners really do react negatively to them because they stutter, the less likely they should be to signal to them that they are embarrassed or ashamed because they stutter and, consequently, the less likely their listeners should be uncomfortable while talking to them. When listeners react negatively to them while they are stuttering, the listeners may be reacting more to the "discomfort" they evince than to their stuttering per se.

How persons who stutter believe others view them also affects their stuttering severity. The more certain they are that a listener reacts negatively to them when they stutter, the more likely they are to try to conceal their stuttering and, as a consequence, stutter relatively severely while talking to him or her (see Chapter 2). There is some evidence, incidentally, that nonstutterers tend to perceive the intelligence and personality of stutterers more positively if they acknowledge their stuttering rather than attempt to conceal it (Collins & Blood, 1990).

It should be evident from the information presented in this section that many persons who stutter tend to have relatively poor self-concepts. This, of course, contributes to the severity of their stuttering problem and the extent to which they are handicapped by it. It may also contribute to the likelihood that they will recover from stuttering. Perkins (1993, p. 11) has hypothesized that "prevention of a self-image of stutterer [in children] would be equivalent to prevention of stuttering as a chronic clinical problem."

The fact that some stutterers do not have relatively poor self-concepts is important. *It indicates that it is possible for persons to stutter and still have a relatively good self-concept.* It may be possible, therefore, to improve your clients' self-concepts at least a little without first improving their fluency. In fact, doing so may help to improve their fluency because the better they feel about themselves, the less severely they are likely to stutter (see Chapter 2).

LANGUAGE SKILLS

Thus far, we have considered persons who stutter from the perspectives of physiological and psychological functioning. One perspective from which we have not yet done so is speech-language functioning other than stuttering. Do persons who stutter, as a group, tend to differ from their peers in any aspects of this? While some investigators (such as Seider, Gladstein, & Kidd, 1982) did not report finding any such group differences, the majority of those who have compared attributes of their speech-language functioning have done so. There is some evidence that children who stutter are late in passing some of their speech milestones: The extent of delay has been reported to be about six months (Andrews et al., 1983). Also, they appear to make more articulation/phonological errors than do their peers (Andrews et al., 1983; Andrews & Harris, 1964; Blood & Seider, 1981; Bloodstein, 1987; Conture & Edwards, 1994; Conture, Louko, & Edwards, 1993; Louko, Edwards, & Conture, 1990; Nippold, 1990; Ryan, 1992; St. Louis & Hinzman, 1988; Williams & Silverman, 1968; Wolk, Edwards, & Conture, 1993). Furthermore, their expressive language skills do not appear to be as highly developed as those of their peers (Andrews et al., 1983; Blood & Seider, 1981; Bloodstein, 1987; Byrd & Cooper, 1989; Ryan, 1992; St. Louis & Hinzman, 1988; Wall, 1980; Watson et al., 1991; Westby, 1979). However, their receptive language skills (Byrd & Cooper, 1989), their narrative ability (Nippold, Schwartz, & Jescheniak, 1991; Weiss & Zebrowski, 1994), and their reading ability (Nippold & Schwartz, 1990) appear to differ little, if at all, from those of their peers.

Is there any reason to believe that a linguistic performance deficit can contribute to the onset and development of stuttering? Some speech-language pathologists believe that the demands that language places on the speech motor planning and execution capacities of persons who have such a deficit can contribute to the disorder's etiology (see Watson et al., 1991, for a review of the literature supporting this point of view).

ASSIGNMENTS

Eye Contact

Many adults who stutter do not maintain normal eye contact, particularly while they are stuttering. Talk to three persons and, at times, stare at the ceiling or the floor while doing so. How did you feel while your eye contact was abnormal? Were your listeners aware when you failed to maintain eye contact and if they were, did they react differently to you when you did so? If you are uncertain, ask them.

Impact of Set on Perception of Self

Some adults who stutter expect people to react negatively to them because of their impairment. Consequently, they often enter speaking situations with a set that causes them to perceive such reactions when they aren't there. ("Seek and ye shall find.") For a period of several hours, assume that the people whom you engage in conversation are going to react negatively to you. While doing so, keep the following questions in mind: Is there anything in their behavior that could be interpreted as supporting your expectation ("certainty")? If there is, do you think you would have interpreted it in this way if you hadn't had this set?

▶ 4

The Onset and Development of Stuttering

The symptomatology and phenomenology of stuttering at or near onset not only differs from that of the "typical" adult who has the disorder, but also that of the "typical" school-age child who has it (Brady & Hall, 1976). The disorder, following onset, tends to develop over a period of years in a fairly predictable way along a continuum or track. Some authorities (see Van Riper, 1982) believe that there is more than one track along which it can develop. Regardless of the track along which it develops, the stuttering of the typical school-age child would tend to be more like that of the typical adult than would that of the typical preschool child. The manner in which the symptomatology and phenomenology of stuttering are likely to change as the disorder develops is addressed in this chapter.

ONSET

Although stuttering can begin at any age, its onset, in most cases, is *reported* to be between the ages of 2 and 5 years (Darley, 1955; Johnson & Associates, 1959; Yairi, 1993). The mean ages of onset that have been reported range from 32 (Yairi & Ambrose, 1992c) to 46 months (Darley, 1955). Age of onset here refers to the age at which an informant (usually a parent) reports that he or she first concluded that a child's repetitions and/or other hesitations probably were abnormal. Unfortunately, very few children have been evaluated by speech-language pathologists within days or even weeks of the time the disorder was reported to have begun. Consequently, almost all the information we have about stuttering at onset is from reports by informants who are not speech pathologists made months (or even years) after the disorder probably began. However, the fact that data from thousands of such reports from many different countries tend to agree fairly well makes it probable that at least some of the information we have from this source is reliable.

Our information about the onset of stuttering also is incomplete because much of it is based on what can readily be observed by a layperson through vision and hearing. There are undoubtedly associated physiological and psychological events that either cannot be observed without instrumentation or that a layperson after observing would be unlikely to regard as being related to the onset of the disorder. This has one, or possibly two, implications. First, it means that the onset of stuttering as described here is incomplete, possibly in some important ways. And second, it *could* mean that the onset of stuttering occurs at an earlier age than a layperson's reports would suggest. That is, it *could* mean that the presence of relatively high levels of syllable and word repetition and/or other disfluency behaviors is not the first stage in the development of the disorder—it is just the first one about which laypersons are likely to become concerned.

Symptomatology and Phenomenology of Stuttering at or near Onset

The questions discussed in this section are the following:

- Does the onset of stuttering tend to be sudden or gradual?
- What are the speech characteristics of early ("primary") stuttering?
- How similar is early stuttering to normal childhood disfluency?
- How aware of and concerned about their stuttering do young children tend to be?
- To what extent do children at the initial stage in the disorder's development do things to avoid stuttering?
- How well are children at the beginning stage of the disorder able to predict their moments of stuttering?
- To what extent does stuttering at (or near) onset tend to vary on a situational basis? How representative does stuttering observed in the "therapy room" tend to be of that in other situations?
- What impact is stuttering during its initial stage likely to have on a child's self-concept? How are reactions to the child's stuttering likely to influence this?

Does the Onset of the Disorder Tend to be Sudden or Gradual?

This question is difficult to answer because most of the relevant data (such as Johnson & Associates, 1959) are from reports by parents and other laypersons months (or even years) after the disorder is thought to have begun. Such reports may be inaccurate because the persons making them classified at least some of the child's normal repetitions and other hesitations as the beginning of stuttering. This would tend to make the onset of the disorder appear to have been more gradual than it really was. The reports may also be inaccurate because the persons making them either were not aware of the child's earliest moments of stuttering or considered them to be normal hesitations. This would tend to make the onset of the disorder appear more *sudden* than it really was.

Though the relevant data have to be interpreted with caution for the reasons indicated earlier, they do seem to indicate that the onset can be either sudden or gradual (Yairi, 1983), with a gradual onset being more usual (Van Riper, 1982). Levina (1968) states:

> *Our [Russian] studies have confirmed that stammering usually begins between the ages of three and four. In almost all cases of stammering among children it sets in gradually, beginning with slightly interrupted speech similar to the physiological difficulties accompanying the transition to phraseological speech. (p. 28)*

The percentages of cases reported by other investigators in which the onset was gradual are 86 (Ajuriaguerra, Diakine, Gobineau, Narlian, & Stambak, 1958), 92 (Morley, 1957), 76 (Preus, 1981), 69 (Berlin, 1954), and 90 (Van Riper, 1982).

What Are the Speech Characteristics of
Early ("Primary") Stuttering?

When children begin to stutter, what is the nature of their hesitations? Of what behaviors do their moments of stuttering tend to consist? In other words, what are they doing that causes someone (usually a parent) to first decide that something is wrong with their speech? Almost all reports of their speaking behavior (see Bloodstein, 1987; Bloodstein & Grossman, 1981; Hoepfner, 1911; Froeschels, 1943; Johnson & Associates, 1959; Meyers, 1986; Taylor, 1937; Wyatt, 1969; Van Riper, 1982; Yairi, 1993; Yairi & Ambrose, 1992c; Yairi & Lewis, 1984) agree that what these children are most likely to be doing is repeating single-syllable words and the first syllables of multisyllable ones (particularly the latter). Since a single-syllable word is also a syllable, the repetition of such a word can be classified as a syllable as well as a word repetition. What they are repeating, therefore, is syllables. Their syllable repetitions may not only call attention to themselves because they are judged to occur frequently, but also because the number of units per instance of repetition is considered to be excessive (Yairi & Lewis, 1984). For example, they might say "I-I-I-I-I want..." rather than "I-I want...."

The repetitions evinced by at least a third of the children who are diagnosed as beginning to stutter show signs of tension at least some of the time (Johnson & Associates, 1959; Yairi, 1993). Whether such signs usually are present from the moment they begin to stutter or whether they tend to develop after a few days, or weeks, or months has not been established empirically.

While the first type of disfluency that usually causes someone to become concerned about a child's speech is sound, syllable, and/or single-syllable word repetition (Yairi, 1993), in some cases it is complete stoppages, or rather, prolonged articulatory postures, which may be silent or accompanied by prolonged sounds (Schwartz, Zebrowski, & Conture, 1990; Yairi, 1993; Yairi & Lewis, 1984). These usually occur on the initial sounds of words. When they occur within words, they may not be at syllable boundaries—for example, "v---ery." When such blockages occur within a word, the word is referred to as broken. The blockages almost never occur on the final sounds of words. Some of them are accompanied by behavioral events usually associated with developed stuttering such as eyelid opening and closing, eyeball movement (lateral or vertical), head movement, limb movement, torso movement, audible inhalation, vocal intensity change, audible exhalation, lip movement, or some combination of these (Schwartz et al., 1990).

The percentage of children who evince prolonged articulatory postures during the first few weeks after the onset of the disorder is not known for certain. However, Van Riper (1982, pp. 69–70) has shed some light on this. Over a period of years he evaluated sixty-one children within three weeks of the reported onset of the disorder. Of these children, approximately one-third evinced articulatory postures that lasted at least two seconds.

How Similar Is Early Stuttering to Normal Childhood Disfluency?

Some of the data referred to in the previous answer indicate that what young children usually are doing when someone becomes concerned about their speech fluency is repeating single-syllable words and/or the first syllables of multisyllable ones in a relatively relaxed manner. To what extent do their normal-speaking peers repeat single-syllable words and/or the first syllables of multisyllable ones? Since most cases of stuttering are reported to begin between the ages of two and five, the data used here for answering this question were obtained from preschoolers. Most normal-speaking preschool children repeat single-syllable words and the first syllables of multisyllable ones (Johnson & Associates, 1959; McLaughlin & Cullinan, 1989; Silverman, 1972; Yairi, 1981, 1982). Hence, the fact that a child repeats these does not, *by itself,* indicate that he or she is beginning to stutter.

While the presence of syllable repetition does not allow one to differentiate children beginning to stutter from their normal-speaking peers, perhaps the amount and/ or the manner in which they do so would allow one to distinguish between them. Do children beginning to stutter tend to repeat syllables more often than their normal-speaking peers? The most comprehensive study of the syllable repetitions of both groups of preschoolers was reported by Johnson & Associates (1959). These data (see Table 1-1) show considerable overlap between the groups. While most children who are thought to be beginning to stutter repeat syllables more often than the majority of their normal-speaking peers, not all appear to do so. In fact, there are children about whose fluency no one seems to be concerned who repeat more often than some children who are thought to be beginning to stutter (see Table 1-1). The overlap between the groups was confirmed by Yairi and Lewis (1984) and Meyers (1986), though the degree to which it occurred in their subjects was considerably less than reported by Johnson & Associates (1959). Consequently, if a clinician decides whether children are beginning to stutter *solely* on the basis of whether they repeat syllables, he or she is likely to misdiagnose some of them. And according to the diagnosogenic theory (see Chapter 5), such a misdiagnosis can precipitate stuttering.

Do children who stutter differ from their normal-speaking peers with respect to the number of times they are likely to repeat the first syllable of a multisyllable word or a single-syllable word? When they repeat, do they tend to have more *units* of repetition per instance of repetition than do their normal-speaking peers? Would an instance of repetition such as "I-I-I-I-I-I want..." ever occur in the speech of a normal-speaking child? The available data (Johnson & Associates, 1959) indicate that there is overlap between groups. While the typical preschool-age child who stutters tends to produce more units of repetition per instance of repetition than his or her normal-speaking peers, there are normal-speaking preschool-age children who produce more of them than some of their peers who have the disorder. In fact, normal-speaking four-year-olds have been observed repeating a syllable as many as seven times (Silverman, 1972). Hence, it would not be safe to conclude that a child is beginning to stutter solely because he or she *occasionally* repeats a syllable a large number of times.

Some children who are beginning to stutter evince prolonged articulatory postures—which may be silent or accompanied by prolonged sound. Do normal-speaking preschool-age children ever evince such postures? The available evidence (see Johnson & Associates, 1959) indicates that they do. However, the "typical" child who stutters evinces them more often and for longer periods of time than does his or her "typical" normal-speaking peer. There appears to be less overlap between groups for prolonged articulatory postures than for syllable repetitions. Nevertheless, an *occasional* prolonged articulatory posture—particularly when a child is upset or seems to have a great deal to say—is not necessarily indicative of early stuttering.

While the data indicate unequivocally that syllable repetitions and prolonged articulatory postures occur in the speech of normal-speaking children as well as in those beginning to stutter, this does not necessarily mean that information about such disfluencies should be ignored when deciding whether a child is beginning to stutter. There are some children for whom the amount of repetition, the number of units per instance of repetition, the frequency and duration of prolonged articulatory postures, or some combination of these, is clearly abnormal. To deny this would be playing the "Emperor's New Clothes" game. If their disfluency is abnormal, they are in need of help.

For further information about the differentiation of early stuttering from normal childhood disfluency, see Gordon and Luper (1992a, b) and Onslow (1992b).

How Aware of and Concerned about Their Stuttering Do Young Children Tend to Be?

Most young children who are judged to be beginning to stutter because they are repeating excessively and/or have frequent prolonged articulatory postures do not usually seem to be aware that there is anything abnormal about their speech fluency. And even if they are aware of their hesitations, most of the time they tend to evince much less concern about them than do adults who have the disorder. Van Riper (1982, pp. 95–107) reported that the stuttering of 68 percent of the 300 children he studied developed along Track I or Track II (see Tables 4-1 and 4-2 for descriptions of these tracks). A characteristic of both is "no awareness" of stuttering during the beginning stage of the disorder. Yairi (1993) reported, based on parental question-naire data, that 77 percent of the children in his sample did not seem to be aware of their stuttering when it first began. Bloodstein (1987, p. 42) concluded, after exam-ining the clinical case histories of 418 children who stutter, that "Most of the time children in the first phase of stuttering show little evidence of concern about the interruptions in their speech." He described the awareness and concern that they do show as follows:

> *It is commonplace for children as young as two or three to show acute frus-tration when they stutter by refusing to speak, crying, beating the wall with their hands, or saying, "Why can't I talk?" Such reactions are usually brief and sporadic, however, in contrast to the chronic fear and embarrassment of many older stutterers. Furthermore, the characteristic reaction of the Phase I stutterer may be epitomized by saying that when there is any reac-tion at all, it is apparently in response to the immediate experience of being thwarted in efforts to communicate rather than to the ramified implications of the knowledge on the part of the child that he or she "is a stutterer." (Bloodstein, 1987, p. 42)*

However, some children do appear to be highly aware of and concerned about stuttering almost from the moment of the onset of the disorder. Twenty-seven (9 per-cent) of the 300 children Van Riper (1982) studied appeared to evince such aware-ness and concern. And of few of the twenty preschool-age children studied by Ambrose & Yairi (1994) did also.

To What Extent Do Children at the Initial Stage of the Disorder's Development Do Things to Avoid Stuttering?

Since most children at the initial stage of the disorder's development usually do not seem to be concerned about (or even aware of) their moments of stuttering, they

TABLE 4-1 **Onset Characteristics.**

Track I	Track II
Begins 2½ to 4 years.	Often late. At time of first sentences.
Previously fluent.	Never very fluent.
Gradual onset.	Gradual onset.
Cyclic.	Steady.
Long remissions.	No remissions.
Good articulations.	Poor articulations.
Normal rate.	Fast; spurts.
Syllabic repetitions.	Gaps, revisions, syllable and word repetitions.
No tension; unforced.	No tension.
No tremors.	No tremors.
Loci: First words, function words.	Loci: First words; long words; scattered throughout sentence; content words.
Variable pattern.	Variable pattern.
Normal speech is well integrated.	Broken speech with hesitation and gaps even when no disfluency.
No awareness.	No awareness.
No frustration.	No frustration.
No fears; willing to talk.	No fears; willing to talk.

Track III	Track IV
Any age after child has consecutive speech.	Late, usually after 4 years.
Previously fluent.	Previously fluent.
Sudden onset, often after trauma.	Sudden onset.
Steady.	Erratic.
Few short remissions.	No remissions.
Normal articulation.	Normal articulation.
Slow, careful rate.	Normal rate.
Unvoiced prolongations.	Unusual behaviors.
Laryngeal blockings.	
Much tension.	Variable tension.
Tremors.	Few tremors.
Beginning of utterance after pauses primary.	First words; rarely on function words; content words especially.
Consistent pattern.	Consistent pattern.
Normal speech is very fluent.	Normal speech is very fluent.
Highly aware.	Highly aware.
Much frustration.	No frustration.
Fears speaking; situation and word fears.	No evidence of fear; willing to talk.

Source: Reproduced from Van Riper, 1982, p. 106 with permission of the publisher.

TABLE 4-2 **Developmental Characteristics.**

Track I	Track II
Repetitions of syllables increase in frequency and speed and become irregular.	Behaviors remain the same but the speed increases; their number also increases.

Then:

Track I	Track II
Repetition of syllables begin to end in prolongations.	Little change in form.

Then:

Track I	Track II
Prolongations show increased tension, tremors, struggle. Evidence of frustration.	Little change; little awareness; little frustration.

Then:

Track I	Track II
Overflow of tension; facial contortions; retrials; speech output decreases; signs of concern.	Duration of nonfluencies increases; more syllabic repetitions; little awareness.

Then:

Track I	Track II
Word fears and avoidance occur. Fears of certain sounds arise. Then situation fears develop. Repetitions and prolongations turn into silent fixations with struggle (blocking). Poor eye contact and tricks to disguise the difficulty are observed. Shows hesitancy, embarrassment.	Occasional fears of situations, not of words or sounds. Long strings of syllabic repetitions at fast speed are added to other behaviors. Some fears of situations. Good eye contact. No disguise. Output of speech increases. Little avoidance. Primarily repetitive. Unorganized.

Track III	Track IV
An increase in the frequency but the behavior at first changes little. Signs of frustration.	The number of instances increases, and they are shown in more situations.

Then:

Track III	Track IV
More retrials are seen; lip protrusions, and tongue fixations appear; prolongations of initial sounds.	Little change in form; monosymptomatic and symbolic.

Then:

Track III	Track IV
Tremors; struggling; facial contortions; jaw jerk, gasping; marked frustration.	Little change.

Then:

Track III	Track IV
Interruptor devices become prominent; rate slows; more hesitancy; more refusals to talk.	Little change in type but duration and visibility increase; no interruptors or new forcings; increased output of speech.

continued

TABLE 4-2   *Continued*

Track III	**Track IV**
Then:	
Intense fears of words and sounds; many avoidances; patterns change in form and grow more bizarre; much overflow; output of speech decreases; will cease trying to talk. Poor eye contact; the normal speech becomes hesitant. Nonvocalized blockings are frequent. Primary tonic blocks with multiple closures.	Very few avoidance or release behaviors. Not much evidence of word fears. Few consistent loci. Very aware of stuttering. Stutters very openly. Good eye contact. Little variability in the stuttering behavior. Normal speech very fluent. Talks a lot. Consistent pattern; few silent blockings. Either tonic or clonic.

Source: Reproduced from Van Riper, 1982, p. 107 with permission of the publisher.

would not be expected do things to avoid them. Those who are aware of and concerned about them, however, sometimes seem to do things to avoid stuttering. Van Riper (1982) reported evidence of such avoidance by approximately 9 percent of the 300 children in his sample who were at the initial stage in the development of the disorder. Children who appear to be trying to avoid stuttering definitely are in need of professional help.

The presence of avoidance behavior can provide useful information when trying to determine whether children are aware of and concerned about stuttering. If they try to avoid stuttering, this means that they are aware of and concerned about it at least *some* of the time.

How Well Are Children at the Beginning Stage of the Disorder Able to Predict Their Moments of Stuttering?

Those children who are not aware of their moments of stuttering are unable, of course, to predict them with greater-than-chance accuracy. Those children who are aware of them—like the 9 percent in Van Riper's (1982) sample—*may* be able to do so. However, even by elementary-school age most children's ability to predict them is not nearly as good as that of most adults who have the disorder (Silverman & Williams, 1972).

To What Extent Does Stuttering at (or near) Onset Tend to Vary on a Situational Basis? How Representative Does Stuttering Observed in the "Therapy Room" Tend to Be of That in Other Situations?

Many (perhaps most) children in the initial stage do not stutter the same amount in all situations. Bloodstein (1987, p. 41), for example, included the following two among his six characteristics of the beginning of stuttering:

1. The difficulty has a definite tendency to be episodic.
2. The child stutters most when excited or upset, when seeming to have a great deal to say, or under other conditions of communicative pressure.

The tendency for stuttering to vary on a situational basis also is a characteristic of the disorder in adults (see Chapter 2).

The stuttering observed in the therapy room may not be representative of that in other situations. When it is not representative, in most cases the child is more fluent there than in other situations (Silverman, 1975). The reason may be that children are less likely to be excited, upset, or under communicative pressure in this situation than in some others. Regardless of the reason, it is not safe to assume that a child's speech in the therapy room is representative of that in other situations, particularly if it is quite fluent. Some children who stutter may not do so at all in a therapy room environment (Silverman, 1975)!

What Impact Is Stuttering during Its Initial Stage Likely to Have on a Child's Self-Concept? How Are Reactions to a Child's Stuttering Likely to Influence This?

The disorder during its initial stage is unlikely to affect significantly the self-concepts of children who have it if those with whom they interact do not express concern about it (Johnson & Associates, 1959). However, the disorder can, during its initial stage, adversely affect the self-concepts of children who are often aware of and concerned about their stuttering. This is particularly likely to happen if someone whom they respect gives them the message that what they are doing when they hesitate is "bad" and that they could stop doing it if they really wanted to or tried (Johnson & Associates, 1959). Children may communicate in several ways that they have accepted the judgment that their hesitations are "bad" and, hence, something about which to be embarrassed or ashamed. One is maintaining poor eye contact during moments of stuttering. (We have already mentioned research that shows how "looking away" expresses feelings of embarrassment or shame [Atkins, 1988]). Another way is by doing things to avoid these moments, such as the avoidance of talking in some situations and use of the devices employed by older children and adults—such as word substitution (Van Riper, 1982).

Reactions of Parents and Others to a Child's "Stuttering" at (or near) Onset

This section deals with how people tend to react to young children whom they believe are beginning to stutter. Our primary focus will be on the parents of the children, since they are the ones who usually are the first to become concerned about their speech fluency.

Most parents will react in some manner if they believe that something about their child is abnormal. However, they differ with respect to both what they consider abnormal and how they react when they classify something as such. A behavior that will cause one parent concern may not come to the attention of another (may not be abstracted) or if it does, it does not cause concern (he or she does not classify the behavior as abnormal). Also, while one parent will react to believing a behavior is abnormal by remaining calm and seeking professional help, another will do so by becoming anxious or depressed.

Are parents of children who stutter more likely than those of their peers to be aware of and to classify repetitions and prolonged articulatory postures as abnormal? The answer to this question is not certain (Johnson & Associates, 1959; Zebrowski & Conture, 1989). If they are, perhaps it is because they are more likely to have a set to see and hear them as stuttering. The findings of a number of studies (such as Berlin, 1960; Williams & Kent, 1958) indicate that whether repetitions and other types of speech hesitations are classified as stuttering is a function, in part, of whether the person doing the classifying has a set to hear it. If there is a history of stuttering in their family, for example, parents may be more likely to have a set to hear stuttering in their children's speech than they would otherwise. And, as has been pointed out earlier in this chapter, families of persons who stutter are more likely to have a history of stuttering than those of their normal-speaking peers.

Once parents have classified their children's hesitations as stuttering, they may react to them in a number of ways, including the following:

- They may try to ignore them or not communicate concern about them to the child. There are several reasons why they may do so. First, they may be grieving for the loss of their child's ability to speak normally. The first stage of the grieving process is denial (Tanner, 1980). Second, they may hope that by not communicating concern about them to the child, stuttering will just be a phase through which he or she will pass.
- They may react to the hesitations in a way that is likely to increase the child's awareness of and concern about them. Among the ways they may do this are using body language—such as looking away (Atkins, 1988)—when the child hesitates, which communicates that they are embarrassed by it or by saying things that communicate this feeling.
- They may give the child advice about what to do to be more fluent (Johnson & Associates, 1959). The advice is likely to reflect why they think he or she is stuttering. If they think the reason is speaking too rapidly, they are likely to tell the child to slow down. If they suspect that the child is not adequately formulating the message before beginning to speak, they are likely to tell him to "think of what he is going to say before he says it" or to "stop and start over again." And if they think the stuttering is caused by inadequate breath support, they are likely to tell the child to "take a deep breath before speaking."

The persons, other than parents, who probably spend the most time with preschool children are those who provide them with day care. Since many children are raised in either a single-parent family or one in which both parents work at least part of the time, they are likely to spend a great deal of time with persons who provide them with day care. These can range from family members (such as grandparents or older siblings) to professional day-care workers. Their reactions to the hesitations of children beginning to stutter are likely to influence both how the children view them and how they view themselves (their self-concept). Therefore, it is important when evaluating a child who is thought to be beginning to stutter to determine how those who take care of the child during the day react to his or her hesitations.

Onset of Stuttering in Adults

Stuttering tends to be regarded as a disorder of childhood because the relevant data indicate that its onset almost always occurs before the age of eighteen, usually before the age of five. However, there are a number of reports in the literature of persons who began to stutter after the age of eighteen (see Van Riper, 1982, pp. 44–46). While some of these may be cases in which the person stuttered for at least a short time during childhood (but doesn't remember doing so), stopped, and then began again as an adult, it seems unlikely that they all are. It seems probable, therefore, that stuttering can have its onset during adulthood.

DEVELOPMENT

Thus far in this chapter we have considered how the symptomatology and phenomenology of stuttering at (or near) onset differs from that in adults. In this section we will consider how the symptomatology and phenomenology of the disorder at (or near) onset evolve into their adult form. That is, the process through which stuttering *increases* in complexity (severity) is addressed. In not all cases, however, do the symptomatology and phenomenology of the disorder increase in complexity. In some the opposite seems to occur: The person eventually recovers completely or almost completely. Consequently, in this section we also will consider how the symptomatology and phenomenology of the disorder evolve into normal (or near normal) speech fluency. That is, we will consider the process through which persons have been reported to recover from the disorder.

Stages Through Which the Disorder Evolves into Its Fully Developed Adult Form

There have been several attempts to describe how the symptomatology and phenomenology of stuttering in preschool children evolves into that evinced by most adults. Three of them are discussed in this section. These are the ones that appear to have had the most impact on how the development of the disorder is currently viewed.

Bluemel's "Primary" and "Secondary" Stages
One of the first attempts to describe the development of the disorder was by Dr. Charles Bluemel (1932, 1957). He referred to the stuttering evinced during the first stage as "primary" stuttering and that evinced during the second as "secondary" stuttering. He described primary stuttering as consisting of relatively effortless repetitions and prolonged articulatory postures ("blocks"). This is the type that would be exhibited by most children at (or near) onset. According to Bluemel (1957) secondary stuttering

> ...*is marked by the conscious physical struggle to articulate while the mental process of speech is momentarily halted. The stammerers' [Bluemel used the term* stammerer *instead of* stutterer.] *breathing is disturbed; likewise his vocalization and articulation. He uses starters and wedges to get the speech going. He becomes conditioned against difficult words and difficult situations, and he develops speech aversion and avoidance. He resorts to synonyms and circumlocutions to avoid his stammering. He remains silent when he should speak. Confusion and phobia enter into the speech situation. (p. 128)*

Bluemel's scheme has been criticized for several reasons. One is that much, if not all, of the behavior he indicates as being symptomatic of primary stuttering can be observed in the speech of normal-speaking preschool-age children.

A second basis on which Bluemel's scheme has been criticized is that stuttering does not always begin with relatively relaxed hesitations of which the person is unaware. Cases have been reported in which children exhibited behaviors characteristic of secondary stuttering immediately following the onset of the disorder.

A third basis on which Bluemel's scheme has been criticized is that it is not sufficiently detailed. It does not describe in sufficient detail the transition between beginning stuttering and the fully developed form of the disorder.

Bloodstein's "Four Phases" in the Development of Stuttering
One of the limitations of Bluemel's two-stage scheme (as previously noted) is that it does not describe what occurs during the transition between the preschool and the fully developed (adult) form of the disorder. That is, Bluemel's scheme does not adequately describe the symptomatology of the disorder in school-age children, particularly in those of elementary-school age. Bloodstein (1960) proposed a four-stage scheme that includes aspects of the symptomatology of the disorder in school-age and preschool children and adults. While, as he appropriately points out, there is considerable variation in the age at which a person evinces the symptomatology associated with each phase, the "typical" person who stutters will evince that associated with *Phase I* while a preschooler, that associated with *Phase II* while in elementary school, that associated with *Phase III* during late childhood and early adolescence, and that associated with *Phase IV* by late adolescence or adulthood.

Not all persons who stutter, incidentally, will eventually reach Phase IV: the symptomatology evinced by some adults is that of Phase II or III.

According to Bloodstein (1960), the symptomatology associated with each phase is at follows:

Phase I

1. *The difficulty has a distinct tendency to be episodic.* One of the best indications that stuttering is still in its most rudimentary form is that it appears for periods of weeks or months between long interludes of normal speech. During this phase there is apparently a high percentage of spontaneous recoveries from stuttering that consist essentially of cases in which episodes of stuttering have failed to recur. How high this percentage is would be very difficult to determine. It is not improbable that single episodes of stuttering so mild and brief that they are overlooked or soon forgotten are exceedingly common during these years.

2. *The child stutters most when excited or upset, when seeming to have a great deal to say, or under other conditions of communicative pressure.*

3. *The dominant symptom is repetition.* This must be hastily qualified. Practically any of the integral or associated symptoms of stuttering may be seen in some of the youngest stutterers, and in some cases there seems to be little or no repetition. For the most part, however, the more severe symptoms appear briefly and intermittently in these children, and relatively simple repetition is far more common. In some cases repetition is practically the only symptom to be observed. While much of it consists of repetition of initial syllables, as it does in older stutterers, there is also usually a conspicuous tendency to repeat whole words.

4. *There is a marked tendency for stutterings to occur at the beginning of the sentence, clause, or phrase.* In some of the youngest children stuttering seems to be limited almost entirely to the first word of the sentence.

5. *In contrast to more advanced stuttering, the interruptions occur not only on content words, but also on the function words of speech—the pronouns, conjunctions, articles, and prepositions.* Stuttering on such words often tends to consist of whole-word repetitions. In short, there is frequent repetition of such words as "like," "but," "and," "so," "he," "I," and "with."

6. *Most of the time children in the first phase of stuttering show little evidence of concern about the interruptions in their speech.* This is not to say that they are completely unconscious of them. It is commonplace for children as young as two or three to show acute frustration when they stutter by refusing to speak, crying, beating the wall with their hands, or saying, "Why can't I talk?" Such reactions are usually brief and sporadic, however, in contrast to the chronic fear and embarrassment of many older stutterers. Furthermore, the characteristic reaction of the Phase I stutterer may be epitomized by saying that when there is any reaction at all it is apparently in response to the immediate experience of being thwarted in efforts to communicate rather than to the ramified implications of the knowledge on the part of the child that he or she "is a stutterer."

Phase II

1. *The disorder is essentially chronic.* There are few, if any, intervals of normal speech.
2. *The child has a self-concept of a stutterer.*
3. *The stutterings occur chiefly on the major parts of speech—nouns, verbs, adjectives, and adverbs.* There is much less tendency to stutter only on the initial words of sentences and phrases, and whole-word repetitions are no longer quite as common.
4. *Despite a self-concept as a stutterer, the child usually evinces little or no concern about the speech difficulty.* There is an absence of such features of more advanced stuttering as conscious anticipations of stuttering, substitution, circumlocution, avoidance of speaking, and word, sound, and situation fears.
5. *The stuttering is said to increase chiefly under conditions of excitement and when the child is speaking rapidly.*

Phase III

1. *The stuttering comes and goes largely in response to specific situations.* Among the situations the person often reports to be especially difficult are classroom recitation, speaking to strangers, making purchases in stores, and using the telephone.
2. *Certain words or sounds are regarded as more difficult than others.*
3. *In varying degrees, use is made of word substitutions and circumlocutions.* This tends to be done only occasionally and more often as a reaction to frustration, or its imminence, than to actual fear of stuttering.
4. *There is essentially no avoidance of speech situations and little or no evidence of fear or embarrassment.*

Phase IV

1. *Vivid, fearful, anticipations of stuttering.*
2. *Feared words, sound, and situations.*
3. *Very frequent word substitutions and circumlocution.*
4. *Avoidance of speech situations, or other evidence of fear and embarrassment.*

While Bloodstein's scheme provides a more complete description of the development of the disorder than that of Bluemel, it does have one of the same limitations. Five of the six "symptoms" characteristic of Phase I stuttering also are exhibited by many normal-speaking preschool-age children. That is, the amount they repeat (or otherwise hesitate) tends to vary considerably from day to day (Yairi, 1981, 1982); they tend to hesitate most "when excited or upset, when seeming to have a great deal to say, or under other conditions of communicative pressure"; they frequently repeat syllables and whole words (Johnson & Associates, 1959; Yairi, 1981, 1982); they tend to hesitate frequently at the beginnings of sentences, clauses, and phrases; their hesitations occur on both content and function words; and most of the time they "... show little evidence of concern about the interruptions in their speech." The only one that may differentiate the groups is the tendency to hesitate most when excited or upset, when seeming to have a great deal to say, or under conditions of communicative pressure. There is some evidence that normal-speaking preschool-age children, as a group, do not tend to hesitate more frequently in "stress" than in "neutral" situations (Wexler, 1982).

Van Riper's Four Tracks along Which Stuttering Can Develop

Van Riper (1982) agreed with Bloodstein that the process through which the symptomatology of the disorder in preschool children evolves into the adult form is not dichotomous. However, he concluded that the continuum (track) along which it developed was not the same for all persons. He indicated that there are at least four continua, or tracks, along which it can develop (see Tables 4-1 and 4-2). Their existence has been verified by two other investigators (Daly, 1981; Preus, 1981). Track I, which his data suggest more than 50 percent of cases follow, is quite similar to the continuum defined by Bloodstein's four phases. As such, it has the same limitation as the scheme proposed by Bloodstein—the symptoms that define the beginning of this track also are exhibited by some normal-speaking preschool-age children.

Is the disorder that develops along tracks II, III, and IV the same as that which develops along track I? Though all are labeled "stuttering," they may not be the same disorder. The symptomatology evinced by the children on track II (see Tables 4-1 and 4-2), for example, seems to be that of cluttering.

Development of Stuttering during Middle Age and Beyond

In the schemes that have been reviewed thus far there is an implicit assumption that once stuttering has reached its most severe form—usually during adolescence or early adulthood—it ceases to develop in a predictable manner. Research pertaining to this assumption began during the 1980s (Manning et al., 1984; Manning & Monte, 1981; Manning & Shirkey, 1980). Does the severity and symptomatology of the disorder tend to change during middle age and beyond? There is some evidence that personality and attitudes tend to change in predictable ways during the adult life cycle (Sheehy, 1976). Since personality attributes and attitudes influence stuttering severity (see Chapter 2), it would not be particularly surprising if stuttering did change during middle age and beyond. There is a little evidence that this does, in fact, happen. According to Peters and Starkweather (1989), the following changes tend to occur after the age of thirty:

> *During this period, a gradual decline in the severity of stuttering usually is seen. New behaviors are no longer acquired, and although the tendency for a reduction of abnormality has largely stopped, the increased self-*

confidence and maturity seem to reduce the frequency with which all stuttering behaviors occur. Occasionally, there is complete remission. (pp. 316–317)

In addition, older stutterers tend to perceive their stuttering as less of a handicap than they did when they were young adults (Manning et al., 1984).

Recovery from Stuttering

Considered thus far in this chapter is how the symptomatology of the stuttering problem, following onset, evolves into a more severe (complex) form. There is a second way in which the disorder can evolve. The person can recover. According to Ainsworth and Fraser-Gruss (1981):

It has been estimated that for every person who stutters today, there are three other people who have stuttered at some point in their development. The reasons these people and their parents give for their recovery [incidentally] are extremely varied.... (p. 10)

Such a recovery apparently can occur at any age from preschool to adulthood.

How do we know that some persons—estimates range between 32 percent and 79 percent (Andrews, 1984; Johnson & Associates, 1959)—recover from stuttering? The evidence comes from several sources. One is anecdotal reports from persons who claim to have stuttered and no longer do so. I have met more than ten people during the past thirty years who claim to have recovered from stuttering whom I am fairly certain really did stutter at one time. Various explanations were offered by them for their recovery. For example, one attributed it to manipulation by a chiropractor; another to learning diaphragmatic breathing; a third to the healing power of a television evangelist; a fourth to learning to talk slower; a fifth to having his lingual frenum cut; and a sixth to elocution lessons. All indicated directly or indirectly that they had had confidence in the ability of the technique and/or the person who administered it to cure their stuttering and that they no longer thought of themselves as having a stuttering problem.

Further evidence that some persons recover from stuttering comes from surveys in which participants (mostly high school and college students) were asked whether they had stuttered at any time during their life (Cooper, 1972; Culton, 1986; Porfert & Rosenfield, 1978; Seider, Gladstein, & Kidd, 1983; Sheehan & Martyn, 1970). The percentages of persons in these surveys who reported to have stuttered ranged from less than 1 percent to more than 10 percent. And the percentages of those who reported that they had stuttered but recovered in all of them exceeded 35 percent. While this percentage may be somewhat inflated because it is likely to include some persons who considered their normal repetitions and/or other hesitations to be stuttering, it nevertheless provides strong evidence that some persons do recover from the disorder.

A third source of evidence that some persons recover from stuttering is longitudinal research. Yairi and Ambrose (1992b) have reported data that are consistent with this conclusion on twenty-seven preschool-age children who were followed for a period of from two to twelve years after they began stuttering.

Assuming that recovery from stuttering is possible, at what ages does it tend to occur? The available data suggest that it can do so at any age. Seider et al. (1983), for example, reported ages of recovery that ranged from three to thirty-eight years. However, younger persons appear more likely to recover than older ones (Seider et al., 1983). Andrews, et al. (1983), from an analysis of the findings of several studies, estimated that approximately three times as many who are stuttering by age four than are stuttering by age ten will have recovered by age sixteen. Of course, some of those who were looked upon as stuttering at age four may actually have been normally disfluent. However, it is unlikely that enough were misdiagnosed to account for the probability of recovery in them declining as a function of age.

If some children recover before reaching adulthood, the prevalence of the disorder in preschool and elementary-school-age children would be expected to be higher than in high-school-age children and adults. While this has not been demonstrated unequivocally to be the case, the available data (Brady & Hall, 1976; Louttit & Halls, 1936; Schindler, 1955) suggest that it is.

Is there any relationship between the severity of a person's stuttering and the likelihood that he or she will recover? There is some evidence that there is a negative relationship between them (Dickson, 1971; Sheehan & Martyn, 1970). That is, the more severe the stuttering, the less the likelihood of recovery.

Another factor that may influence how likely a person is to recover is the degree to which he or she is perfectionistic. According to Amster (1994):

> *A young stuttering child who is perfectionistic may react more strongly to disfluency and, in order to control his or her speech, use more effort, tension, struggle, and avoidance, making the disorder more severe and less likely to spontaneously remit. (p. 150)*

Once a person has recovered from stuttering, how likely is it that he or she will begin to stutter again? That is, how likely is it that the person will relapse? There is considerable anecdotal evidence that suggests that relapse is very common within the first five years following "recovery." Relapse can occur after this period, but it seems to be less likely. Richter (1982), a German speech pathologist, reported beginning to stutter again after a period of recovery that lasted twenty-eight years. One of my clients began to stutter again after a period of recovery that he reported had lasted forty years. Unfortunately, there is insufficient data available to estimate the probability of relapse for persons who have been "recovered stutterers" for more than five years.

ASSIGNMENTS

Preschooler Disfluency

Record the spontaneous speech of a three- or four-year-old child who is not regarded as having a fluency disorder. Describe the disfluencies. To what extent are they similar to those of Bloodstein's Phase I stuttering?

Stuttering Set

Listen to the syllable repetitions of a three- or four-year-old child who is not regarded as having a fluency disorder with the set that his or her repetitions are abnormal. Did you hear beginning stuttering? If you heard it, do you think that you would have if you hadn't had this set?

▶ 5

Etiology of Stuttering

The cause of stuttering is unknown (Boehmler & Boehmler, 1989). While there have been many attempts during the past 2,500 years to explain why people stutter (see Chapter 1), there is currently no theory, or hypothesis, that is generally accepted as being adequate to provide a conceptual framework for doing so (Perkins, 1994; Zimmermann et al., 1981). The fact that authorities disagree about its etiology has several implications for clinicians. First, it suggests that clinicians are going to have to reach their own conclusions or formulate their own hypotheses about what causes stuttering. They are going to have to decide which explanations are the most plausible, which ones are the most consistent with both research on the disorder and information they have received from their clients (Perkins, 1990a). This means that competent clinicians can differ on how they explain aspects of its etiology. For example, Cooper and Rustin (1985) reported that 32 percent of a sample of 371 speech-language pathologists in the United States agreed with the statement that stuttering is the result of an underlying physiological impairment. The others either were "undecided" or disagreed. Unfortunately, there is no way to know for certain who is "right." This situation, incidentally, can make clinicians uncomfortable, particularly if "on a gut level" they do not accept the principle of the scientific method—that all knowledge is *tentative* and subject to change as new information becomes available (Silverman, 1993, Chapter 3). If applied here, this principle would result in a statement similar to the following: "Based on the information I currently have available, the most plausible explanation for this aspect of my client's disorder is...." New information could either strengthen the clinician's confidence in the plausibility of the explanation or cause him or her to change it.

Second, it results in a lack of agreement about how to treat the disorder. The approach a clinician uses to treat a disorder should be based, at least in part, on the assumptions he or she makes about its etiology (Williams, 1968). If, for example, a clinician believes that a client's stuttering is a symptom of psychopathology, he or she should treat the disorder (or have someone else do so), at least in part, by means of psychotherapy. On the other hand, if a clinician believes that an aspect of a client's stuttering is learned behavior, he or she should treat it (at least in part) by learning-theory-based behavior modification strategies. Deciding which particular strategies would be appropriate to use, incidentally, would depend on how one assumed the behavior was learned. Clinicians who assume that it was an instrumental response probably would treat it differently than would those who assume it was a classically conditioned one (Brutten & Shoemaker, 1967).

A third implication is that each clinician has to decide how best to answer the question: "Why do I (or why does someone else) stutter?" This is a question that clients who stutter are likely to ask their clinician. It is also a question that others (particularly parents) are likely to ask clinicians, either with regard to stutterers in general or to particular persons who stutter. This question is particularly difficult to answer if it is being asked about stutterers "in general." Authorities disagree not only about the cause of stuttering, but about whether it *always* has the same cause (Van Riper, 1982).

The manner in which the question is answered can affect the person asking it in various ways. If this person is someone who stutters, the answer can affect his or her self-concept and the extent to which he or she experiences shame, embarrassment, or guilt about having the disorder. For some, the answer is more likely to have a negative impact if it indicates a psychological cause rather than a physiological one. Diagnosing a disorder as psychological in our society implies that a person can overcome it, if he or she really wants to and tries hard enough.

If the parents of someone who stutters are asking the question, the answer can affect both their self-concept and their reaction to their child. If it suggests that something they did may have caused the child to stutter, it could adversely affect their self-concept. One explanation (discussed later in chapter) for why persons begin to stutter—the diagnosogenic theory—can have this effect since it suggests that parental reactions to normal hesitations contribute to precipitating the disorder.

The answer to why a person stutters can also affect how the parents of a child who does so reacts to him or her. If they are reacting in a way that is unlikely to be helpful to the child (as in telling him or her to "stop stuttering"), the answer could cause them to stop doing so, or to do so less often. This, of course, would be a desirable outcome. The answer also can affect how they view the person and, thereby, how they react to him or her. If the answer suggests that the child is emotionally disturbed, they are likely to react differently to him or her than they would if it suggests that he or she has some type of neurological dysfunction.

If those asking the question are members of the general public, the answer can affect how they view and react to persons who stutter. That is, it can influence their stereotypes of such persons and, thereby, their reactions to them. A considerable amount of research indicates that many persons have such stereotypes and that they tend to be negative (Bloodstein, 1987). For example, many tend to treat persons who stutter in ways that suggest that they regard them as being childlike or not particularly intelligent. Consequently, an answer indicating that intelligence is not adversely affected by what causes the disorder may help to promote more beneficial reactions.

An answer to the cause of stuttering can also impact in another way on how persons who stutter (particularly children) are treated by others. If, for example, the answer suggests that stuttering can be acquired through imitation or fails to indicate that it cannot be acquired in this manner, parents may resist having persons who stutter (particularly children who do so) spend time with their children.

This chapter deals with what have been referred to as *theories* of stuttering. Some attempt to explain why people begin to stutter or the factors that cause them to be at greater or lesser risk for doing so. Others attempt to explain the symptomatology and phenomenology of moments of stuttering. And still others attempt to explain why the disorder persists after it has begun.

The term *theory,* in this context, refers to an explanation for some aspect of the disorder. Such explanations range from hypotheses that have been tested fairly extensively to ones that have been tested little, if at all. The latter can be classified as speculations, or hunches. Such classification does not necessarily mean the latter are wrong: It just means that these ideas have not been tested sufficiently to judge how likely they are to be true.

What factors should you consider when deciding how likely it is that such hypotheses are true? Perhaps the main thing to consider when evaluating the cogency of such a hypothesis is how well it can explain what is known about the disorder. If, for example, the hypothesis is one that attempts to explain the nature of moments of stuttering, it should be able to account for why they tend to increase and decrease in the way they do (see Chapter 2) and why some of the words spoken by almost all stutterers appear to be spoken normally. A hypothesis that cannot account for these instances in a reasonable manner (one that is counterintuitive) is less likely to be true than one that can do so. This is not the same as concluding the former to be false, because new information may become available that will allow it to account for "facts" in a way it was not able to previously.

Since it is not possible either to prove or disprove any hypothesis with absolute certainty, what is a clinician to do? As I indicated previously, one of the "rules" of the scientific method can be helpful here—the one stating that all conclusions are *tentative* and subject to change as new information becomes available (see Silverman, 1993, Chapter 3). Hence, the clinician could decide which explanation is most consistent with what he or she knows about the disorder and make clinical decisions based on it until receiving information that causes it to no longer be the most viable.

CATEGORIZATION OF STUTTERING HYPOTHESES

Many hypotheses have been proposed to explain stuttering. Some deal with a single aspect of the disorder and others more than one. They have been categorized in a number of ways. Several that are of interest to clinicians are described in this section.

Predisposing Cause versus Precipitating Cause versus Maintaining Cause

The word *cause* in the question "What is the cause of stuttering?" can have three meanings. Each of the following questions illustrates one of them:

1. What factors *cause* one person to be at greater risk than another for beginning to stutter?
2. What actually *causes* a person to begin to stutter?
3. What *causes* a person to continue to stutter after the disorder has begun?

Answers to the first question are hypotheses concerning the *predisposing* cause(s) of stuttering; those to the second are hypotheses concerning the *precipitating* cause(s) of stuttering; and those to the third are hypotheses concerning the *maintaining* cause(s) of the disorder. Some explanations attempt to answer only one of them and others two or three.

Etiology of Stuttering versus Moment of Stuttering

This scheme, which was proposed by Bloodstein (1987), has a somewhat different focus than the one just outlined. It is based on the aspect of the disorder being explained rather than its etiology. His *etiology of stuttering category* is a combination of the predisposing and precipitating cause categories in the preceding scheme with a little of the maintaining cause category thrown in. Any hypothesis that attempts to explain an aspect of the cause of stuttering can be placed in the etiology of stuttering category.

Bloodstein's *moment of stuttering category* includes a number of hypotheses, some of which can be placed in the maintaining cause category of the preceding scheme. Any that suggest answers to questions such as the following can be placed in this category:

- What abnormal physiological events result in moments of stuttering?
- Why are moments of stuttering more likely to occur on some words than on others?
- Why does stuttering tend to be more severe in some situations than in others?
- What psychological factors can influence the frequency and severity of moments of stuttering?
- Why does reading in chorus cause moments of stuttering to disappear?
- What behaviors (if any) that occur during moments of stuttering are learned? If any are learned, how are they learned?
- What is the role of expectancy in precipitating moments of stuttering?

Breakdown versus Repressed Need versus Anticipatory Struggle

This scheme, which was also proposed by Bloodstein (1987), categorizes hypotheses on the basis of *theme* rather than on that of the aspect of the disorder being explained. Hence, explanations with similar themes are included in a category regardless of whether they attempt to explain the cause of stuttering (predisposing, precipitating, or maintaining) or the symptomatology and phenomenology of the disorder.

There are three general themes that have appeared over and over again in explanations of both the cause of stuttering and the moment of stuttering. The first of these is the *breakdown* theme. Hypotheses having this theme attribute the aspect of the disorder being explained to some sort of physiological breakdown, which may or may not be stress related. Explanations that attribute stuttering to abnormal functioning of the central nervous system would fit into this category.

The second of these themes is *repressed need*. Hypotheses based on this theme view the aspect of the disorder being explained as a symptom of an abnormal psychological process, of which the person is probably not aware on a conscious level (Columbus, 1992; Porret, 1993). One hypothesis that has a theme of this type is the Freudian one, which views the disorder as a symptom of a fixation at the oral or anal stage of infant sexual development (Glauber, 1982).

The third of these themes is *anticipatory-struggle*. Hypotheses having this theme view the disorder as either resulting or worsening from the person *anticipating* with dread the occurrence of stuttering and *struggling* to avoid it. Explanations of this type for both the etiology of stuttering and the moment of stuttering have greatly influenced how the disorder has been managed during the past forty years.

IS THE CAUSE OF STUTTERING PHYSIOLOGICAL OR PSYCHOLOGICAL?

There have been many attempts to answer this question. Some who have attempted to do so believe the evidence indicates that the cause is "physiological" (e.g., genetic) and others believe it indicates that the cause is "psychological" (learned behavior). And still others believe it indicates that the cause is some combination of the two—neuropsychological. The latter view appears to be the most accepted one at present, with the main focus being on the physiological (Ingham, 1993; Siegel, 1993; Smith, 1990a).

Why have persons knowledgeable about stuttering reached such different conclusions? There are several reasons why they may have done so. One is that they have different beliefs about the most likely cause for abnormal behavior. Each of us has a belief about this based on the totality of our life experience. That is, we accept a particular cause unless the evidence to the contrary is so strong that we would feel we were being "irrational" to continue doing so. The beliefs of persons who attempted to answer this question, not surprisingly, have been influenced by their professional training. Psychoanalytically trained psychiatrists, for example, have tended to conclude that the cause is psychological (Glauber, 1982).

A second reason why persons knowledgeable about stuttering have reached different conclusions about its "organicity" is that they weigh the evidence bearing on it differently. While the findings of some studies suggest that the physiological functioning of persons who stutter differs in some way(s) from that of their normal-speaking peers, those of others do not (see Chapters 2 and 3). Persons who give greater weight to the former are more likely to conclude that the cause is physiological than those who do so to the latter. A person's beliefs about the cause of abnormal behavior undoubtedly will influence how he or she weighs such evidence.

During the past sixty years, the beliefs held by the majority of speech-language pathologists about the organicity of stuttering have changed several times (Bloodstein, 1987). As this book is being written, most appear to believe that the cause is, in large part, physiological. During the forties, fifties, and sixties, most seemed to believe that the cause was, in large part, psychological. Yet during the thirties, most seemed to believe that the cause was, in large part, physiological. Such opinion shifts also occurred prior to 1930.

Why would persons knowledgeable about stuttering change their belief from the cause being psychological (functional) to it being physiological (or vice versa) and back again? One reason would be the publication of research reports indicating that the physiological functioning of persons who stutter differs in some way from that of their normal-speaking peers. For example, publication of such reports during the seventies and eighties (see Chapter 3) changed the minds of many of those who previously had believed the cause to be psychological.

The cause of stuttering appears to be both physiological and psychological (Smith, 1990a). Some aspects of its symptomatology and phenomenology appear to result from physiological factors and others from psychological ones (see Chapters 2 and 3). Also, a cause that can be viewed as psychological also can be viewed as physiological. If, for example, you believe that the desire to avoid stuttering contributes to precipitating it (a psychological belief), it follows that such a desire causes persons who stutter to function abnormally physiologically. It would be this disturbance in physiological functioning that precipitates moments of stuttering. Hence, based on this belief the cause of moments of stuttering would be *both* physiological and psychological!

WHAT FACTORS CAUSE ONE CHILD TO BE MORE "AT RISK" FOR ACQUIRING THE DISORDER THAN ANOTHER?

Some children appear to be at greater risk than others for beginning to stutter (Andrews et al., 1983). That is, they appear to be more vulnerable to the condition, or conditions, that *precipitate* stuttering. A number of factors are discussed in this section that may influence the probability that a child will begin to stutter. Some of these factors have been referred to as *predisposing causes* of stuttering. While the presence of more than one probably increases the likelihood of a child beginning to stutter, the degree to which it does so has not been established. However, even if a number of these factors do apply to a particular child, the odds still appear to be greater that he or she will *not* begin to stutter than that he or she will begin doing so (Andrews et al., 1983).

The Sex of the Child

The likelihood of a boy beginning to stutter is greater than that of a girl. The sex ratio that has been reported by investigators in a number of countries ranges from 3:1 to 5:1 (Andrews & Harris, 1964; Beech & Fransella, 1968; Bloodstein, 1987; Van Riper, 1982). Since the prevalence of stuttering in the population has been reported to be approximately 1 percent, this means that fewer than 1 percent of girls stutter and more than 1 percent of boys do so.

Why are boys more likely than girls to stutter? While the reason has not been established empirically, there has been considerable speculation about it. Some writers (such as Schuell, 1946) have pointed out that boys are more vulnerable than girls for developing a number of disorders, possibly indicating that they are "weaker" than they are in some ways or are less able to tolerate stress. We know, for example, that boys tend to develop (mature) at a somewhat slower rate than girls in a number of ways, including language acquisition.

A second reason suggested for why more boys than girls begin to stutter is that the *environment* in which boys grow up tends to differ from that for girls in ways that make them more vulnerable to developing the disorder. One difference mentioned is in how parents and others tend to perceive, evaluate, and react to boys. According to Ainsworth and Fraser-Gruss (1981):

> *Some psychologists feel that part of this difference comes from our cultural expectations for boys. A boy is expected to act like a man too soon. If he cries for reasons not approved of for boys, [a parent] may think that he is not measuring up. (p. 22)*

Some of these explanations assume that the manner in which a child's speech hesitations are perceived, evaluated, and reacted to influences the probability that he or she will begin to stutter and that parents and others are more likely to perceive, evaluate, and react to those of boys than those of girls in a manner that could precipitate stuttering. Research bearing on such explanations is summarized in this chapter in the section dealing with the diagnosogenic theory for the onset of stuttering.

A third reason that has been suggested for this phenomenon is that a specific biologic sex-related difference contributes to making boys more vulnerable. It has been suggested, for example, that the sex ratio in stuttering is due to higher levels of testosterone in the male than in the female fetus, which affects the development of the central nervous system in a way that makes males more vulnerable to developing the disorder (Geschwind & Galaburda, 1985).

A fourth reason that has been suggested for it is a genetic predisposition for stuttering (some type of sex-modified inheritance) that is more likely to affect males than females (Ambrose, Yairi, & Cox, 1993; Kidd, Kidd, & Records, 1978; Ludlow & Dooman, 1992; MacFarlane, Hanson, Walton, & Mellon, 1991). While such a predisposition would cause a child to be more likely to begin to stutter, it probably would not precipitate the disorder. The actual precipitating cause probably would be "environmental" in nature (Kidd et al., 1978).

The Age of the Child

While a person can begin to stutter at any age, the likelihood of doing so is greater before the age of five than after the age of five. According to Andrews (1984), "On the basis of the data presently available, half the risk of stuttering is passed by age four, three-quarters by age six, and virtually all by age twelve."

Very few cases of stuttering that began during adulthood have been reported (Van Riper, 1982). Some persons who claim to have begun to stutter as an adult may actually have stuttered occasionally and/or mildly during childhood. However, they either don't remember doing so or they don't consider it to be the same disorder because they remember their hesitations as being much less tense than those they are presently experiencing. Several persons who initially told me they began to stutter while an adult reported episodes of mild stuttering in childhood after I questioned them about their fluency during this period. Some persons who report that they began to stutter when an adult may actually have one of the other fluency disorders (see Chapter 8).

While some cases of stuttering reported to have begun during adulthood may not have done so or may not be stuttering, there undoubtedly have been cases that began during this period. Actually, there is evidence (see Silverman, 1988 and the discussion of the "monster" study elsewhere in this chapter) that suggests that a person of almost any age can be made to stutter by reacting to his or her fluency in a negative manner.

Whether Any Members of the Family Stutter

The probability that a person will begin to stutter if he or she has relatives who stutter (or who had the disorder and recovered) is greater than it is for one who has no such relatives (Cox, Seider, & Kidd, 1984; Hedges, Umar, Mellon, Herrick, Hanson, & Wahl, 1995; Johnson & Associates, 1959; Kidd, 1977; Pauls, 1990; Poulos & Webster, 1991; Sheehan & Costley, 1977; Yairi, 1993). The fact that stuttering tends to run in families has been established by investigators in many countries, including the United States. The percentages of persons in these studies who had relatives on the maternal or paternal side who stuttered ranged from 30 to 69 (Bloodstein, 1987,

Table 7). The comparable percentages for normal speakers in these studies ranged from 5 to 18 (Bloodstein, 1987, Table 7).

While a child who is born into a family in which there is a history of stuttering is at greater risk for acquiring the disorder, this does not necessarily mean that he or she is going to do so. All that these data really indicate is that the probability of a child beginning to stutter is greater than 1 in 100 if he or she is born into a family in which there is a history of stuttering.

It is important to note that stuttering does occur in families in which there is reported to be no previous history of the disorder (Poulos & Webster, 1991). The data referred to earlier in this section (Bloodstein, 1987, Table 7) suggest that the families of at least 25 percent of the persons who stutter do not have such a history.

Why does stuttering tend to run in families? While authorities do not agree on the answer to this question, they have speculated about it a great deal. Reasons suggested include the following:

• A predisposition for stuttering may be inherited (MacFarlane, Hanson, Walton, & Mellon, 1991; Pauls, 1990; Poulos & Webster, 1991; West, Nelson, & Berry, 1939). Hence, stuttering (like diabetes and certain types of cancer) would be more likely to occur in families in which there is a history of the disorder.

• Stuttering can be caused by imitation. Young children, according to this explanation, are likely to imitate the speech of persons with whom they spend time. Hence, having someone in the family who stutters increases the odds that a child will spend time with a person who has the disorder. While some authorities during the first half of this century believed that stuttering can be caused by imitation, few (if any) do now (Bloodstein, 1987; Van Riper, 1982). One reason why this explanation has been rejected is that the symptomatology of beginning stuttering tends to differ from that evinced by older children and adults. Hence, if young children were imitating family members who stutter, they probably would be exhibiting the symptomatology of an advanced stage of the disorder, rather than the beginning one.

• Concern about a child stuttering can cause him or her to stutter. If there is a history of stuttering in the family, parents are more likely than otherwise to monitor their children's fluency and communicate to them that they are concerned about their repetitions and other hesitations. Some authorities (see Johnson & Associates, 1959) believe that such expressions of concern can be a precipitating cause of stuttering (see the discussion of the diagnosogenic theory in this chapter).

Socioeconomic Status of the Family

While stuttering occurs in families of all socioeconomic classes, there is a little evidence suggesting that it does so more often in those that are middle or upper-middle class than in those that are lower class (Morgenstern, 1956). The evidence for this, however, is not clear cut (Andrews & Harris, 1964). Assuming that there is a tendency for stuttering to occur more frequently in middle- and upper-middle-class families, what might be the reason? One reason suggested is that there tends to be a greater drive for achieving a higher status in middle- and upper-middle-class families than in those of other classes. This, of course, does not mean that persons in other socioeconomic classes do not have such a drive: It only means that there tend to be more status-oriented people in middle- and upper-middle-class families. Such persons usually want their children to achieve at least as high a status as did they themselves, and they are likely to believe that doing so requires excellence in a number of areas, including speaking. These parents, therefore, would be likely to become concerned if their children's speech appeared to be defective and would likely communicate their concern to them. Some writers, as mentioned previously, have suggested that this can precipitate stuttering (see the discussion of the diagnosogenic theory in this chapter).

Nationality of the Family

The prevalence of stuttering in some cultures appears to be higher than that in others. While that in Western and other "technologically developed" cultures (including the Japanese) has been reported to be approximately 1 percent, there are cultures in which it appears to differ from this. In some of these, fewer than one percent have been reported to have the disorder. Among them are the Mundugumar, Arapesh, Tchambuli, Manus, Dobuan, New Hanover, Tabor, and Kamamentira tribes of New Guinea; the aborigines of Australia; Polar Eskimos; the Bannock and Shoshone tribes of American Indians; and Polynesians (Bullen, 1945; Lemert, 1962; Snidecor, 1947). Those in which the prevalence of stuttering has been reported to exceed 1 percent include the population of Korea; the Kawakiutl, Nootka, and Salish Indians of Canada; the Idoma and Ibo peoples of West Africa; and school children in Dakar and the Accra district of the Gold Coast (Lemert, 1953; Morgenstern, 1953).

Why might the prevalence of stuttering be higher in some cultures than in others? To answer this question, anthropologists and others have attempted to determine what those with a high rate of stuttering have in common that differentiates them from those with a relatively low rate of stuttering. Bloodstein (1987) summarized their findings as follows:

> *To say that there are many stutterers in a given society is very possibly to say that it is a rather competitive society that tends to impose high standards of achievement on the individual and to regard status and prestige as unusually desirable goals, that it is sternly intolerant of deviancy, and that, as a by-product of its distinctive set of cultural values, it in all likelihood places a high premium on conformity in speech. (p. 119)*

Hence, the reason for cultural variation in stuttering prevalence may be the same as that based on the socioeconomic status of the family. Reread the above quotation from Bloodstein substituting *socioeconomic class* for *society*. He seems to be describing attitudes that are common in middle and upper-middle class families.

Whether the Child Is a Twin

A child who is a twin appears more likely to stutter than one who is not (Howie, 1981). Studies of the prevalence of stuttering in the twin population have consistently yielded percentages that are higher than the 1 percent in the general population.

If one member of a twin pair stutters, is the other likely to do so? The answer appears to depend on whether the pair is identical or fraternal. While the available evidence of identical twin pairs indicates that it is more common for both twins to stutter than only one doing so, that on fraternal twin pairs indicates that it is more common for only one member of a pair to stutter (Howie, 1981). It should be noted, however, that there are a significant number of identical twin pairs in which only one member stutters. In the studies reviewed by Bloodstein (1987, p. 112) this number exceeded 25 percent.

Why are children who are twins more likely to stutter than those who are not? Several explanations have been suggested. One is that a tendency toward twinning and a predisposition to stuttering are genetically linked in some families (Howie, 1981; West & Ansberry, 1968). A second is that an environmental factor (such as the competitive pressures members of a twin pair often encounter as a result of comparisons made between them) can make them more likely to stutter (Bloodstein, 1987).

Whether the Child Is Brain Injured

The incidence of stuttering that has been reported in most studies among children who are brain injured—particularly among those who have cerebral palsy or epilepsy—considerably exceeds 1 percent (Van Riper, 1982). It is uncertain, however, in how many of them the disorder is stuttering. Dysarthrias, apraxias, and word-finding problems (dysnomias), for example, can cause higher than normal levels of speech disfluency (see discussion of neurogenic-acquired stuttering in Chapter 8).

Whether the Child Is Mentally Retarded

A relatively high incidence of stuttering has been reported among children who are mentally retarded, particularly among those who have Down syndrome. The percentages of such children who have been reported to stutter in almost all studies considerably exceeds 1 percent (Bloodstein, 1987, Table 20; Van Riper, 1982, Table 3.1). The question arises (as it does with children who are brain injured) whether the disorder they evince is stuttering or something else. While the abnormal disfluency of some mentally retarded children undoubtedly is cluttering, disfluency associated with neuropathology, and/or developmentally delayed "normal" disfluency, that of others does appear to be beginning stuttering (Lerman, et al., 1965; Preus, 1972). Some mentally retarded persons, incidentally, have been reported to exhibit symptoms of advanced (secondary) stuttering including word fears, avoidances, and facial grimaces (Lerman, et al., 1965; Preus, 1972).

Whether the Child Is Bilingual

A child who is bilingual appears to be more likely to stutter than one who is unilingual (Travis, Johnson, & Shover, 1937; Stern, 1948). The reason for this has not been established.

Whether the Child Is Delayed in Language Development

Most studies of the language development of children who stutter indicate that they are more likely than their peers to be delayed in saying their first words, phrases, and sentences and in acquiring speech sounds (see Chapter 3). The reason for this relationship between stuttering and delayed speech and language development has not been established. Several interpretations have been suggested:

- Both are caused by the same thing. It has been suggested, for example, that they can be caused by a common genetic predisposition (West, Kennedy, & Carr, 1947) or developmental apraxia (Yoss & Darley, 1974).
- Children who are delayed in speech and language development are likely to acquire a sense of failure as speakers and learn to struggle with their speech attempts (Bloodstein, 1987).

While there undoubtedly is a tendency for stuttering and delayed speech and language development to occur together, most children who stutter do not have a history of delayed speech and language development and most children who do have such a history do not stutter.

Other Factors

A number of other conditions have been investigated because it was thought that they might influence the probability that a child will stutter. Some of these are listed below.

- Abnormalities in physiological functioning, particularly neurophysiological functioning (see Chapter 3)
- Abnormalities in emotional adjustment (see Chapter 3)
- Abnormalities in sensory and perceptual functioning (see Chapter 3)

- Medical conditions, including diseases and events associated with birth, that could cause brain damage. The findings of most studies suggest that stutterers are not more likely than their peers to have abnormal medical histories (Accordi et al., 1983; Andrews & Harris, 1964; Cox et al., 1984)
- Abnormalities in physical and social development. Children who stutter appear to compare favorably to their peers with respect to the ages at which they teethe, are weaned, dress and feed themselves, acquire bowel and bladder control, sit, creep, stand, and walk (Accordi et al., 1983; Andrews & Harris, 1964; Cox et al., 1984).

WHY DO PEOPLE BEGIN TO STUTTER?

A number of factors were mentioned in the preceding section that could cause one person to be more likely to begin to stutter than another. However, the mere presence of one or more of these factors does not appear to cause someone to do so. Something has to *precipitate* the disorder. There has been considerable speculation about what this "something" is. Unfortunately, persons knowledgeable about the disorder do not agree on it. We will consider in this section the three major types of explanations (hypotheses, theories) that have been mentioned in the literature for why persons begin to stutter: breakdown, repressed need, and anticipatory struggle. We also will consider several explanations that do not fit neatly into one of these categories. None of these appear to be widely accepted at present.

Breakdown Hypotheses

These hypotheses are of two types. One suggests that stuttering is precipitated solely (directly) by some sort of breakdown in physiological functioning. The other suggests that the breakdown precipitating it is a joint product of some sort of abnormality in physiological functioning and an environmental condition (or conditions) producing stress. Some writers (e.g., Bloodstein, 1987) refer to the physiological abnormality as the predisposing cause and the condition (or conditions) producing stress as the precipitating one. However, regardless of how one refers to these, such hypotheses indicate that both have to be present before someone will begin to stutter.

Hypotheses of the first type attribute the onset of stuttering directly to some abnormality in physiological functioning that may or may not be genetic in origin. The abnormality is said to interfere with the ability of the speech mechanism to produce normally fluent speech. There has been speculation about the nature of this abnormality for thousands of years. Hippocrates, for example, in the fifth century B. C. explained it as being a disturbance in the harmonious mingling of the four humours: blood, bile, phlegm, and the "watery humour" (see Chapter 1). If Hippocrates were stating this hypothesis today in contemporary language, he probably would indicate that the abnormality is some sort of biochemical imbalance.

The second type of hypotheses attribute the onset of the disorder to a combination of an abnormality in physiological functioning and an environmental condition that produces stress. The physiological abnormality may or may not be regarded as genetic. Most present-day breakdown hypotheses are of this type.

Hypotheses of both types that have been suggested during this century are discussed in this section. While these are not the only such hypotheses, they include the ones that have been most influential. For further information about breakdown hypotheses, see Bloodstein (1987), Hahn (1956), Luchinger & Arnold (1965), and Van Riper (1982).

A Disturbance in Cerebral Dominance for Speech Production

One half of the cerebral cortex (usually the left) normally is dominant over the other for various aspects of speech production. If such dominance is not present to a sufficient degree or if the "wrong" hemisphere is dominant for a particular aspect (or aspects) of speech production, it has been suggested that this could result in a *breakdown* in speech production manifested as stuttering. According to these explanations, the person could either have been born with or acquired this anomaly. If the person acquired it, the cause sometimes was attributed to being forced to write with the nondominant hand. During the first half of this century many people believed that forcing a left-handed child to write with his or her right hand could precipitate stuttering. While most authorities now do not believe that switching handedness *by itself* can precipitate stuttering, the evidence on this is inconclusive and conflicting. For example, while Haefner (1929) reported that 24 percent of the forty-one children whose handedness he had shifted stuttered, Ojemann (1931) reported that none of the twenty-three children he had shifted did so.

Because our society does not consider it more desirable to be left-handed than right-handed, few (if any) able-bodied right-handed children probably have been forced to write with their left hand (Haefner, 1929). Therefore, if switching handedness is a factor in precipitating stuttering, we do not know whether it is so simply because handedness is switched or because switching handedness affects lateral dominance in a specific way. In this regard, Van Riper (1982) has reported three cases of boys who began to stutter after their handedness was purposefully switched from right to left to be more like their fathers (who were left-handed). Also, Oates (1929) reported an experiment in which twelve "subnormal" right-handed children were shifted to the left hand: All were reported to be stuttering after five months of such training. It would appear, then, that the act of shifting probably is more significant in precipitating stuttering than the direction in which the shifting is done.

If switching handedness does contribute to precipitating stuttering, perhaps it does so indirectly. Forcefully switching a child's handedness may cause him or her to become upset and, as a consequence, more disfluent than usual. This increases the probability that someone will become concerned about the child's fluency and communicate this concern to him or her. On the other hand, switching handedness may not make a child more disfluent, but instead may cause an adult to become concerned about the child's "normal" disfluency because he or she has heard that switching handedness can cause stuttering. Here, expecting stuttering causes the person to listen to the child's fluency through a different "filter" than he or she would be likely to use otherwise (Johnson, 1946). Based on the diagnosogenic theory (discussed elsewhere in this chapter), either scenario could precipitate stuttering.

A Biochemical Imbalance or Difference

These hypotheses are of the second type. They suggest that persons can begin to stutter because of a biochemical imbalance or difference that makes their speech mechanism more vulnerable than normal to the fluency-disrupting effects of emotional stress. One explanation of this type views the moment of stuttering as a kind of miniature seizure somewhat similar to that evinced by those who have a childhood form of epilepsy known as pyknolepsy. Such seizures affect mainly the speech mechanism and are precipitated by emotional stress (West, 1958). According to this hypothesis, children who begin to stutter are seizure-prone persons who would evince more severe epileptiform seizures if it were not for the fact that they had a biochemical imbalance, such as a relatively high blood sugar level (West, 1958). In other words, these children have epilepsy, but are kept from evincing the usual symptomatology of the disorder by their relatively high blood sugar levels. While some studies suggest that persons who stutter have relatively high blood sugar levels, others do not.

Another explanation of this type for why persons begin to stutter—particularly for why more males than females do so—is based on a biochemical *difference* between the sexes, that is, the level of the male sex hormone testosterone to which they were exposed as fetuses (Geschwind & Galaburda, 1985). There is some evidence that the neuronal development of the fetal brain, particularly that of the left cerebral hemisphere, tends to be retarded if the level of testosterone to which it is exposed is relatively high (Geschwind & Galaburda, 1985). Since the male fetus is exposed to higher levels of testosterone than the female, males are more prone to disturbances in left hemisphere functioning for speech and language than females, which could make them more prone to use their right hemisphere for processing speech. Since the right hemisphere is less adequate than the left for doing this, the result could be an increase in hesitation, particularly in stressful situations.

Stress

Stress, by itself, can produce a breakdown in speech fluency. Both normal speakers and persons of all ages who stutter tend to be more disfluent when feeling stressed or anxious (see Chapter 2). There have been a number of reports of persons beginning to stutter after a traumatic experience. Such an incident is likely to result in a relatively large increase in the amount of stress or anxiety a person is experiencing.

Stress, or anxiety, has been hypothesized to contribute to precipitating stuttering in three ways. The first is *directly* precipitating the disorder *by itself*. Reports of persons beginning to stutter after extremely traumatic experiences support such an explanation. The second is *directly* precipitating the disorder *in conjunction with some type of abnormality* in physiological functioning, for example, a disturbance in cerebral dominance for some aspect of speech production. This explanation differs from the first by suggesting that stress, by itself, cannot precipitate stuttering and that a particular level of stress can precipitate the disorder in some persons (those with a particular physiological anomaly) but not in others. The third way is *indirectly* precipitating the disorder by causing the person to repeat more often or otherwise be more disfluent. This would make it more likely that someone would become concerned about the person's speech fluency and "diagnose" it as abnormal. Some persons—including myself—believe that such a diagnosis can precipitate stuttering (see the discussion of the diagnosogenic theory in this chapter). This explanation differs from the other two by suggesting that stress does not directly precipitate stuttering, but does so indirectly by increasing the probability that someone will diagnose a person's hesitations as stuttering and react to them accordingly.

Auditory Feedback Defect

The fluency of people who stutter improves under altered conditions of auditory perception, such as those produced by delayed auditory feedback devices (see Chapter 2). Based on this observation, a number of theories have been proposed that attribute stuttering to aberrant auditory feedback during speech production (see Postma & Kolk, 1992, for a review of these theories). A common theme in these theories seems to be that the disturbance in auditory feedback causes the stutterer to detect errors that probably do not exist: The stutterer's attempts to overcome them produce the types of breakdowns in speech fluency that are classified as stuttering-type disfluencies. One example of such a theory is the covert repair hypothesis (see Postma & Kolk, 1993). These theories do not appear to widely accepted at present (Postma & Kolk, 1992).

Repressed-Need Hypotheses

These hypotheses, which view stuttering as a type of neurosis, state that children begin to stutter because they attempt to cope with some type of repressed (unconscious) "neurotic" need in a way that causes them to be disfluent (Glauber, 1982). These hypotheses look upon stuttering as being both a symptom of an unsatisfied repressed emotional need and purposeful behavior. Because it is repressed, the child is usually not consciously aware of this need nor is he or she aware of attempting to cope with it. Such explanations assume that behaviors occurring during moments of stuttering are symbolic of (have meaning with regard to) the repressed need. Their meaning is interpreted differently, therefore, depending on what the repressed need is assumed to be. If, for example, it is assumed to be an infantile one for oral erotic gratification, behaviors occurring during the moment of stuttering may be interpreted as symbolizing "the immature sexual pleasures of nursing, biting, and oral incorporation of objects that the person enjoyed as an infant..." (Bloodstein, 1987, p. 49). Those who explain stuttering in this manner assume that the person's need for oral erotic gratification was not fully satisfied while he or she was an infant, possibly because of a disturbance in the mother-child relationship.

What repressed needs has stuttering been interpreted as symbolizing? The following are ones that have been mentioned frequently in the literature:

- An unconscious mental conflict or disequilibrium. According to Glauber (1982, p. 57), when it "threatens to emerge in consciousness, the stutter worsens and/or becomes a major concern."
- An infantile need for oral erotic gratification (Glauber, 1982).
- An infantile need for anal erotic gratification (Glauber, 1982). Those who claim that stuttering satisfies this need interpret aspects of the moment of stuttering as symbolically representing anal movements (which have been "displaced upward"). Hence, persons stutter because their need for anal erotic gratification was not fully satisfied while they were an infant, possibly because of a disturbance in the mother-child relationship.
- An aggressive expression of hostile feelings that the person is afraid to express openly. Stuttering has been equated with aggression in several ways. One is that it allows the person to make those with whom he or she speaks "uncomfortable" without fear of retaliation. The assumption here is that stuttering is "painful" to the listener, particularly if he or she is a parent or other family member. It is well known, incidentally, that the severity of stuttering tends to increase when a speaker who has the disorder is angry at the listener, but not openly acknowledging it. For a discussion of other ways in which stuttering has been equated with (interpreted as symbolizing) aggression, see Bloom (1978).
- A conflict between a conscious desire to speak and an unconscious desire to be silent. Several reasons have been suggested for why persons may experience such a conflict. One is that they may be afraid if they speak they will reveal certain desires or feelings or use words (such as obscene "anal" ones) that their listeners will find unacceptable. Another is that the act of speaking itself means something to them that they feel should be suppressed. For example, they may secure oral gratification (pleasure) from speaking, and because they do not believe they deserve to be happy they may have guilt feelings for doing so. Also, they may view speaking as an act that will cause others to react negatively to them. They may have had people react negatively to them because of how they spoke (e.g., how they pronounced words), what they had to say, or both. For further information about this type of conflict, see Fenichel (1945, Chapter 15).

For further information about stuttering viewed as a childhood neurosis satisfying a repressed need, see Bloodstein (1987), Bloom (1978), Coriat (1933), Glauber (1958, 1982), Hahn (1956), Perkins (1979), and Van Riper (1973, 1982).

Anticipatory-Struggle Hypotheses

These hypotheses view stuttering (at least in part) as *learned behavior* (Bloodstein, 1958, 1975).

The Diagnosogenic Theory

The most influential hypothesis of this type was formulated by Professor Wendell Johnson of the University of Iowa during the 1940s. This hypothesis, which usually is referred to as the *diagnosogenic theory* for the onset of stuttering (Johnson & Associates, 1959), suggests one set of circumstances (not necessarily the only one) that can precipitate the disorder. This hypothesis also has been referred to as the *semantogenic theory* and the *interactional theory* for the onset of stuttering (Perkins, 1990a).

What does the term *diagnosogenic* refer to in this context? A diagnosogenic disorder is one that is caused (precipitated) by its diagnosis (Johnson, 1946). A person's normal behavior is labeled "abnormal" and as a consequence he or she begins to behave abnormally. The person begins doing this, at least in part, because he or she wants to *avoid* behaving in the way that has been labeled abnormal and/or because of *fear* of doing so. Trying not to behave in a particular way or fearing doing so can cause you to behave abnormally more often (Frankl, 1985). For example, desiring to avoid perspiring excessively and fearing doing so can increase the frequency at which it occurs (Frankl, 1985). As the behavior that was labeled abnormal increases in frequency, both the person(s) who initially labeled it such and the one who is exhibiting the behavior are likely to become more concerned about it. This is likely to strengthen both their desire to avoid it and their fear of it occurring, and as a consequence it is likely to occur even more often. In this manner a *vicious circle* is established: The fear of behaving in a particular way and the desire to avoid doing so causes the behavior to occur even more often, and the more frequently it occurs, the stronger becomes both the desire to avoid it and the fear of not being able to do so.

According to the diagnosogenic theory, there are three events that have to occur before a child will begin to stutter (Johnson & Associates, 1959):

1. The child repeats or otherwise hesitates while he or she speaks. The frequency of occurrence of these behaviors does not have to be high: However, the higher it is, the more likely someone is to become concerned about it. Most, if not all, young children occasionally repeat sounds, syllables, and words and hesitate in other ways (see Chapter 4). The amount that they do so appears to be related to a number of factors, including their cognitive stage of development (Lindsay, 1989).

2. A person with whom the child interacts "diagnoses" his or her repetitions and/or other hesitations as being abnormal and reacts to them accordingly. The person may be a parent, a grandparent, a teacher, a day-care giver, or anyone who spends time with the child. Most often, it is a parent. He or she does, however, have to be someone whom the child respects and would like to please.

The person may make the child aware of the disfluencies by occasionally saying one or more of the following when they occur:

- "Stop and start over again."
- "Think of what you are going to say before you say it."
- "Take a deep breath before you talk."
- "Talk more slowly."
- "Stop repeating (or stuttering)."

The person may also communicate that the disfluencies are undesirable by doing one of the following when they occur:

- Looking at (having eye contact with) the child while he or she is being disfluent (LaSalle & Conture, 1991).
- Having a pained or concerned expression.
- Refusing to acknowledge their presence when the child indicates awareness of them (in other words, playing the "Emperor's New Clothes" game).

3. The child becomes concerned about them and tries not to be disfluent. He or she attends more to the disfluencies than previously and tends to become upset when they occur. Any strategy the child uses to keep them from occurring (such as "thinking of what he or she is going to say before saying it") is likely to fail because repeating is not under one's voluntary control. The more he or she tries to avoid them, the more frequently they tend to occur. And the more frequently they do so, the more he or she tries to avoid them. This vicious circle causes an increase in both the frequency at which the child repeats (or otherwise hesitates) and his or her desire to avoid doing so. As the child's repetitions increase, expressions of concern about them from listeners also tend to increase. This, in turn, reinforces the child's desire to avoid them. It is in this manner, according to the diagnosogenic theory, that stuttering begins.

When the diagnosogenic theory was originally formulated, one of the main pieces of evidence used to support it was the finding that in several tribes of American Indians (e.g., the Bannock-Shoshone) in which there appeared to be no word for stuttering, there appeared to be no stutterers (Snidecor, 1947; Stewart, 1960, 1985). Evidence has been reported relatively recently suggesting both that these tribes have a word for stuttering and stutterers (Zimmermann, Liljeblad, Frank, & Cleeland, 1983). While the presence in a culture of both a word for stuttering and stuttering is consistent with the diagnosogenic theory, it also could be consistent with other theories. Consequently, such data can no longer be interpreted as providing strong support for it.

What evidence is there then that a child can begin to stutter in the manner specified by the diagnosogenic theory? There are a number of research findings that directly or indirectly support aspects of this theory, including the following:

- Some normal-speaking preschool-age children, particularly those between the ages of two and four, tend to repeat sounds, syllables, and single-syllable words a great deal (see Johnson & Associates, 1959; Silverman, 1972b; Yairi, 1981, 1982).
- The repetitions that initially caused the parents of some young stutterers to become concerned about their speech do not appear to have been abnormal (Johnson & Associates, 1959). Hence, it seems quite likely that normal repetitions sometimes are diagnosed as stuttering. It should be noted, however, that for some such children the amount of repetition they were exhibiting at the time someone first became concerned about their speech fluency probably exceeded that exhibited by most of their normal-speaking peers (Yairi & Lewis, 1984).
- After parents diagnose their child's repetitions as being abnormal, they say things or react in a manner that would tend to increase their child's awareness of and concern about them (Johnson & Associates, 1959). There are data that suggest that parent-child interactions can influence children's disfluencies (see Guitar, Schaefer, Donahue-Kilburg, & Bond, 1992, for a review of the literature in which they are reported).
- Some children appear to accept their parents' "diagnosis" that their hesitations are abnormal and react to them in ways suggesting that they are both concerned about them and attempting to avoid them (Johnson & Associates, 1959).
- There is some evidence (Johnson & Associates, 1959) that counseling parents who recently have diagnosed their preschool-age children as beginning to stutter who do not perceive their hesitations as abnormal and react to them as such can reduce the probability that the child will continue to be regarded as having a stuttering problem.

While these findings are consistent with major assumptions of this theory, none provide a direct test of it. To do such a test, it would be necessary to take some children who are normally fluent, cause them to become concerned about their hesitations, and see if they begin to stutter. Even better, children would be selected who are at low risk for beginning to stutter—those over the age of ten who are exceptionally fluent speakers. While their beginning to stutter certainly would not prove that all children begin doing so in this manner, it would certainly provide strong evidence that a child can begin to stutter in the manner specified by this theory.

The results of an unpublished master's thesis (Tudor, 1939), completed more than fifty years ago, can serve as a direct test of the diagnosogenic theory. This investigation, which is reported to have resulted in normal-speaking children being turned into stutterers, was referred to by those who knew of its existence as the "monster" study (Silverman, 1988b). Because of embarrassment about the outcome (and possibly also because of fear of litigation), the study was not reported in print until almost fifty years after it was completed (Silverman, 1988b).

This study was conducted *before* the diagnosogenic theory was formulated, at a time when the prevailing belief was that stuttering resulted from a lack of unilateral cerebral dominance. Hence, the results of the study probably could not have been predicted. It is unthinkable that the study would have been done had the investigator known there was a possibility that stuttering could be precipitated in the manner specified by this theory. The study was *not* a part of a stuttering research program. It was one of a series of at least five master's theses intended to assess the validity of certain general semantics formulations (Johnson, 1946, pp. 517–518). One of these formulations was *evaluative labeling,* the tendency "to evaluate individuals and situations according to the names we apply to them" (Johnson, 1946, p. 261). None of the other theses dealt with stuttering.

One of the primary objectives of Tudor's study was to determine whether labeling a person, previously regarded as a normal speaker, as a stutterer would have any effect on his or her speech fluency. Tudor screened the children in an orphanage and selected six who were regarded as normal speakers to serve as subjects. Their chronological ages were five, nine, eleven, twelve, twelve, and fifteen. She made the following statement to each child at the beginning of the experiment:

> *The staff has come to the conclusion that you have a great deal of trouble with your speech. The types of interruptions which you have are very undesirable. These interruptions indicate stuttering. You have many of the symptoms of a child who is beginning to stutter. You must try to stop yourself immediately. Use your will power. Make up your mind that you are going to speak without a single interruption. It's absolutely necessary that you do this. Do anything to keep from stuttering. Try harder to speak fluently and evenly. If you have any interruptions, stop and begin again. Take a deep breath whenever you feel you are going to stutter. Don't ever speak unless you can do it right. You can see how [the name of a child in the institution who stuttered rather severely] stutters, don't you! Well, he undoubtedly started the same way you are starting. Watch your speech every minute and try to do something to improve it. Whatever you do, speak fluently and avoid any interruptions whatsoever in your speech. (Tudor, 1939, pp. 10–11)*

In addition, she made the following statements to the teachers and matrons who interacted with these children:

> *The staff has come to the conclusion that these children show definite symptoms of stuttering. The types of interruptions they are having very frequently turn into stuttering. We have handled a number of cases very similar to these children. You should impress upon them the value of good speech, and that in order to have good speech one has to speak fluently. Watch their speech all the time very carefully and stop them when they have interruptions; stop them and have them say it over. Don't allow them to speak unless they can say it right. They should be made very conscious of their speech, and also they should be given opportunities to talk so that*

their mistakes can be pointed out to them. It is very important to watch for any changes in the child's personality, in his attitude toward his school work, in his attitude toward his playmates, etc. (Tudor, 1939, pp. 12–13)

Tudor spoke to the children and their teachers and matrons at least once a month for a semester to attempt to reinforce the label "stutterer." She reported the following description of the children's speech at the end of the semester:

All of the subjects . . . showed similar types of speech behavior during the experimental period. A decrease in verbal output of all six subjects; that is they were reluctant to speak and spoke only when they were urged to. Second, their rate of speaking was decreased. They spoke more slowly and with greater exactness. They had a tendency to weigh each word before they said it. Third, the length of response was shorter. The two younger subjects responded with one word whenever possible. Fourth, they were more self-conscious. They appeared shy and embarrassed in many situations. Fifth, they accepted the fact that there was something definitely wrong with their speech. Sixth, every subject reacted to his speech interruptions in some manner. Some hung their heads; others gasped and covered their mouths with their hands; others laughed with embarrassment. In every case the children's behavior changed noticeably. (Tudor, 1939, pp. 147–148)

She concluded that her findings supported the hypothesis that evaluative labeling can influence behavior.

Judging by information I received from four persons who were knowledgeable about the outcome of the study (including the late Dean E. Williams of the University of Iowa), some time following its completion her advisor (Wendell Johnson) was notified by the orphanage that the changes in the children's communicative behavior had not only persisted, but there was concern that at least some of them had become stutterers. Tudor, of course, was concerned about the children and visited them periodically for at least several years. Letters she wrote her advisor about her visits with the children suggest that at least some of them continued to stutter. For additional evidence that at least some of the children continued to do so, see Silverman (1988b).

The findings of the Tudor study provide strong evidence that diagnosing normal disfluency as stuttering can cause stuttering. What is particularly impressive about the findings is that fact that five of the six children were considerably beyond the age at which stuttering ordinarily begins. They had experienced being normal speakers for a number of years. The implications of the findings seem clear—asking a child to monitor his or her speech fluency and attempt to be more fluent may lead to increased disfluency and possibly stuttering!

While, to the best of my knowledge, nobody has attempted to do a direct replication of the Tudor study, an experiment has been reported by Newman (1987) providing further evidence that reacting negatively to normal speech repetitions can result in the development of stutter-like behaviors. She had ten normal-speaking adult males speak spontaneously for fifteen minutes. While repetitions decreased when the stimulus "you repeated" was said immediately after each occurrence of repetition, several behaviors surfaced that were judged by her to be stutter-like in nature. According to Newman (1987):

> *Every subject responded to the situation with behavioral changes that included both speech behaviors...as well as other behaviors (facial expressions, posture changes, etc.). In general, speech movements seemed to become overcontrolled and speech was uttered with restrained and precise movements that resulted in a halting, hesitant performance.*
>
> *A wide variety of behavioral alterations were noted as each subject tried to speak without repeating. At the start of conditioning, most subjects responded to the instructions by changing their posture in the chair from a relaxed to a more formal position. The subjects sat upright immediately and began to fidget. They started to laugh or smile nervously when reminded of their repetitions. They also began to use their hands more frequently, doing things such as playing with the table edge, the topic cards, or the microphone cord. Other behavior changes noted among the subjects included looking down or away while speaking, closing their eyes after delivery of the adversive stimulus, increasing their depth of inhalation, increasing their vocal intensity, and using a rising vocal inflection at the ends of sentences. These behaviors appeared to be similar to superstitious behaviors in that the subjects behaved as though these behaviors would help them talk without repeating...It may be assumed that the responses just described are not unlike those of the stutterer as he or she attempts to speak without being disfluent. (pp. 60–61)*

Newman did not report whether any of these behaviors persisted after the experiment ended. However, regardless of whether they did so, the findings of this study provide further evidence that reacting negatively to normal speech repetition can result in the development of stutter-like behavior.

While it seems likely that the conditions specified by the diagnosogenic theory contribute to precipitating some cases of stuttering, *the evidence reviewed here does not prove that they contribute to precipitating all such cases or that they will always do so.* A number of writers (such as Van Riper, 1982) have argued quite cogently that stuttering may have more than one cause.

For critiques of the diagnosogenic theory, see Onslow (1992a) and the papers in the first issue of the *Journal of Fluency Disorders* for 1992, particularly the two by Hamre (1992a, 1992b). When reading them, note that none of the authors who claim there isn't any evidence that supports the diagnosogenic theory refer to either the Tudor (1939) study or to my report of it (Silverman, 1988b). They, of course, would find it difficult to make this claim if they acknowledged the existence of the Tudor study. The diagnosogenic theory, incidentally, appears to be used by many (perhaps the majority of) pediatricians when making management decisions about young children whose parents believe they are beginning to stutter.

The Continuity Hypothesis

This theory, which was proposed by Oliver Bloodstein (1961, 1987), also states that stuttering develops from the disfluency exhibited by most young children. However, it does not assume that the reason is someone's misdiagnosis of normal disfluency. According to it:

> *Stuttering develops when speech tensions and fragmentations become magnified by communicative pressure. In this view, stuttering develops along a continuum as the child struggles increasingly in the face of a mounting conviction that speaking is difficult. It does not occur... as the child's effort to avoid the normal disfluency that was being mislabeled as stuttering.... It originates from the child's effort to speak. (Perkins, 1990a, p. 373)*

When the speech tensions and fragmentations are magnified to the point that they are severe and chronic, they tend to be identified as episodes of stuttering (Bloodstein, 1961).

> *One of the main differences between this hypothesis and the diagnosogenic one is in how they explain the similarities between normal childhood disfluency and that exhibited by children thought to be beginning to stutter. According to the diagnosogenic theory: If one child's speech repetitions are normal there is little justification for calling another child's speech repetitions anything else just because there are more of them. By contrast, the continuity hypothesis says that if one child's speech repetitions are stuttering there is little reason to call another child's repetitions anything else merely because there is a relatively normal amount of them. While these two statements appear to represent only differences in definition of stuttering there is a vast distinction between them in their ultimate implications for theory and therapy. In the first instance we must look for the source of the child's problem largely in the perceptual distortions of a listener by reason of which the child comes to regard disfluencies as a matter of concern and to struggle to avoid them. In the second case we must look for the causes of the problem largely in the nature of the stutterings that are latent in almost all children's speech and in the variety of possible factors that might tend to increase them. (Bloodstein, 1987, pp. 352–353)*

While these hypotheses disagree about whether childhood disfluency is normal or abnormal and what initially causes the "tension and fragmentation" in a child's speech to increase, they are not necessarily incompatible. Sooner or later both will result in a child becoming aware of the behavior and desiring to avoid it. Whether a child does so because of the negative reactions of listeners to his or her disfluency (diagnosogenic theory), or the child's own awareness and dislike of it (continuity hypothesis), or both of these, the consequences will be the same.

Other Hypotheses

A number of "old" and "new" hypotheses pertaining to the etiology of stuttering that do not fit neatly into one of the other three categories are discussed in this section.

Shocks and Fright

Some persons relate the onset of their stuttering to a particular event—usually a traumatic one. They either remember beginning to stutter after it occurred or were told that they did so by someone.

It is necessary to exercise caution when interpreting such reports. In some cases, for example, the onset of the disorder actually preceded the event. We do not know how often this happens because it usually is extremely difficult to document that the person was stuttering before the event occurred. Van Riper (1982) has reported a case in which he was able to do so:

> *A sixteen-year-old stutterer was brought to us by his mother with a clear history of onset at the age of eight years. Both the mother and the boy remembered the event vividly. The boy was on his way home in the early darkness of a winter evening and stumbled across the body of a dead man on the sidewalk in front of the boy's home. (They had the newspaper clipping to prove it.) The boy rushed into the house, opened his mouth to speak, and was unable to do so for some minutes despite repeated attempts. His stuttering dated from this time, so they said, and it was interesting that his major stuttering behavior was this same wide gaping mouth. The mother was absolutely convinced that the boy had been completely fluent previously. Nevertheless, we were able to find school records, and to get the testimony of his first grade teacher who remembered the boy because of his speech difficulty. It was clearly established that he had been stuttering fairly frequently and severely, though repetitively, before the incident. (p. 72)*

While such events may not cause children to stutter, they may contribute indirectly to the onset of their stuttering. That is, they may cause them to repeat more often or otherwise be more disfluent than they were previously (Irwin & Duffy, 1955). This increases the probability that others will become concerned about their speech fluency. Persons with whom they interact who believe that stuttering can be caused by a traumatic incident are particularly likely to do so ("Seek and ye shall find.''). As I have indicated previously, some writers have suggested that communicating to children that their hesitations are abnormal is an event that can precipitate the disorder.

The early twentieth-century literature on stuttering contains many reports of children beginning to stutter after a shock or frightening experience. For example, Makuen in 1914 reported that 28 percent of the stutterers in his sample and Gutzmann in 1900 reported that 14 percent of his stutterers (see Luchinger & Arnold, 1965) had suffered shocks or fright prior to onset. The event causing the shock or fright, however, usually was not as dramatic as the one reported by Van Riper—finding a dead body. According to Luchinger and Arnold (1965, p. 745), "In most cases minor physical or emotional mishaps are incriminated: a dog barked suddenly; a rooster flew into the child's shoulder; or the child stumbled over a carpet in a department store."

The evidence that a shock or frightening experience can cause stuttering is both anecdotal and circumstantial. It is based on reports that a shock or frightening event preceded the moment when someone first concluded that the child was stuttering. Even if the disorder really began after such an event, this does not necessarily mean that the event precipitated the disorder.

Illness

There are a number of reports in the literature of children beginning to stutter following an illness. Gutzmann (1939) reported that in almost 10 percent of his cases the onset of stuttering followed severe attacks of infectious diseases and other illnesses. West, Nelson, and Berry (1939) reported that between 16 and 20 percent of their stutterers began to stutter after an illness such as a severe respiratory infection, rheumatic fever, whooping cough, bronchitis, pneumonia, epilepsy, and encephalitis. Goda (1961) reported a case of a seven-year-old boy who began to stutter following an attack of spinal meningitis.

Do children who stutter tend to be ill more often during early childhood than their peers? Perhaps if illness can be a factor in precipitating stuttering, the likelihood of it being one is a function of the amount of time a child is ill rather than the specific illness that he or she has. This does not seem to be the case. The available data indicate that children who stutter do not tend to have more illnesses during early childhood than their peers (Andrews & Harris, 1964; Johnson & Associates, 1959).

Assuming that some children do begin to stutter after an illness, why do they do so? There are several possible explanations. The first is coincidence. With the number of illnesses that many young children tend to have, it would not be particularly surprising if one occurred before the presumed onset of the disorder.

A second possible explanation is that the illnesses resulted in physiological changes that precipitated stuttering. Such changes presumably would involve the central nervous system.

A third possible explanation is that the stress resulting from such illnesses causes children to be more disfluent than usual. In this regard, Luchinger and Arnold (1965) state that:

The causative influence of infections . . . should not be construed to repre-
sent a specific neurological damage. What is important is the general debil-
itation and the reduction of physical and mental resistance. Following such
a breakdown of psychophysical well-being, stuttering may develop as a
psychic reaction. (p. 745)

If children because of "general debilitation" become more disfluent following an illness, the concern of persons in their environment about it may be communicated to
them. Some authorities believe that his can precipitate the disorder (see the discussion of the diagnosogenic theory in this chapter).

Imitation

The onset of stuttering has been attributed to imitation of another person's stuttering.
Mygind (1898), for example, reported that imitation was the important precipitating
cause in 13 percent of his cases: In most of them there were other family members
who stuttered. Otsuki (1958), in Japan, reported it to be a significant causal factor
in 70 percent of his cases. Two other writers claimed it to have been one in 4 percent
(Katsovskaia, 1962) and 12 percent (Froeschels, 1943) of their cases.

How likely is it that a child's stuttering could be caused by imitation? The available data are insufficient for answering this question with a high degree of confidence. With regard to this, Van Riper (1982) reported the following:

For many years we have sought evidence for imitation as a precipitant of
the onset of stuttering in every case we examined. Though we never counted
up the cases we saw in those years, they constitute a substantial number.
We tried to trace every account of imitation as a source of stuttering and
only in one single stuttering child did we feel confident that the disorder
was triggered in this way. (p. 75)

Perhaps the most compelling argument against imitation, by itself, causing stuttering is that the symptomatology of the disorder at onset almost always differs from
that in its developed form. Consequently, if a young child's stuttering resulted from
imitating that of an older child or adult, his or her symptomatology would be
expected to be that of the developed form of the disorder, including facial grimaces
and associated movements.

Conflicts (Emotional and Communicative)

These probably have been regarded as precipitating causes of stuttering more often
than any of the other factors mentioned in this section. The following four excerpts
from case reports illustrate what is meant by a conflict in this context. The conflict
in the first three is emotional and in the fourth it is communicative.

The boy, in constant fear lest one of his obscene terms may slip out in the
wrong company, and having experienced this dangerous tendency of words

to go astray, soon begins to hesitate over every word which begins in the same way as do those dangerous words; and as the hesitations become a more and more fixed and noticeable habit, it extends to other types of words also. (Dunlap, 1917, p. 46)

Patty was referred to the clinic at the age of three and a half by her mother who was concerned about the child's stuttering. This symptom had started three months earlier following a spanking administered by the mother after the child had run into the street and narrowly missed being run over by a car. Shortly afterward the stuttering had cleared up but a few weeks later, after a second spanking for running into the street, she again began to stutter. (Harle, 1946, p. 156)

The onset of Nana's stuttering occurred at a time when her mother, because of an acute illness, had become inaccessible to the child. Nana consequently experienced a break in a previously well-established speech chain. This disruption coincided with a critical period in Nana's language development.... (Wyatt, 1969, p. 93)

When I was four years old my mother took a job and put me in a day nursery....We moved to an apartment at about that time which was located on the top floor and we were required to run up five flights of stairs to get up to it. One of my habits was to run up the five flights and upon getting into the house I would try to speak while out of breath. This is the first time I can remember "stumbling" in my speech. (Duncan, 1949, p. 258)

The conflict in the first involves the boy's approach-avoidance urges to say "dirty" words and not to say them; that in the second and third involves a disturbance in the mother-child relationship; and that in the fourth involves a desire to speak before having adequate breath support to do so fluently.

According to Van Riper (1982), emotional conflicts that have been reported to precipitate stuttering occur on three levels: word, situation, and relationship. Those on the *word level* to which the onset of the disorder has been attributed include conflicting urges to say something and not to say it, trying to say unfamiliar words, and trying to think of and say the "right" word without being sure that it is the right (appropriate) one.

Events resulting in emotional conflicts on the *situation level* that have been reported to precipitate stuttering initially cause the disorder to manifest itself in (be confined to) only one situation. In one case, for example, the situation was talking on the telephone and in another it was talking to a puppy (Van Riper, 1982, p. 77).

Conflicts on the *relationship level* that have been reported to precipitate stuttering involve a disturbance in the relationship between the child and someone else.

Most often the "someone else" is reported to be the child's mother. The excerpts in this section from the case studies by Harle and Wyatt illustrate such conflicts.

Emotional conflicts on word, situation, or relationship levels that have been reported to precipitate stuttering may not have actually done so. The fact they occurred at the time the disorder was thought to have begun may have been a coincidence. Also, children who stutter do not appear to differ from their normal-speaking peers with regard to the number of emotional conflicts that they have (Andrews & Harris, 1964; Johnson & Associates, 1959). Finally, many children experience emotional conflicts similar to those reported to precipitate stuttering without developing the disorder.

While emotional conflicts, by themselves, may not precipitate many cases of stuttering, they may contribute to doing so by making a child more disfluent. As Van Riper (1982, p. 79) has stated, "It is at least tenable that the motor sequencing of speech breaks down when communication is overloaded by stress of any kind. . . ." Certainly, conflicts on word, situation, and relationship levels can produce a great deal of stress. Hence, some children while experiencing such conflicts may tend to be more disfluent than they were previously. This would increase the probability that someone would become concerned about their speech fluency and communicate this concern to them. According to the diagnosogenic theory, such an expression of concern can contribute to precipitating stuttering. This same scenario could result in communicative stress contributing to precipitating the disorder.

Demand for Fluency Exceeding Capacity

This hypothesis has been referred to as the "demands and capacities" model (Adams, 1990; Andrews et al., 1983; Kelly & Conture, 1992; Starkweather, 1987; Starkweather & Gottwald, 1990; Weiss & Zebrowski, 1992). According to Starkweather (1987):

> *In this model, the capacities for fluent speech—the motoric, cognitive, and linguistic skills that make easy speech possible for most children—interact with demands for fluency placed on the child by the external communicative environment and by the child himself. As the capacity for fluency grows, the expectations of parents and of the child will also increase. Very young children are expected to be hesitant and stumbling in speech. Older children are expected to produce more words more quickly and more easily. In this way, capacities and demands for fluency are simultaneously increasing. If the environment demands more fluency than the child can produce, stuttering will begin. Whether the stuttering will continue or remediate depends on whether a growing capacity to produce fluent speech can catch up with the world's accelerating demands. (p. 144)*

This model, because it is of relatively recent origin, has not been evaluated sufficiently empirically to judge its cogency.

Reduced Ability to Generate Temporal Patterns
Kent (1983) has posited that stuttering results (at least in part) from a central nervous system disturbance, the nature of which "is a reduced ability to generate temporal patterns, whether for sensory or motor purposes, but especially the latter" (Kent, 1983, p. 252). Stutterers, according to this hypothesis, do not have as much ability as their nonstuttering peers to "smoothly" sequence the movements (gestures) of which spoken words consist. While the reason for their deficit is physiological (possibly genetic), the degree to which their capacity for temporal regulation is reduced at a particular moment while speaking is likely to be a function of social and psychological variables. This hypothesis, like the preceding one, being of relatively recent origin, has not been evaluated sufficiently on an empirical level to judge its cogency.

Linguistic and Paralinguistic Components Being Dyssynchronous When the Speaker Is under Time Pressure
Perkins, Kent, and Curlee (1991) have proposed a theory of neuropsycholinguistic function to explain the production of fluent speech, normal disfluency, and moments of stuttering. They have summarized their theory as follows (Perkins, Kent, & Curlee, 1991):

> *Speech involves linguistic and paralinguistic components, each of which is processed by different neural systems that converge on a common output system. Fluent speech requires that these components be integrated in synchrony. When they are dyssynchronous, the result can be either nonstuttered disfluency or stuttering, depending on time pressure. Time pressure is defined as the speaker's need to begin, continue, or accelerate an utterance. Nonstuttered disfluency results when the linguistic and paralinguistic components are dyssynchronous and the speaker is not under time pressure. Stuttering results when the speaker is under time pressure and is relatively unaware of the cause of dyssynchrony. Both of these factors are necessary for the identification of the phenomenon of stuttering. Stuttering is defined as a disruption of speech that is experienced by the speaker as a loss of control. (p. 734)*

There is considerable evidence that stuttering severity tends to increase when a stutterer speaks while experiencing time pressure (see Chapter 2). While this hypothesis appears to explain the moment of stuttering, at least in part, it is of relatively recent origin and has not been tested sufficiently to judge its overall cogency and heuristic value. With regard it the latter, it has generated some strong reactions (see Christensen, 1992; Smith, 1992) and counterreactions (see Perkins, 1992a, 1992b).

WHY DO PEOPLE CONTINUE TO STUTTER?

Thus far in this chapter, two of the three levels at which attempts have been made to explain the etiology of stuttering have been explored: those dealing with the predisposing cause and the precipitating cause. In this section the third of these levels is explored, that dealing with the *maintaining* cause of stuttering. Specifically, we will consider "answers" that have been given to the following questions:

- Why do moments of stuttering occur when they do and what is their nature?
- Why do people continue to stutter after they have begun doing so?

Hypotheses are categorized, as done previously, on the basis of whether they indicate some type of *breakdown, repressed-need,* or learned *anticipatory-struggle* response. For further information about these and other hypotheses about maintaining causes of stuttering see Bloodstein (1987), Freund (1966), Hahn (1956), and Van Riper (1982).

Breakdown Hypotheses

While these hypotheses are concerned primarily with predisposing and precipitating causes of stuttering, some do offer answers to the questions posed in this section. Some of those who attribute the moment of stuttering at onset to some type of physiological breakdown (e.g., Nudelman, Herbrich, Hoyt, & Rosenfield, 1989; Zimmermann, 1980; Zimmermann et al., 1981) probably would assume that people continue to stutter because the physiological anomaly in speech motor control processes is still present. Further, they probably would regard moments of stuttering as being a symptom of this physiological anomaly, the occurrence of which may be influenced by stress and variables that are not physiological, such as sociocultural and behavioral ones (Smith, 1990b).

Repressed-Need Hypotheses

These hypotheses view the moment of stuttering as a *symbolic* expression (symptom) of a repressed emotional need. It is symbolic in the sense that movements that occur during moments of stuttering communicate the nature of this need. For example, those who believe that the repressed need involves fixation at the oral stage of infantile sexual development as a consequence of inadequate mothering, interpret movements that occur during moments of stuttering as symbolizing infantile sucking behavior (Glauber, 1982). According to these hypotheses, people continue to stutter after they have begun doing so (at least in part) because the repressed need that precipitated the disorder has not been dealt with adequately.

Anticipatory-Struggle Hypotheses

These hypotheses view the moment of stuttering as learned behavior that is somehow precipitated by it being anticipated and feared. They indicate that what maintains the disorder is *anticipating* stuttering and *struggling* to avoid it. Some of those who advocate such hypotheses (such as Bloodstein, 1987) refer to the moment of stuttering as "struggle behavior." Theoretically, if a person who had the disorder stopped fearing and desiring to avoid stuttering (could develop a "don't care" attitude about it), he or she would become more fluent, perhaps even normally fluent. Better yet, if such a person could be made to *want* to stutter (somehow to be made to view it as advantageous to do so), he or she would be even more likely to experience increased fluency.

While many persons knowledgeable about stuttering agree that anticipation of stuttering contributes to both precipitating moments of stuttering and maintaining the disorder, there is no general agreement on the nature of the mechanism by which this occurs. Specifically, there is no agreement on the answer to the following question: How do events associated with the anticipation and occurrence of moments of stuttering serve to reinforce (maintain) the behavior? Among the answers that have been suggested are the following:

- The "unpleasantness" of stuttering reinforces the desire to avoid it and, thereby, reinforces the behavior (Van Riper, 1982).
- Because the presence of a stimulus (words or situations) that tends to give rise to anticipation of stuttering is not always followed by stuttering, the behavior is reinforced on a *partial reinforcement schedule* (Brutten & Shoemaker, 1967). As a consequence, the experience of being fluent a number of times in the presence of such a stimulus (words or situation) does not extinguish the fear of stuttering when encountering it. This may partially explain why some persons who have recovered from the disorder relapse after months, or even years, of being normally fluent. That is, relatively long periods of being normally fluent may not extinguish the fear of stuttering nor do they necessarily result in an unshakable anticipation of fluency. The occurrence of only a few instances of disfluency that the person judges to be abnormal may be sufficient to cause him or her to again anticipate stuttering and precipitate a relapse.
- The success that most persons who stutter experience when communicating reinforces the struggle behavior (Silverman, 1976a). Even while stuttering severely, they usually are able to make themselves understood.

TO WHAT EXTENT IS STUTTERING LEARNED BEHAVIOR?

Many types of behaviors can occur during, or accompany, moments of stuttering (see Chapter 2). Which of these are learned and how are they learned? Is there more than one type of learning involved? These questions are addressed here.

Perhaps the first question we should ask here is the following: How well do authorities agree that at least some behaviors associated with moments of stuttering are learned? They appear to do so fairly well. In a recent review of factors in the etiology of stuttering Smith (1990a) stated that:

> *For many years the debate raged whether stuttering was a "learned" or "organic" disorder. Happily this debate has passed, and at present I do not think anyone would argue with the statement that learning plays a role in the development of stuttering. (p. 43)*

In the previous section we dealt with hypotheses that regard stuttering as anticipatory-struggle behavior. Those who accept them view the moment of stuttering—at least in part—as learned behavior. However, these hypotheses are not accepted by all of those who believe aspects of it are learned.

There are behaviors associated with moments of stuttering that almost everyone agrees are learned. These are the so-called secondary behaviors, or secondary symptoms (see Chapter 2). They include facial grimaces, "starters," and lack of eye contact (Van Riper, 1982). Facial grimaces consist of gestures that the person uses to avoid or reduce the severity of moments of stuttering that had become habitual by the time they ceased being effective. "Starters" are gestures and/or words that are used before moments of stuttering to either avoid them or reduce their severity. They are thought to initially have been learned because at the times when they occurred before words on which stuttering was anticipated, the stuttering either did not occur or its severity was judged by the person to have been considerably less than expected. The outcome, of course, could have been the same if the "starter" had not been used. Nevertheless, the person's belief in at least the occasional efficacy of the starter may cause him or her to continue using it even when he or she regards it as not having been effective for a while. This is particularly likely to happen if there were periods in the past during which it did not seem to work followed by ones during which it did.

A third type of behavior associated with moments of stuttering that most persons knowledgeable about the disorder agree is learned is poor eye contact. Embarrassment and shame are signaled in our culture by looking away (Atkins, 1988). The person has *learned* to be embarrassed or ashamed about stuttering.

While there appears to be fairly good agreement among persons knowledgeable about stuttering that secondary symptoms (see Chapter 2) are learned, this is not the case for the disfluency behaviors themselves (the primary symptoms). Some believe that the latter are learned either because they can be *manipulated* in the same manner as behaviors that are known to be learned or because they are *distributed in a nonrandom manner* that can be explained by learning theory (Starkweather, 1987). For example, some believe they are learned because their frequency of occurrence can be manipulated by response-contingent reinforcement in a manner that would be expected if they were learned (Curlee, 1993a; Ingham, 1993a; Prins & Hubbard, 1988). That is, they would be expected to be reduced by response-contingent punishment. Some persons do not accept this as proof that stuttering is learned either because they feel that the available data are not sufficiently compelling to support this conclusion or that there are other possible explanations for the variations in stuttering severity that occur after response-contingent reinforcement.

A second reason why people may believe that disfluencies that occur during moments of stuttering are learned is because they are distributed in the speech sequence in a manner that can be explained by learning theory (Starkweather, 1987). They are, for example, more likely to occur on words on which moments of stuttering have occurred previously than would be expected by chance (see the discussion of the consistency effect in Chapter 2). A plausible explanation for this phenomenon is that they have learned to stutter on these words.

Thus far, we have dealt with the question: Which behaviors associated with moments of stuttering are learned? Assuming that some are learned, how are they learned? Is there more than one type of learning involved (are they all learned in the same way)? Persons knowledgeable about the disorder who believe that some behaviors are learned do not agree very well on how they are learned. This is unfortunate because the strategy a clinician would use to modify a behavior (response) would be based, at least in part, on his or her assumption about how it was learned (Williams, 1968).

One particularly influential answer to the questions raised in the preceding paragraph utilizes a two-process theory to explain how behaviors associated with moments of stuttering are learned (Brutten & Shoemaker, 1967). It stipulates that some are *classically conditioned* responses and others are *instrumental* ones. According to this theory, the disfluencies (repetitions, disrhythmic phonations, and tense pauses) that occur during moments of stuttering are probably classically conditioned responses and most of the other behaviors that do so (e.g., poor eye contact) are likely to be instrumental ones. The stronger a person's desire to avoid a classically conditioned response, the *more* likely it is to occur. On the other hand, the stronger his or her desire to avoid an instrumental one, the *less* likely it is to occur. If, for example, a person is told before performing a speaking task that he or she will be administered an electric shock after completing the task for each time he or she evinces a certain behavior during it (e.g., syllable repetitions), the effect of this information on the frequency of occurrence of the behavior will be determined by whether it is a classically conditioned response or an instrumental one. The behavior would tend to occur *more frequently* if it was a classically conditioned response, and it would tend to occur *less frequently* if it was an instrumental one.

For a lively discussion of the implications of learning theory for explaining and modifying stuttering, see the papers in the March 1993 issue of the *Journal of Fluency Disorders.*

IS STUTTERING REALLY A DISORDER OF SPEECH?

Stuttering traditionally has been viewed as a disorder of speech. It is not particularly surprising, therefore, that most of the theorizing about its etiology has focused on the speech mechanism. People have attempted to explain why the speech mechanism malfunctions to give rise to moments of stuttering. Proponents of breakdown hypotheses have theorized about physiological anomalies that either alone or in combination with stress could disrupt the functioning of this mechanism. Proponents of repressed-need hypotheses have theorized about how certain psychological anomalies can disrupt its functioning. And proponents of anticipatory-struggle hypotheses have theorized about how anticipating stuttering and desiring to avoid it can do so.

In this section stuttering is viewed from a somewhat different perspective. Rather than viewing it as a disorder of speech per se, we are going to view it as *one member of a class of disorders* that are characterized by the anticipation of "difficulty" increasing the likelihood of it occurring. This perspective, therefore, is a generalization of the anticipatory-struggle one.

The notion that stuttering is one member of a class of disorders characterized by fearful expectancy of "difficulty" causing it to occur is not a new one. Approximately one hundred years ago the kinship of stuttering with a great many similar disturbances in other areas was detected (Denhardt, 1890) and later, as a consequence, stuttering was classified by some psychiatrists as an *expectancy neurosis* (Freund, 1966). According to Freund (1966) expectancy neuroses are

> *disturbances of learned and automatized skills, of simple motor and vegetative functions, and even of elementary perceptual acts, manifesting themselves as "stuttering," e.g., in the playing of any musical instrument, as stutter-like disturbances in artistic singing,... writer's cramp, erythrophobia, stage fright,... some forms of sexual impotence, etc.... All these forms of expectancy neurotic disturbances have as a common characteristic that they are based upon actual "primary" traumatic experiences of failure in the performance of a learned skill or a simple motor or sensory act, often though not necessarily, in socially embarrassing situations. The anticipation of their dreaded recurrence leads then ... to the establishment of a* vicious spiral *[italics mine].... A further common feature is that dread, anticipation and the whole hypercompensatory mechanism are in the beginning on a completely unconscious level, and that awareness and conscious anticipation are usually later developments. (pp. 37–38)*

The vicious spiral (or vicious circle) referred to in the preceding paragraph is displayed graphically in Figure 5-1. The experience of "failure" leads to anticipating the recurrence of "failure," which leads to the recurrence of "failure" which leads to again anticipating its recurrence, et cetera. As long as the person continues to anticipate, with dread, the recurrence of failure in the performance of the skill or act, the vicious circle (spiral) will not be broken. A similar expectancy/anticipation phenomenon has been reported by psychologists (see Miller & Turnbill, 1986, for a review of the psychological literature on this phenomenon).

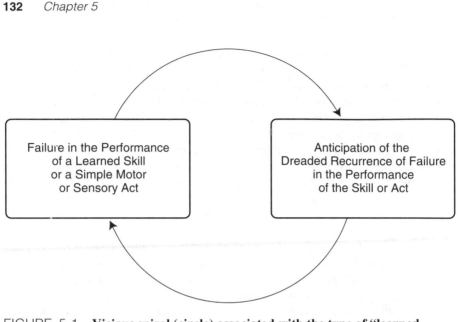

FIGURE 5-1   **Vicious spiral (circle) associated with the type of "learned maladjustive behavior" disorder that has been referred to as an expectancy neurosis.**

Is the expectancy neurosis viewed by psychiatrists as being learned behavior? The answer to this question appears to be "yes." According to Freund (1966), the terms *neurosis* and *learned maladjustive behavior* define the same set of phenomena.

Are some persons more likely than others to develop the type of "learned maladjustive behavior" disorder referred to as an expectancy neurosis? Some authorities believe that there are genetic-constitutional, psychodynamic, psychosocial, and/or psychophysiological factors that make some persons more likely than others to develop such a disorder (Freund, 1966). These, then, would function as predisposing causes for them.

Is stuttering a member of the class of learned maladjustive behavior disorders that have been referred to as expectancy neuroses? This question probably would not be answered in the same way by all persons who are knowledgeable about stuttering. The answer would be determined, at least partially, by their belief about the precipitating and maintaining causes of the disorder. A person who accepted an anticipatory-struggle explanation for these probably would be more willing to classify stuttering as this type of disorder than one who accepted a breakdown or repressed-need explanation. The answer to this question also would be influenced by their belief regarding the degree of similarity between the symptomatology and phenomenology of stuttering and that of other disorders looked upon as being precipitated and maintained by the type of vicious spiral depicted in Figure 5-1. These *may* include the following:

- Stutter-like disruptions in the playing of a musical instrument. Several investigators (Freund, 1966; Meltzer, 1992; Nadoleczny, 1926; Silverman & Bohlman, 1988) have reported disruptions in "fluency" during the playing of such musical instruments as the flute, French horn, piano, violin, and trumpet that there is reason to believe were precipitated and maintained by such a vicious spiral.
- Stutter-like disruptions in manual communication. Silverman and Silverman (1971) surveyed teachers at residential schools for the deaf in the United States to determine whether they had ever observed "disruptions" during manual communication that appeared to be similar to stuttering during speech. Several responded that they had seen such cases and from their descriptions of them there is reason to believe that they could have been precipitated and maintained by such a vicious spiral. Montgomery and Fitch (1988), in a recent survey of schools for the hearing-impaired, also received reports of stutter-like disruptions in manual communication.
- Agoraphobia. Most persons with this disorder have anxiety attacks if they stray too far from their home, and these attacks are thought to be precipitated (at least in part) by their recurrence being anticipated with dread.
- Diarrhea. Some persons precipitate episodes of diarrhea by anticipating their recurrence with dread.
- Headaches. Some persons develop severe headaches by anticipating their recurrence with dread.
- Impotence. Some men frequently are unable to achieve or maintain erection because they anticipate, with dread, being unable to do so.
- Insomnia. Some persons, at times, are unable to sleep because they anticipate, with dread, being unable to do so.

These are only a few of the disorders that are thought to be precipitated by anticipating, with dread, their recurrence. Since almost any aspect of functioning can be disrupted in this manner, the list probably is quite long.

What would be the implications—both theoretical and clinical—of viewing stuttering as a member of this class of disorders rather than as a disorder of speech per se? Theoretically, it would present a challenge to those who attribute stuttering to a physiological anomaly specific to the functioning of parts of the speech mechanism (such as the larynx) because comparable breakdowns in performance can occur that do not involve these structures. It also could add to our understanding of the symptomatology, phenomenology, and etiology of stuttering because information about other disorders in this class may provide some valuable insights into them.

Viewing stuttering in this way may also have clinical implications. For example, it could enable our clients to benefit from the clinical research and experience on other disorders in this class. That is, intervention strategies that have been helpful to persons who have one of these disorders also may be helpful to persons who stutter.

IS THE MYSTERY OF STUTTERING SOLVABLE?

After hundreds—perhaps thousands—of years of attempts to determine the cause of stuttering, there is still no general agreement. The prevailing view has cycled periodically between constitutional and environmental explanations (see Perkins, 1994). For at least two reasons it is particularly surprising that there is still no consensus about its etiology. A huge amount of information about the symptomatology and phenomenology of the disorder and about persons who have it that has been gathered and published during the past seventy years. And fantastic advances have been made in establishing the etiologies of many other disorders during this period.

While the reason for our lack of success in determining the etiology of stuttering is uncertain, it may be—at least in part—a consequence of the approach that has been used to test theories about it. There are two basic strategies that can be used for this purpose. The first is to gather evidence to prove a theory "true" and the second is to do so to prove a theory "false." Almost all investigators who have have attempted to test theories of stuttering have used the first strategy and almost all of those who have been successful in explaining other phenomena—including other disorders—have used the second.

While it is possible to prove that a theory is "false," it is impossible to prove that one is "true" (Perkins, Kent, & Curlee, 1991). Even if a theory can explain everything that is known about a phenomenon, it is possible that something will be learned about it in the future that the theory cannot explain. On the other hand, one fact about a phenomenon that a theory cannot explain proves it to be "false."

Almost all attempts that have been made to prove a theory about the etiology of stuttering "true" consist of reports of data that are consistent with it. These data may have been generated by the person testing the theory, taken from the literature, or both. Data that were not consistent with the theory were either ignored, declared to be uncertain with regard to validity, reliability, and/or generality, or interpreted as indicating that stuttering does not have a single cause and, consequently, there are one or more subgroups of stutterers to which the theory does not apply. In most scientific fields such data would cause a theory to be rejected. If it becomes fashionable to be more hardnosed when evaluating theories about the etiology of stuttering—that is, to do it like it's done in other scientific fields—perhaps the mystery of stuttering will be solved!

For other discussions of this issue, see Perkins (1994) and Perkins, Kent, and Curlee (1991).

ASSIGNMENTS

Cause Survey

Survey at least five young adults who have not had any training in speech-language pathology about what they believe to be the cause of stuttering. Did they tend to view the disorder as primarily a physiological or a psychological one? Did any of them mention causes that are no longer widely accepted, such as imitation? If they were the parents of children who stutter, would any of their beliefs be likely to impede therapy? Why?

Relaxation

Several times when you are feeling tense or anxious, tell yourself to relax within the next ten seconds. What effect did doing this have on your tension or anxiety level? If it did not reduce, what do you think was the reason?

► 6

Evaluation: Principles and Methods

My primary objective in this chapter is to provide you with a methodology for determining whether clients have a fluency disorder and if they do, for identifying the set of behaviors that define it. It consists of asking questions that are both relevant and answerable and of making the observations needed to answer them. The methodology described here is appropriate for both children and adults. However, the specific questions that would be asked and the tasks that would be used for making the observations needed to answer them would, of course, be influenced by the age of the client.

REASONS FOR EVALUATING SPEECH FLUENCY

There are a number of reasons why a speech-language pathologist may be asked to evaluate a child's or adult's speech fluency. Those discussed in this section include the most common ones.

To Determine Whether the Client Has a Fluency Disorder or Is at Risk for Developing One

One reason for undertaking such an evaluation is to determine whether the amount of repeating (or being disfluent in other ways) that a client is doing is abnormal. A clinician is more likely to be asked to evaluate a preschool-age or elementary-school-age child to determine this than an older child or adult. One reason is that such children often have to be evaluated to assess the need for developing an Individualized Training Program (IEP) (Cooper, 1978). This determination is often difficult to make for preschool-age children because many of them who are normally fluent do a lot of repeating (see Chapter 4). Guidelines have been developed to assist clinicians in making it. Riley and Riley (1989), for example, have devised a data-based screening protocol—*Physician's Screening Procedure for Children Who May Stutter*—that can be used by physicians and others (including speech-language pathologists) for assessing the degree of abnormality of a child's disfluency and reactions to it (see Appendix C).

If a child is currently stuttering, the clinician must decide if the child is likely to recover without therapy. Many children have been reported to do so (see Chapter 4). One device that is helpful when making this decision is the *Stuttering Prediction Instrument for Young Children* (SPI) (Riley, 1984). It yields a score that is based on both parental responses to a questionnaire and clinician observations of selected aspects of the child's disfluent speech. If a child's score is 9 or below, he or she would be judged likely to stop stuttering without intervention. For further information about this device and other measures that have been proposed for making this determination, see Yaruss & Conture (1993).

If a person's speech fluency appears to be within normal limits, the clinician should then attempt to determine if the person is at risk for developing a fluency disorder. That is, the clinician will attempt to determine whether there are any existing conditions that could directly or indirectly precipitate one. If, for example, a clinician believed that stuttering could be precipitated in the manner posited by the diagnosogenic theory (see Chapter 5), he or she probably would regard persons at risk if they were reacting negatively to their hesitations and attempting to avoid them. Persons who do not have a fluency disorder but are at risk for developing one, may be in need of intervention (see Chapter 7).

A discussion of considerations and procedures for determining whether a preschool-age child is beginning to stutter is found elsewhere in the chapter.

To Determine the Type of Fluency Disorder

After a clinician has determined that a client has a fluency disorder, he or she usually will attempt to identify the type. This is important to do, in part, because intervention programs for the various types are not the same (see Chapters 7 and 8).

To Identify the Set of Behaviors That Define the Client's Fluency (Stuttering) Problem

A client's fluency problem is defined by a set of behaviors. The set for a particular client is likely to include some that are not components of his or her abnormal disfluency behavior. These would include behaviors associated with (motivated by) attitudes and feelings toward speaking abnormally. The term *behavior*, as used here, includes what traditionally have been referred to as attitudes and feelings because both have behavioral components. For further information about this approach to describing fluency problems, see Chapter 1.

Information about this set of behaviors can be used clinically in several ways. First, it can be used to judge the severity of both a client's *abnormal disfluency behavior* and of his or her *fluency problem.* For example, scales for rating stuttering severity in specific situations—such as the *Iowa Scale of Severity of Stuttering* (see Appendix C)—use information about behaviors that occur during moments of stuttering that are a part of this set.

A second way that this information can be used clinically is to establish a prognosis for achieving specific goals. The presence and/or absence of certain behaviors can influence how likely they are to be achieved. For example, the absence of a strong desire to conceal stuttering from a client's set should result in the client being more willing than otherwise to "work on" his or her speech outside of the clinic environment, which should increase the likelihood of achieving goals that necessitate him or her doing so (Van Riper, 1973).

A third way such information can be used clinically is to establish goals for therapy. To reduce the severity of a client's fluency problem it is necessary to eliminate or modify behaviors in the set that defines it. Since the goals for a particular client are determined by the behaviors in this set, it is essential that they be identified.

To Assess Progress

Clients are reevaluated periodically to determine whether there is any change in the set of behaviors that define their problem. They are judged to have improved if there are fewer behaviors in this set or if some of those in it have been modified in desirable ways. If there has been little or no change, the clinician is likely to do further evaluation to determine the reason. Among the possibilities that he or she is likely to consider are the following:

- The assumption being made about why the client is exhibiting the behavior(s) is *wrong* and, hence, the intervention (which is based on it) is *inappropriate.*
- The assumption being made about why the client is exhibiting the behavior(s) is *correct,* but the intervention is *inappropriate.*
- The assumption is *correct* and the intervention is *appropriate,* but the client is not sufficiently motivated to do what is necessary to improve.

To Assess the Severity of the Problem for Funding Eligibility, Litigation, and Other Purposes

Speech-language pathologists occasionally are asked to evaluate speech fluency for a reason other than rehabilitation. They may be asked to testify as a expert witness about the severity of the person's disorder and/or the extent to which he or she is handicapped by it (Silverman, 1992). Such an expert opinion may be requested by

ney, an insurance company, or an organization to whom the person has
J for funding. For example, persons who stutter have applied to and received
ung from state vocational rehabilitation agencies for educational purposes.
.pert opinion also may be requested by a court in a criminal case (see Shirkey,
1987; Bloodstein, 1988).

AN OVERVIEW OF THE EVALUATION PROCESS

The evaluation process for persons who stutter or have another fluency disorder consists mainly of the *asking and answering of questions*. The clinician formulates
"answerable" questions and then makes the observations (gathers the data) needed
for answering them. Answerable questions are ones that can be answered by making
observations and that indicate the observations needed to answer them (Johnson,
1946). Questions that are answerable differ in the extent to which they are so. Consider the following questions:

1. Has the client improved during the past six months?
2. Have any of the behaviors in the set that define the client's stuttering problem
   been eliminated or changed "for the better" during the past six months?

The second is more answerable than the first because it indicates the observations
needed to answer it less ambiguously.

While the specific questions asked during an evaluation are determined by the
reason it is being conducted, there are several that are likely to be asked regardless
of the reason. These include the following:

1. Does the client have a fluency disorder?
2. If the client has a fluency disorder, what type is it?
3. How severe is the disorder? The answer to this question would be based on
   answers to more specific ones, such as these two:
   • To what extent does the client's fluency disorder interfere with communication?
   • How much impact does the disorder have on the client's life (i. e., to what
     extent is he or she handicapped because of it)?
4. What is the prognosis for a meaningful reduction in the severity of the disorder?

These questions probably should be answered whenever a client is being seen for
the first time even if he or she has recently been evaluated by another clinician and
a report is available. There are at least two reasons. First, all clinicians do not use
the same data to answer these questions and, hence, they could arrive at different
answers (Van Riper, 1982). And second, some answers could have changed since the
last time the client was evaluated. That is, behaviors could have been eliminated
from or added to the set that defines the client's fluency problem or behaviors still
included in it could have changed in some way.

Some of the questions clinicians attempt to answer during an evaluation are formulated before it is begun. Others are formulated during the evaluation from information they obtain.

We have dealt, thus far, with the "question asking" part of the evaluation process. We will now deal with the "question answering" one.

There are three approaches that are used for gathering data to answer questions. The first is observing the client's behavior under conditions that were purposefully created, or structured, by the clinician. That is, the clinician asks the client to do a task and observes certain aspects of his or her behavior while it is being done. The behaviors that are observed, or attended to, may be related to the client's speech, body language, physiological functioning, something he or she has written, or some combination of these. An example of a task in which the behavior attended to is likely to be an attribute of speech is reading in chorus: The clinician would observe the effect of this condition on the client's speech fluency. An example of a task in which a behavior attended to is likely to be an attribute of body language is asking the client questions: The clinician could observe whether the client maintained normal eye contact while answering them. An example of a task in which the behavior attended to could be an aspect of physiological functioning is having the client say syllables on command and observing through the use of instrumentation whether his or her phonatory initiation and termination times are abnormally long (see Chapter 3). And an example of a task in which the behavior attended to would be an attribute of what a client has written is having him or her complete a questionnaire: Certain of the responses would be analyzed.

The second of these approaches is observing aspects of a client's behavior under conditions that were *not* created (structured) by the clinician. In this situation he or she does not attempt to manipulate the behavior. With the first, the clinician does attempt to do so by having the client perform a task. For example, if a clinician wanted to use the first to observe behaviors that occur during moments of stuttering, he or she could have the client do the Job Task (Johnson, 1961)—have the client talk for a few minutes about his or her present job or one for which he or she is being trained. On the other hand if the clinician wanted to use the second for this purpose, he or she could observe the client while the client is having a conversation with someone.

The third of these approaches is interviewing an informant. The informant could either be the client or someone (such as a parent, spouse, or teacher) who had information about particular aspects of his or her behavior. The interview could be conducted face-to-face, on the telephone, or in response to written questions (such as a case-history questionnaire). This is the most frequently used approach for obtaining information about the symptomatology and phenomenology of the disorder outside of the therapy room. Since the abnormal disfluency exhibited by a client during an evaluation may not be typical of that in most other situations (Silverman, 1975), it is necessary to establish whether it was or not by asking the client and/or another informant who was present.

After the necessary data have been gathered, the questions are answered, the answers are interpreted, and recommendations are made. This information is usually communicated in a written report. The report may consist of a paragraph or two in a client's chart, or it may be a formal, multipage document. It usually includes information about the reason for the evaluation, the questions asked, how they were answered, the answers obtained and interpretations made of them, and recommendations for future action ("Where do we go from here?"). Its purpose is communication—both to other professionals and to the person who wrote it. Without a written report to jog your memory, you are unlikely to remember very much about an evaluation you did even a month or two earlier.

QUESTIONS TO ASK

The first step in the evaluation process is formulating one or more answerable questions. There are many that could be asked when evaluating a client who has (or is suspected of having) a fluency disorder. Which ones were formulated would be determined by the reason for the evaluation.

A number of questions are mentioned in this section that could be asked when evaluating a client who has, or is suspected of having, a fluency disorder. It is unlikely that all of them would be asked during an evaluation or that all of those that could be asked are mentioned here. This list was formulated, in part, by examining representative evaluation reports of persons who have fluency disorders submitted to me by clinicians who specialize in their treatment (see Appendix A).

Does the Client Have a Fluency Disorder?

This is the first question a clinician probably would ask when evaluating a client who is suspected of having a fluency disorder. If the answer was "yes," the clinician would attempt to determine the type of disorder and identify the set of behaviors that define it.

Is the Client at Risk for Developing a Fluency Disorder?

If the answer to the preceding question was "no," this is the second question a clinician would be likely to ask. If a client did not appear to have a fluency disorder, but seemed to be at risk for developing one, some type of intervention probably would be needed.

What Type of Fluency Disorder Does the Client Have?

Once it is established that the client's speech fluency is not within normal limits, the next task is deciding what type of fluency disorder he or she has. The differential diagnostic process used for doing so is described in Chapter 8.

What Behaviors Are in the Set That Defines the Client's Fluency (Stuttering) Problem?

To identify the behaviors in the set that defines the client's fluency problem, the clinician asks a series of questions. The answers indicate whether particular behaviors are present and if they are, to provide the information needed to describe them. Some questions that might be asked for this purpose about specific behaviors are the following:

- *Amount of disfluency.* Is the client ever normally fluent? How frequently does the client usually exhibit abnormal disfluency behavior?

  To what extent does the amount of disfluency exhibited by the client vary on a *situational* basis, that is, are there some situations in which the client almost always is more fluent than in others? To what extent does the amount of disfluency exhibited by the client vary on the basis of *content* (e.g., is the likelihood of the client being disfluent greater during oral reading than during spontaneous speech)? To what extent does the amount vary on the basis of his or her *emotional state,* for example, does the client tend to hesitate less frequently than usual when angry? To what extent does the amount vary on the basis of *how important it is for him or her to be fluent,* that is, does the client tend to be most disfluent when he or she wants to be most fluent? Does the client become more fluent when he or she speaks in a *nonhabitual manner* (for example, at a slower than usual rate)? Is the client normally fluent while reading in chorus? Does the client tend to be less fluent while talking to someone on the telephone than while talking to him or her face-to-face? Does the client tend to be more fluent while talking to some persons than while talking to others? If the answer to the preceding question is "yes," who are the persons with whom he or she tends to be most and least fluent?

  Has the amount that the client tends to be disfluent in most situations changed since the onset of the disorder? If the answer to the preceding question is "yes," how has it changed?

  Does the client do things to avoid being disfluent? If the answer to the preceding question is "yes," what does the client do? How much confidence does the client appear to have in its fluency-enhancing capability? Has a speech-language pathologist or other clinician ever suggested to the client specific techniques or strategies for becoming more fluent? If the answer to the preceding question is "yes," what techniques or strategies were suggested and how well does the client feel that they have worked?

  How important does it appear to be to the client to become more fluent? How confident does the client appear to be in his or her ability to achieve this goal?

- *Behaviors that occur during moments of abnormal disfluency.* Does the client tend to repeat sounds, syllables, and/or single-syllable words more often than his or her peers? If the answer to the preceding question is "yes," approximately how much more often? What is the average and maximum number of units of repetition (the number of times a particular sound, syllable, or word is repeated)? Are the phonemes (particularly vowels) repeated during syllable repetitions ever not the appropriate ones for the word that follows? How often are the repetitions accompanied by tension? How aware does the client appear to be of his or her repetitions?

Does the client ever exhibit blocks (prolonged sounds, broken words, tense pauses, and/or abnormally long silent pauses)? If the answer to the preceding question is "yes," how often do they occur? What are the average and longest times that blocks tend to last? Do the majority of the client's blocks tend to be audible or silent? Do the behaviors that occur when the client "blocks" almost always tend to be the same? If the answer to the preceding question is "yes," in what sequence do they tend to occur? Do both repetitions and blocks ever occur on the same word? How aware does the client appear to be of his or her blocks?

Do extraneous movements and vocalizations (secondary symptoms) ever occur while the client is being disfluent? If the answer to the preceding question is "yes," describe them and indicate approximately how often each occurs. Why does the client appear to be making them? How aware does the client appear to be of them?

Does the speed of the client's speech appear to be excessive? If the answer to the preceding question is "yes," does the client appear to be aware that it is? Does the amount of disfluency tend to decrease when the client speaks at a rate that is slower than his or her habitual one?

Is there any evidence of word-finding difficulty, dysarthria, or apraxia while the client is being disfluent? If the answer to the preceding question is "yes," does a slower-than-habitual-speaking rate affect his or her disfluency behavior and if it does, how?

Does the client exhibit the "consistency" effect (see Chapter 2)? If the answer to the preceding question is "yes," what words or sounds (if any) does the client report being particularly difficult for him or her to say?

Does the client usually maintain normal eye contact while being disfluent? If the answer to the preceding question is "no," can the client do so for at least a few minutes if requested? To what extent does this lack of normal eye contact appear to result from feelings of shame and/or embarrassment about being disfluent?

• *Avoidance of disfluency.* Does the client ever reduce verbal output (not talk) to avoid being disfluent? If the answer to this question is "yes," in what situations and with what persons is he or she most likely to do it? Does the client appear to avoid using the telephone for this reason? Are there persons from whom the client has been able to conceal his or her disorder by doing so? If there are, what does the client believe would happen if they learned "the truth"? Does the client appear to have considered the possibility that his or her interpersonal relationships are hurt more than they are helped by avoiding talking?

Can the client predict with better-than-chance accuracy some of the words on which he or she is going to be disfluent? If the answer to the preceding question is "yes," what strategies, if any, does the client use to avoid being disfluent? Does the client ever substitute words for ones on which disfluency is anticipated? If the client does this, are the words substituted ever inappropriate? Does the client ever answer questions incorrectly or incompletely to avoid being disfluent? Does the client ever choose not to revise errors (mispronunciations and "wrong" words) because of fear of being disfluent while doing so? Does the client ever use circumlocution as a device to avoid being disfluent? If the client does this, are the phrases (utterances) substituted ever inappropriate?

Does the client ever use devices (e.g., syllables, words, and/or gestures) that function as "starters"? If the answer to the preceding question is "yes," which ones does the client use? What devices does the client report having used in the past for this purpose? Are any behaviors observable while the client is being disfluent that in the past could have been "starters"?

• *Client's attitude toward his or her disfluency.* To what extent does the client react negatively to his or her disfluency? Does the client react more negatively to it than most listeners are likely to?

Does the client appear to feel ashamed or embarrassed about speaking disfluently? Does the client behave in a manner that is likely to signal listeners that he or she is ashamed or embarrassed about doing so (such as having poor eye contact)?

To what extent does the client judge his or her performance in speaking situations on the basis of how fluently he or she spoke rather than on how well he or she communicated? Has anyone previously attempted to encourage the client to base such decisions more on the latter?

How strong is the client's desire to conceal his or her fluency disorder? If it is relatively strong, how does the client believe people would react differently if they were aware of it? Does the client ever purposely bring his or her fluency disorder "out into the open"? If the answer to the preceding question is "yes," how does the client do it?

In what ways does the client appear to be handicapped by the fluency disorder? How frequently does it keep him or her from being understood?

If the fluency disorder were to disappear tomorrow, how much impact does the client appear to believe it probably would have on his or her life? What things would the client begin doing that he or she does not do now? Does the client appear to believe that he or she would have more friends? That dating would be more enjoyable? That his or her marriage probably would be better? That he or she probably would be happier? Respected more by people? Better off financially? More outgoing and/or have a better self-concept? More effective as a communicator? Would the client be likely to change jobs? If the answer to this last question is "yes," what field(s) might the client enter (or go to school to get the training to enter)? Does the client appear to believe that his or her speech at present is not good enough for entering these fields? Is the client's present job one that does not require him or her to talk much? Does the client appear to believe that becoming more fluent might, in some way, be disadvantageous?

• *Impact of the disorder on the client's self-concept.* In what ways (if any) has the disorder adversely affected the client's self-concept? Is the client a "people pleaser"? Is the client chronically depressed? Is the client suicidal? Does the client often appear to be a "wimp"? Do the client's body language, grooming, and/or clothing frequently suggest that he or she has a poor self-concept? Does the client tend to be more fluent when he is feeling good about himself? Does the client openly express anger when he or she feels it or is the client usually passive aggressive? How assertive is the client? Does the client's orientation toward life tend to be optimistic or pessimistic? Does the client tend to be a risk taker? What are some things that make the client feel good about himself or herself? Achieving what goals, other than fluency, does the client believe would improve his or her self-concept?

Does the client appear to overvalue fluency? Does the client's orientation toward it tend to be two-valued (success is perfect fluency and failure is anything else)? Do the client's disfluencies tend to call less adverse attention to him or her than he or she seems to believe?

Why Does the Client Appear to Exhibit Each of the Behaviors That Defines His or Her Fluency Disorder?

After the clinician has identified at least some of the behaviors in the set that define the client's fluency disorder, the next task is to formulate a tentative hypothesis (explanation) for each. Such hypotheses are likely to influence both the goals for therapy and the intervention strategies (therapies) selected for accomplishing them (Williams, 1968).

Clinicians are unlikely to have the same degree of confidence in the accuracy of all their hypotheses about why clients are behaving in particular ways. In some cases, they are likely to regard them as being no more than "hunches." Such hunches are more likely to be based on observations than the persons making them may assume. This phenomenon has been referred to as *tacit knowing* (Polanyi, 1967). According to Polanyi:

> *We know more than we can tell. This fact seems obvious enough; but it is not easy to say exactly what it means. Take an example. We know a person's face, and can recognize it among a thousand, indeed among a million. Yet we usually cannot tell how we recognize a face we know. (Polanyi, 1967, p. 4)*

If the Client Has a Fluency Disorder, Is There Any Reason Why He or She Should Not Be Scheduled for Therapy?

Once it has been established that the client has a fluency disorder, some type of intervention *usually* is recommended. There are several reasons, however, why it may not be advisable to do so. These include the following: The client is coping successfully with the disorder; the client lacks adequate motivation; the client is unable to make the necessary investments; the client's intervention needs can be met better by somebody else; or the clinician does not believe that the client's goals are achievable.

Therapy may not be recommended because the client appears to be coping successfully with the disorder. He or she has been functioning and seems capable of continuing to function as his or her own therapist.

A second reason why it may not be advisable to recommend therapy is insufficient motivation. A client is unlikely to make the investments necessary to achieve therapy goals unless he or she is highly motivated to do so (Lanyon, Lanyon, & Goldsworthy, 1979).

Clients who do not invest sufficiently to benefit from therapy waste their time and possibly their financial resources. In addition, *They may develop (or reinforce) a certainty that they cannot be helped by therapy.* Consequently, when they enter therapy in the future, they may have less confidence in it than they had previously. This can reduce the probability of it being effective.

Why might unsuccessful therapy experiences make future successful ones less likely? According to an old saying, "Nothing succeeds like success nor fails like failure." Your previous experiences of success or failure when trying to make a particular type of change influences your *expectation* of success or failure when trying to do so again. This expectation can become a self-fulfilling prophesy. Suppose, for example, that you wanted to lose weight. If this was the first time you attempted to do so and the weight-loss program was recommended by your physician, you probably would begin expecting the program to be successful. On the other hand, if this was your tenth such program and you believed that the previous ones had not been successful, you probably would begin it being less certain of success than you were the first time. While you would hope the result this time would be different, on a gut level you probably would expect it to be the same. As a consequence, after the first few times you stepped on a scale and concluded that you had not lost enough weight, you would be likely to assume the program was not working and go off of it. Perhaps it would have been successful if you had stayed with it longer! Regardless of what the outcome would have been, this additional "failure" experience probably would reinforce your certainty that you cannot lose weight, which would make success at doing so even less likely in the future.

A third reason why it may not be advisable to schedule a client for therapy is that he or she is unable at present to make the necessary investments. The client may, for example, be a full-time student who has a part-time job and must spend a great deal of time studying in order to survive academically. Such a person, even if highly motivated, probably would be unable to make therapy a priority.

A fourth reason is that his or her intervention needs can be met better by someone else. This person is most likely to be another speech-language pathologist or a psychotherapist. There are several reasons why a client who has a fluency disorder may be referred to another speech-language pathologist. First, because this clinician has had more experience with the particular type of fluency disorder the client has. Second, because it would be more convenient and/or affordable for the client to receive therapy from him or her. A speech-language pathologist at a university clinic, for example, may refer a child to one at his or her school. And third, because he or she feels that the clinician to whom the referral is being made is likely to be more effective. A male clinician, for example, may feel that a client is more likely to establish a productive therapeutic relationship with a female one.

If a speech-language pathologist refers a client who has a fluency disorder to a psychotherapist (a psychiatrist, psychologist, or psychiatric social worker), the reason may or may not be directly related to the fluency disorder. Some such clients have emotional problems that do not appear to be directly related to them (Van Riper, 1979). They may, for example, be chronically depressed—perhaps suicidal. Also, there are persons whose abnormal disfluency behavior is thought to be a symptom of psychopathology (see Chapter 8).

A fifth reason why it may not be advisable to schedule a client who has a fluency disorder for therapy is that the clinician does not believe that his or her goal or goals are attainable. The client, for example, may be seeking a complete "cure," and the clinician may not believe that this would be a likely therapy outcome.

ANSWERING QUESTIONS

There are three general approaches that can be used alone or in combination for making the observations (collecting the data) needed for answering the questions asked during an evaluation. These approaches (which were described earlier in the chapter) are informal observation, questioning an informant, and having a client perform a task. The approach or combination that is most likely to yield the information needed at low cost with adequate levels of validity, reliability, and generality is used.

What is meant here by yielding data that have adequate levels of validity, reliability, and generality? An approach (or combination) would yield data that possessed an adequate level of validity if it allowed you to observe *what* you needed to observe to answer a question.

An approach (or combination) would yield data that possessed an adequate level of reliability if it allowed you to observe what you needed to observe to answer a question in a way that is *repeatable*. Repeatable here could have two meanings. First, it could mean that two or more persons viewing an event (e.g., a behavior) would describe it similarly enough that they would answer a question about it the same way. If, for example, a group of clinicians rated the severity of the stuttering in a videotaped sample of a client's speech, their ratings probably would be adequately reliable if the majority indicated that the severity was "mild" and none indicated that it was "severe."

A second meaning that an adequate level of reliability could have in this context is that the client behaves in the same way during repeated observations that occur too close together in time for it to be likely that he or she has changed. If, for example, a client read in chorus with a clinician a number of times and during none of them did he or she stutter, the conclusion that the client does not do so under this condition would appear to be reliable.

An approach (or combination) would yield data that possessed an adequate level of generality if it allowed you to observe what you needed to observe in order to *infer* how the client would be likely to behave under a particular set of circumstances outside of the clinic environment. A client's behavior in the therapy room is not necessarily representative of that in other situations. This is particularly likely to be true for stuttering severity. Many clients, particularly children, tend to be more fluent in the therapy room than they are in most other situations (Silverman, 1975). For this reason, it usually is necessary to determine how representative the sample of a client's fluency observed during an evaluation is of that in other situations. This can be done by questioning the client and/or another informant (e.g., a parent) or by obtaining samples of his or her speech in other situations.

Now that we have considered the concepts of validity, reliability, and generality in this context, we will consider that of *cost*. Cost here refers to both the amount of time it takes to gather the data needed for answering a question and the expense involved in doing so. If two approaches are likely to yield data that possess adequate levels of validity, reliability, and generality and one takes less time and/or involves less expense than the other, that one usually would be selected.

What Types of Information Can Be Obtained by Informal Observation?

The data needed for answering some questions can be obtained through informal observation. Aspects (attributes) of speaking behavior about which information can be acquired in this manner include the following:

- Speaking rate
- Verbal output (including avoidance of talking)
- Amount of disfluency
- Types of disfluency behaviors
- Sequence of behaviors that tend to occur during moments of abnormal disfluency, particularly stuttering
- Duration of moments of disfluency
- Amount of tension accompanying disfluency
- Extraneous movements (gestures) accompanying disfluency
- Use of devices (such as starters, word substitution, and circumlocution) for avoiding disfluency
- Eye contact while being disfluent
- Level of awareness of disfluency

Information also can be acquired by informal observation about aspects (attributes) of a client's functioning other than speech, including the following:

- Physical health
- Mental retardation or other types of cognitive deficits

- The presence of depression
- Self-concept
- Attitudes toward the fluency disorder (such as feelings of shame or embarrassment because of it)
- Willingness to acknowledge openly the disorder ("bring it out into the open")
- Willingness to be assertive
- Tendency to be a "people pleaser"
- Relationships with one or more significant others (such as parents)

Information acquired in this manner can be written down immediately after it is obtained or at some future time from tape recordings of the evaluation session. Some clinicians routinely tape-record their initial evaluation sessions with clients who have fluency disorders. While audiotape recorders can be used for this purpose, videotape ones may be better, particularly if it is desired to describe visual behaviors (such as eye contact while being disfluent) as well as auditory ones.

Abstracting information from a recording rather than writing it down immediately after it occurs can have several advantages. First, it makes it unnecessary to repeatedly interrupt the flow of the evaluation while you record information on a pad or form. As a consequence, you can pay more attention to (be in better rapport with) the client. Second, it may allow you to record information more reliably. You can listen to and/or watch segments of the evaluation as many times as required to describe behaviors accurately. And third, it may allow you to record information more completely. At certain times during an evaluation session, a number of relevant events may be occurring almost simultaneously. Also, certain events that did not appear to be significant when they occurred may take on significance later in the session. If the session was recorded, the clinician could listen to and/or watch the segments containing this information.

The main disadvantage associated with abstracting information from a recording rather than writing it down immediately is that doing so is more time-consuming. The amount of time that a clinician can devote to an evaluation may not be sufficient to do this routinely. One compromise would be to tape-record the evaluation session, but only use the recording when it is absolutely necessary.

What Types of Information Can Be Obtained from an Informant?

Information needed for answering some questions can be obtained most efficiently from an informant. This is particularly likely to be the case for questions concerning behaviors that cannot be observed in the clinic and for those concerning the representativeness of behaviors that can be observed in it. Information needed for answering questions about events that occurred in the past (such as those related to the development of the disorder), of course, can only be obtained in this way. The informant would either be the client or someone who has observed him or her (such as a parent or a classroom teacher).

This approach differs from the other two in that it uses the observations of someone other than a clinician, usually someone who has had no training in speech-language pathology. A person who has not had such training is apt to perceive events differently than one who has. He or she, for example, may not abstract some attributes of the client's speaking behavior that a clinician would be likely to and vice versa. The findings of a number of studies (including Boehmler, 1958; Emerick, 1960; Hoops & Wilkinson, 1973; Tuthill, 1940) suggest that laypersons tend to perceive speech disfluency somewhat differently than do speech-language pathologists. While this does not invalidate the use of information about speaking behavior from informants, it does suggest that it is not safe to assume that an informant's description of such behavior would be the same as yours.

Types of information that can be obtained from an informant include the following:

- The reason(s) why an evaluation is being sought at this time
- The circumstances under which the fluency disorder began
- How the disorder has developed since onset
- Previous attempts to ameliorate the disorder
- The extent to which the client tends to be disfluent in specific situations
- The types of disfluency behaviors about which the client and/or others are concerned
- The client's level of awareness of the disfluency
- The client's attitude toward the disfluency
- How those with whom the client interacts react while he or she is being disfluent
- The amount of talking the client does
- The client's use of word substitution and other devices to avoid stuttering
- The extent to which the client's disfluency usually interferes with communication
- The extent to which the client avoids using the telephone
- The client's willingness to bring the disorder "out into the open"
- The client's physical and emotional health (For example, does he or she tend to be chronically depressed?)
- The client's self-concept and personality attributes
- Ways in which the client is handicapped by the disorder
- The client's level of motivation to invest in therapy
- The client's educational history
- The client's motor, cognitive, and social development
- The client's receptive and expressive speech/language development
- The family history of fluency and other communicative disorders

What Types of Information Can Be Acquired by Having the Client Do a Task?

The data needed for answering some questions can be acquired by having the client do a task and analyzing aspects of his or her behavior. The types of tasks that a client who has or is suspected of having a fluency disorder may be asked to do include the following:

- Talk about a specified topic or read a particular passage
- Speak under a particular condition (such as reading in chorus with the clinician)
- Respond to the items on a questionnaire
- Take a test

Representative tasks of each type are described in this section.

Talk about a Specified Topic or Read a Particular Passage. While you can generate a spontaneous speech sample of adequate length (at least one hundred words) by having a client talk about any of a number of topics, certain topics have been used frequently for this purpose. There are several reasons why a clinician may want to adopt these topics for his or her purposes: They are likely to generate a sample of adequate length; "normative" data are available for various disfluency behaviors; and it is unnecessary in reports to describe them in detail because one can refer to a book or journal article in which this is done.

One task that has been used with adults for generating spontaneous speech samples is known as the *job task* (Johnson, 1961). The client is told to talk for approximately three minutes about his or her present or future vocation. Specifically, the client is told to describe the vocation and indicate why he or she chose it. If the client has not decided on a vocation, he or she is told to talk about previous jobs. The client is allowed a minute or so to think about what to say. If the client stops speaking before the end of two minutes, the clinician can encourage him or her to continue by asking further questions. An effort should be made, however, to avoid formal structuring of the speaking performance. Data on the frequency of occurrence of various types of disfluency behaviors on this task, for male and female adults who stutter as well as for normal speakers of both sexes, are presented in Table 4 of Johnson's (1961) paper.

Another type of task that has been used for generating spontaneous speech samples with adults who have fluency disorders is telling a story about the events depicted in a drawing. The *TAT task* (Johnson, 1961) is representative of this type. The client is shown Thematic Apperception Test (Bellak, 1954) card number 10 (see Figure 6-1) and is told to develop a dramatic story based on the picture. The client is told to speak for about five minutes about what is happening at the moment in the pictured situation, what events preceded those shown in the picture, and what the outcome is likely to be. The client is allowed up to a minute to prepare the story. If the client stopped talking before the end of three minutes, he or she would be encouraged to continue through the use of leading questions. Data concerning the frequency with which various types of disfluency behaviors occur during this task, for both adults who stutter and normal-speaking peers, are presented in Table 5 of Johnson's (1961) paper.

FIGURE 6-1   **Drawing used for the TAT (Thematic Apperception Test) task.**

The *CAT task* provides another another way to elicit a spontaneous speech sample by having the client talk about the action depicted in drawings (Silverman, 1974). It differs from the preceding one in that it can be used with both children and adults and more than one drawing usually is used. The client is presented with the ten Children's Apperception Test (CAT) cards (Bellak, 1954), one after the other, and asked to make up a "once-upon-a-time" story about each. The specific instructions are as follows (Silverman, 1974):

I want you to imagine that you are helping to take care of a very young child. One way to keep a small child sitting still is to tell him or her a story. I am going to show you some cards with pictures on them. I would like you to make up a story, a once-upon-a-time kind of story, about each one that you could tell to a young child. Here is the first card. Let me know as soon as you think of a story and I'll turn on the tape-recorder. (p. 33)

After the client finishes telling a story about the first card, he or she is handed the second. If the first few stories are relatively short (consist of only a few sentences), the client is encouraged to make subsequent ones longer. On the other hand, if the first few stories are relatively long (yield at least a three-minute speech sample), it may not be necessary to use the other cards. Data on how frequently various types of disfluency occur during the performance of this task for male elementary-school-age children who stutter and their normal speaking peers are presented in Table 2 of Silverman's (1974) paper. Somewhat comparable data for male and female pre-school-age children who stutter and their normal speaking peers are presented on pages 206 and 207 in *The Onset of Stuttering* (Johnson & Associates, 1959). The children in this study were simply told to tell stories about the CAT cards.

A third type of task that has been used for eliciting spontaneous speech samples is answering a series of questions. An example that is intended to be used with young children is the Stocker Probe Technique. According to Stocker (1980):

A probe consists of a series of ten questions or requests about two different common objects presented to the child. The questions are presented in random order and represent five graduated levels of demand *on the speaker. The first five questions relate to the first object presented and the second five questions to the second object....*

The different levels of demand *involve different degrees of creativity on the part of the child, and the* level of demand *associated with each question/request is reflected in the type of response the child ordinarily gives.*

A LEVEL I question elicits a short repetition response of a few words to the examiner's question. For example, if you hand the child a ball and ask, "Is it hard or soft?" the answer is implicit in the question and is a low level verbal task.

A LEVEL II question also elicits a short response requiring the name of a common object which is present in the examining situation but the name of the object is not *given in the question, e.g., "What is it?"*

A LEVEL III question elicits a response usually consisting of a propositional phrase, where the referents are not *present in the examining situation and are not named in the question, e.g., "Where would you keep one?"*

A LEVEL IV request elicits a series of attributes not *named in the request. In this task, the child typically responds as follows: "The ball is red, round, bouncy." Furthermore, unlike LEVELS II and III, the syntactic*

form of the response is not *constrained by the nature of the question, e.g.,*
"Tell me everything you know about it."
        At LEVEL V, the highest level *of the* probe, *the child is asked to "Make*
up a story about the object."

The type of speech sample generated by this task at LEVEL V is likely to be similar to that generated by the CAT and TAT tasks.

We have considered thus far in this section tasks for eliciting spontaneous speech samples. A speech sample generated by reading a passage may also be secured.

Why might a clinician want an oral reading speech sample in addition to a spontaneous speech one? One reason is that some persons who have fluency disorders, particularly those who stutter, use word substitution and circumlocution to avoid doing so (see Chapter 2). Hence, an estimate of the amount of disfluency based solely on a spontaneous speech sample could be too low. Since clients cannot substitute words or use circumlocution while reading a passage, they may be more disfluent while doing so than while speaking spontaneously.

Almost any passage that contains at least 150 words with which the client is likely to be familiar can be used for this purpose. The client should be told to read the passage aloud as he or she ordinarily would do. Do not give any more detailed instructions than this. If the client asks specific questions about how it should be read, simply repeat the instruction to read it as he or she ordinarily would.

There are two passages that have been used clinically for a number of years with clients who have fluency disorders. Both are loaded with the types of words on which stuttering tends to occur. The first, the 330-word "Rainbow Passage" (see Appendix C), is intended for adults. The second, the 180-word "Arthur the Young Rat" passage (see Appendix C), can be used with most adults and children above the sixth-grade level.

If a client cannot read, you can elicit a speech sample free from word substitution and/or circumlocution by having him or her repeat a series of fairly short sentences that contain many of the types of words on which moments of stuttering tend to occur (see Chapter 2). A set of such sentences, which total 100 words, is reproduced in Appendix C.

After a speech sample has been elicited, the abnormal disfluency behavior in it is analyzed both quantitatively and qualitatively. Based on the amount (both frequency and duration) and the degree of tension and extraneous behavior accompanying it (see Chapter 2), a judgment is made on its severity. A number of rating (scaling) methods have been used for this purpose (Ham, 1989; Martin, Haroldson, & Wessner, 1988) Two that have been used a great deal clinically are the *Iowa Scale of Severity of Stuttering* (Sherman, 1952; Darley & Spricstersbach, 1978) and the *Stuttering Severity Instrument* (Riley, 1972). Both are reproduced in Appendix C.

The *Iowa Scale of Severity of Stuttering* (Sherman, 1952) has a range from zero to seven, with zero indicating "no stuttering" and seven indicating "very severe" stuttering. Each point on the scale is a composite of several variables, including stuttering frequency and duration, amount of muscle tensing, and conspicuousness of facial grimaces and other extraneous body movements. This scale can be used fairly easily for rating the severity of some persons' stuttering. However, it is difficult to use for rating that of others because the behavioral variables used for defining specific points on the scale are not the same amount for all stutterers (Van Riper, 1982). For example, a person who stuttered on only 1 percent of words, but whose blocks usually lasted for more than four seconds and were accompanied by very conspicuous facial grimaces, could be rated either a two or a seven on this scale.

One approach that has been used for accommodating behavioral variables that do not all increase in the same amount for all stutterers is to rate the variables individually. With the *Stuttering Severity Instrument* (Riley, 1972), for example, frequency of stuttering, duration of moments of stuttering, and physical concomitants (including distracting sounds, facial grimaces, and extraneous movements of the head and extremities) are rated separately. Ratings for frequency can range from zero to eighteen, those for duration from zero to seven, and those for physical concomitants from zero to twenty Also, the individual scores can be totaled and an overall severity rating assigned. A total of zero to five would be labeled "very mild," six to fifteen "mild," sixteen to twenty-three "moderate," twenty-four to thirty "severe," and thirty-one to forty-five "very severe" (Riley, 1972, Table 1).

Another instrument that has been used for individually rating behavioral variables is the *Profile of Stuttering Severity* (Van Riper, 1972, Chapter 9). It is a revision of the *Iowa Scale of Severity of Stuttering* (Sherman, 1952), in which ratings for individual variables—including frequency of stuttering, duration of moments of stuttering, and degree of tension—are plotted on a chart (see Figure 6-2). Such charts can be quite useful for measuring change during therapy.

The devices described thus far for analyzing the abnormal disfluency in speech samples yield quantitative data. They indicate how often in a speech sample abnormal disfluency occurs, how long individual instances tend to last, and the degree to which they are accompanied by tension and extraneous movements. Devices also are available for cataloging the behaviors that occur in a speech sample during moments of abnormal disfluency. One such device, the *Checklist of Stuttering Behavior* (Darley & Spriestersbach, 1978), allows you to describe the presence or absence of twenty-six behaviors during six such moments (see Appendix C). While it may be possible to make such judgments reliably "live" while the client is speaking, it probably would be easier to do so from a videotape.

Speak under a Particular Condition.   These tasks allow you to observe how the frequency of disfluency varies under certain conditions. The information yielded by them can be used in several ways. One is to differentiate stuttering from other types of abnormal disfluency. Persons who stutter tend to behave differently on several of these tasks than do those with other fluency disorders.

Profile of Stuttering Severity

Scale	Frequency	Tension-Struggle	Duration	Postponement-Avoidance
1.	Under 1%	None	Under ½ sec.	None
2.	1 - 2%	Rare but present	Average ½ sec.	Less than 5%
3.	3 - 5%	Usual but mild	Average 1 sec.	5 - 10%
4.	6 - 8%	Severe	Average 2 sec.	11 - 20%
5.	9 - 12%	Very severe	Average 3 sec.	21 - 31 %
6.	13 - 25%	Overflow to eyes and limbs	Average 4 sec.	31 - 70%
7.	More than 25%	Overflow to trunk	Longer than 5 sec.	More than 70%

Name: _Joe P._____ **Date:** _____ **Speaking Situation:** _TAT Pictures_

Scale	Frequency	Tension	Duration	Postponement-Avoidance

———— September 10

‑ ‑ ‑ ‑ ‑ December 10

FIGURE 6-2 **Profile of Stuttering Severity showing changes as a result of therapy. Reproduced with permission from Van Riper, 1982, p. 201.**

A second way this information can be used is for assessing the ability of certain intervention strategies to reduce a client's disfluency. Several of these conditions have been incorporated into intervention strategies, including speaking in the presence of loud masking noise (Moore & Adams, 1985; Silverman & Trotter, 1973a, 1973b, 1974, 1975; Walle, 1980), delayed auditory feedback (Craven & Ryan, 1984; Mueller-leile, 1981), or a metronome beat (Silverman & Trotter, 1973a, 1973b, 1974, 1975).

Tasks are described in this section that allow you to observe how the amount of abnormal disfluency varies under certain conditions. While these are not the only ones that can be used for this purpose, they include those that have been used for it most often.

• *Reading in chorus.* The clinician hands the client a reading passage and reads it in chorus (unison) with him or her. This appears to be one of the best ways to differentiate "ordinary" stuttering from neurogenic acquired stuttering. While persons who stutter usually become normally fluent under this condition, those who have neurogenic acquired stuttering do not (see Chapter 8).

• *Singing.* The client is told to sing a song, such as our national anthem or a hymn. Almost all persons who stutter become normally fluent while doing so (regardless of how well they sing). In fact, several, such as Mel Tellis and Carly Simon, have had successful singing careers. If a client does not become normally fluent while singing, he or she probably has some other fluency disorder.

• *Speaking at a slower than usual rate.* The client is told to speak or read aloud at a slower rate than his or her usual one. Some persons who have a fluency disorder become significantly more fluent while doing so. They may be helped by intervention strategies that result in a reduction in speaking rate (see Chapter 7).

• *Speaking while listening to masking noise.* Masking ("white") noise is presented to the client binaurally through headphones at a level of approximately 90 dB above threshold and he or she is told either to read aloud or to do a spontaneous speech task. The masking-noise generator on many audiometers can be used for this purpose. Some persons who stutter are more fluent than usual while speaking under this condition (see Chapter 2). They may benefit from using a miniature, voice-activated masking noise generator, such as the Edinburgh masker (Dewar, Dewar, & Barnes, 1976; Ingham, Southwood, & Horsburgh, 1981).

• *Speaking under delayed auditory feedback.* The client is interfaced with a delayed auditory feedback device and told either to read aloud or to do a spontaneous speech task. Some persons who stutter become more fluent under this condition (see Chapter 2). They may benefit from the use of intervention strategies for reducing stuttering severity that utilize these devices to teach a slow rate of speech through prolongation of syllables (Craven & Ryan, 1984; Muellerleile, 1981).

• *Pacing speech with a metronome.* The client is told to pace his or her speech while reading aloud or doing a spontaneous speech task with the beats of a metronome—usually one word per beat. Some persons who stutter become more fluent while speaking in this manner (see Chapter 2). There have been attempts to treat such persons by fitting them with miniature electronic metronomes (Silverman & Trotter, 1973a, 1973b, 1974, 1975).

• *Talking on the telephone.* The client is told to make a telephone call—to a store, for example, to find out if they have particular items in stock. Since many persons who stutter do so more severely than usual while talking on the telephone (see Chapter 2), this task is likely to elicit a sample of the client's stuttering that is at the *upper end* of his or her severity range. It is particularly likely to yield useful information if the client does not stutter or does so very little while talking face-to-face during the evaluation session.

• *Attempting to modify behaviors that occur while being disfluent.* The client is told to read aloud or to do a spontaneous speech task and while doing so to try to change a specific behavior that tends to occur while he or she is being disfluent. For example, a client who has poor eye contact while being disfluent might be asked to modify this behavior. This task provides information about the client's ability to modify certain behaviors. It also provides information about whether these behaviors (assuming they are learned) are instrumental or classically conditioned (Brutten & Shoemaker, 1967).

• *Predicting moments of stuttering.* The client is told to predict whether he or she is going to stutter on certain words before saying them. One who was able to predict a high percentage of his or her moments of stuttering probably would benefit more from an intervention program that stressed modification of moments of stuttering while they were occurring than would a person who was not able to do so (Van Riper, 1973).

There are several tasks that have been used for this purpose. In one, the client is handed a copy of a reading passage and asked to underline the words on which he or she expects to stutter. The client then reads the passage and the clinician determines the accuracy of his or her predictions. In another, the client is shown a series of words one at a time and asked to signal before saying each whether he or she expects to stutter while doing so. After making each prediction, the client says the word, and the clinician judges whether it was stuttered. A set of fifty words (nouns, verbs, adverbs, or adjectives that begin with consonants, are five letters or more in length, and are in the client's reading vocabulary) that have been typed on cards can be used here (Silverman & Williams, 1972). This task may provide more useful information than the first about the feasibility of teaching the client to modify moments of stuttering as they occur because it assesses the ability to predict them a few seconds (rather than a few minutes) before they occur.

• *Trying to stutter.* The client is told to stutter "for real" as severely as possible while reading aloud or doing a spontaneous speech task. If the client becomes considerably more fluent, he or she may be a good candidate for a fluency enhancing strategy known as *paradoxical intention* (Frankl, 1985, pp. 145–152), which is described in Chapter 7.

Respond to the Items on a Questionnaire.   Questionnaires are useful for gathering information. They can reduce the amount of time it is necessary to spend during an evaluation session asking questions and writing down answers.

It may be desirable for some questionnaires to be completed and returned before the evaluation session because doing so could help the clinician identify questions that need to be answered during the session. These could either be ones answered incompletely or unclearly or ones suggested by answers to questions.

There are several types of information that usually can be obtained through the use of questionnaires. One is information about the client and the history of his or her disorder. Included here would be information about the client's birth and development during childhood, family, medical history, educational history, social history, as well as a description of the onset and development of the disorder.

Another type of information that can usually be gathered in this manner is the type relevant to the client's abnormal speaking behavior, such as his or her attitudes toward it, and the manner in which he or she attempts to cope with it. A number of questionnaires intended for gathering such information have been published (e.g., Ammons & Johnson, 1944; Andrews & Cutler, 1974; Barber, 1981; Brutten, 1975; Cooper, 1973; Erickson, 1969; Lanyon, 1967; Shumak, 1955; Watson, 1987; Watson, Gregory, & Kistler, 1987). Those described below are representative.

• *The Stuttering Problem Profile.* This task (a copy of which is in Appendix C) can be used both for identifying the set of behaviors that define a client's stuttering problem and for establishing goals for therapy (Silverman, 1980b). Clients are presented with eighty-six first-person statements that reflect behaviors that could be in the set defining their stuttering problem. They are told to circle the numbers of those statements that they would like to be able to make at the termination of therapy but that they do not think they could make now. The following are typical of the types of statements included in the profile:

1. I am usually willing to stutter openly.
6. I am usually willing to use the telephone.
17. I have learned to live with my problem.
38. I have expanded my activities, both business and social.
86. I recite in the classroom as much as most students.

The statements in the Stuttering Problem Profile were abstracted from the responses of 108 adults who stutter, from 17 speech clinics representing various theoretical orientations, to the following: "Would you describe the ways in which you feel your stuttering problem has improved during the past five years?" (Silverman, 1980a). While these persons may not have changed in the ways they indicated, it is reasonable to assume that they considered the behaviors mentioned to be components of their stuttering problem.

The statements a client selects refer to behaviors in the set that defines his or her stuttering problem. If the behavior referred to by a statement is not obvious, the clinician questions the client about what he or she had in mind when selecting it. A set that is defined solely in this manner is likely to be incomplete. Some of the behaviors in it may not be mentioned in any of the statements, and some of the statements that do refer to them may not have been selected.

The statements a client selects also suggest goals for therapy—ones that he or she is interested in achieving. This profile application is discussed in Chapter 7.

• *The S-Scale.* The S-Scale provides information about the attitudes of persons who have fluency disorders toward interpersonal communication (Erickson, 1969, pp. 717–718). It consists of thirty-nine statements (see Appendix C) to which the client gives either a true or false response. A client's score on the S-Scale is the number of the thirty-nine statements to which he or she responded in the manner indicated by the bracketed responses. Hence, S-Scale scores can range 0 to thirty-nine; and the higher the score, the poorer the attitude toward interpersonal communication. Based on Erickson's data (Erickson, 1969), a score over twenty-five suggests that the client's interpersonal relationships are being affected adversely by his or her attitudes. An item-by-item analysis of a client's responses may also provide useful information.

• *Stutterer's Self-Ratings of Reactions to Speech Situations.* This questionnaire (see Appendix C) can be used to gather information about a client's avoidance of speaking situations, particularly from young adults (Shumak, 1955; Darley & Spriestersbach, 1978). The client is asked to give four ratings (between one and five) to each of forty speaking situations. These ratings relate to the amount he or she *avoids* speaking in the situation, *enjoys* speaking in the situation, *stutters* (or is otherwise abnormally disfluent) while speaking in the situation, and *encounters* the situation. The numbers of 1s, 2s, 3s, 4s, and 5s on each of the four scales can be totaled and the mean on each can be compared to that in the normative data reported by Shumak (1955)—which are reproduced in Appendix C.

• *Inventory of Communication Attitudes.* This questionnaire (see Appendix C), which examines affective, cognitive, and behavioral components of attitudes, consists of thirteen subscales representing a variety of types of speaking situations. For each of these subscales, there are three representative examples—a total of thirty-nine. Each of these is rated on five scales. These are judgments concerning (1) the client's enjoyment of speaking in the situation, (2) the clients's speech skills in the situation, (3) other persons' enjoyment of speaking in the situation, (4) other persons' speech skills in the situation, and (5) the frequency at which the client encounters the situation (Barber, 1981; Watson, 1987; Watson, Gregory, & Kistler, 1987). While this questionnaire appears to have been developed primarily for research purposes, responses to it could be used clinically for such purposes as assessing the extent to which a client's enjoyment of speaking in a particular situation is related to his or her fluency level while doing so.

• *Problem Profile for Elementary-School-Age Children Who Stutter about Talking.* This questionnaire (see Appendix C) consists of a series of questions about seven aspects of "talking" intended to provide information about the child's awareness of stuttering, people's reactions to the child's speech, and his or her feelings about them (Williams, 1978, pp. 68–70). The questions are asked by the clinician and the child's responses are either written down immediately or tape-recorded.

Williams also suggests questions that can be asked of the parents and teachers of elementary-school-age clients to obtain information about their attitudes toward and reactions to the child's stuttering problem and the effect they perceive it has had on the child. These questions include the following (Williams, 1978, p. 68):

Why do you believe that he continues to stutter? How serious a problem is it to you or to him? How do you handle it and how do you think it should be handled by other people? In what ways do you feel it has affected your child? What kind of child is he now? In what ways do you think he would be different if he had not stuttered? How does he get along with boys and girls his own age while at school or playing? To what degree has stuttering influenced his relationships with children or with adults (teacher, grandmother, others)? How has it limited what he has achieved socially or educationally? How much help does he need in meeting new situations or new problems? What special allowances do you think he should receive because of his stuttering? How independent is he in comparison with other children? How has be reacted to his stuttering? How has he reacted to your help and concern about it?

• *"Three Wishes" Task.* This task (Silverman, 1970) can be used to determine whether young children are aware of and concerned about their speech disfluency without inadvertently suggesting to them that they should be concerned about it. Clients are asked to imagine that they have a fairy godmother who tells them that she will grant any three wishes. They are asked to tell what their wishes would be. If the client does not make a speech wish, this general three wishes task is followed by a second (more structured) one. The client is told to imagine that his or her wishes were granted and that the fairy godmother returned and said he or she could wish to *change any three things* about himself or herself. The client is then asked to tell what his or her wishes would be.

If a client made a speech-improvement wish on either of these tasks, this would suggest that he or she is both aware of and concerned about being abnormally disfluent and would, incidentally, provide an opportunity to explore his or her feelings about it more directly. On the other hand, if a child did not make such a wish, his or her level of concern would be less certain. While the absence of such a wish would suggest that he or she is not highly concerned about the disorder, it would not by itself establish this.

• *Speech Locus of Control Scale.* This task (McDonough & Quesal, 1988) is intended to determine whether a client tends to believe in an internal or external locus of control for speech. According to McDonough and Quesal (1988):

An individual with an internal locus of control believes that his/her own behaviors, abilities, and attributes determine "reinforcements." Those individuals with an external locus of control believe that reinforcements are under the control of "luck," "chance," "good days," "bad days," "powerful others," etc., rather than under their personal control. (p. 98)

The task consists of eight questions or statements that are either answered "yes" or "no" or to which degree of agreement is expressed. McDonough and Quesal have speculated that clients who score at the "internal" end of the locus-of-control continuum may be able to maintain therapy gains better than those who score at the "external" end; Kroll and De Nil (1994) provide some support for this speculation.

• *Perceptions of Self Semantic Differential Task.* This task (see Appendix C) can be used to assess clients' self-perceptions (Kalinowski et al., 1987). It is based on a semantic differential that was devised by Woods & Williams (1976). Clients' ratings of themselves on each of the twenty-five nine-point, bipolar, adjectival scales can provide information about their self-concepts.

• *Southern Illinois University Speech Situation Checklist.* This questionnaire (see Appendix C) is intended to identify speech-related anxiety (Brutten & Shoemaker, 1974). It consists of fifty-one situations that the client rates on a five-point scale with regard to the amount of negative emotion he or she currently experiences. The higher rating totals, the higher the degree of speech-related anxiety. Preliminary data have been reported (Hanson, Gronhovd, & Rice, 1981) suggesting that a shortened form of this task (twenty-one items) may permit clients who experience an abnormal amount of speech-related anxiety to be identified reliably.

• *Disfluency Descriptor Digest.* The goal of this task (see Appendix C) is to determine which of six fluency-initiating gestures might be used most advantageously with a particular stutterer (Cooper, 1982). These gestures are:

> *(1)* Slow speech, *characterized by a reduction in the rate of speech involving the equalized prolongation of syllables; (2)* easy onset, *characterized by the initiation of phonation with as little laryngeal area tension as possible; (3)* deep breath, *characterized by a consciously controlled inhalation prior to the initiation of phonation; (4)* loudness control, *characterized by a conscious and sustained increase or decrease in the volume of the client's speech; (5)* smooth speech, *characterized by a reduction in phonatory adjustments and by light articulatory contacts with plosive and affricate sounds being modified to resemble fricative sounds; and (6)* syllable stress, *characterized by conscious loudness and pitch variations. (Cooper, 1982, pp. 355–356)*

The digest consists of twenty statements describing behaviors that occur frequently during moments of disfluency. A checkmark is placed in the box preceding each behavior that is observed in the client's speech. Following the twenty statements is a table listing the six gestures and the numbers of the statements that appear predictive of the successful utilization of each. By transferring the checkmarks from the statements at the top of the form to the table at the bottom, a clinician can identify gestures that may be helpful for reducing the client's stuttering severity.

• *Communication Attitude Test.* This is a thirty-five-item questionnaire (see Appendix C) designed to assess the speech-associated beliefs of children (Brutten, 1985; Brutten & Dunham, 1989; De Nil & Brutten, 1990, 1991; Vanryckeghem &

Brutten, 1992). Children respond to the items by circling either the word true or false next to each item. About half the items are indicative of a negative attitude toward speech if the respondent circles the word "true" for them. The score is the total number of statements marked in a way that suggests negativity. This questionnaire has been administered to children as young as six. An attitude modification program—Think-Wise!—that is based partially on this test was developed at the University Hospital Dijkzigt Rotterdam in the Netherlands (Nagel & van Eupen, 1994).

• *The Cooper Chronicity Prediction Checklist.* This checklist (see Appendix C) was designed to assist clinicians in differentiating between those children who are likely to recover without intervention and those who are not (Gordon & Luper, 1992a). It consists of twenty-seven questions that can be answered "yes" or "no." The probability of recovery without intervention is estimated from the number of "yes" responses—the higher the number, the lower the probability of recovery. The authors caution users not to make chronicity judgments solely on the basis of the checklist. (Cooper & Cooper, 1985b)

Take a Test.   Tests have been used to acquire information about a client's *overall functioning* and the possible impacts of the disorder on it. They have been utilized with clients who have fluency disorders to acquire information about their personality (Bloch & Goodstein, 1971; Bloodstein & Schreiber, 1957; Broida, 1963; Craig, 1990; Devore et al., 1984; Goodstein, 1958; Katz, 1966; Lowinger, 1952; Manning et al., 1984; McDonough & Quesal, 1988; Meltzer, 1944; Perkins, 1947; Richardson, 1944; Sermas & Cox, 1982; Shames, 1951; Sheehan, 1979b; Sheehan & Zussman, 1951), intelligence (Andrews et al., 1983; Andrew & Harris, 1964; Okasha et al., 1974; Schindler, 1955), educational achievement (Andrews et al., 1983; Williams, Melrose, & Woods, 1969), speech/language functioning aside from fluency (Andrews et al., 1983; Andrews & Harris, 1964; Blood & Seider, 1981; Bloodstein, 1987; Byrd & Cooper, 1989; St. Louis & Hinzman, 1988; Wall, 1980; Westby, 1979; Williams & Silverman, 1968), and hearing (Anderson et al., 1988; Bonin et al., 1985; Curry & Gregory, 1969; Decker et al., 1982; Hageman & Greene, 1989; Hall & Jerger, 1978; Hannley & Dorman, 1982; Kent, 1983; Liebetrau & Daly, 1981; McFarlane & Shipley, 1981; McLean-Muse et al., 1988; Stager, 1990; St. Louis & Hinzman, 1988; Stromsta, 1957, 1972). Many clinicians routinely screen children that they are evaluating for fluency disorders for other speech, language, and hearing disorders.

MAKING A PROGNOSIS

After it has been established that a client has a fluency disorder, the type has been determined, the set of behaviors that defines it has been identified, and tentative hypotheses have been formulated concerning the etiology of the behaviors, the next step is to decide whether the client is likely to be helped by therapy and if so, how much. There are at least two reasons for this. First, it is a violation of the Code of Ethics of the American Speech-Language-Hearing Association to accept a client for therapy who is highly unlikely to benefit from it. Second, the client needs this information in order for his or her *consent* to participate in therapy to be an *informed* one (Silverman, 1992). It is important that it be "informed" both for the legal protection of the clinician (Silverman, 1992) and to maximize the probability that the client's expectations when entering therapy will be realistic.

A number of factors can influence the likelihood that a client will benefit from therapy. Some are mentioned in this section. The order in which they are discussed is not intended to indicate their importance for establishing a prognosis.

The Length of Time the Client Has Had the Disorder

The longer the client has had the disorder the poorer the prognosis tends to be. For example, the prognosis for significantly reducing stuttering severity in young children tends to be better than that for adults (Cooper, 1987). According to Freund (1966):

> *Age seems to limit the chances for a complete cure. We have as yet not seen an adult who, after successful self-treatment or treatment by a therapist, has lost every trace of stuttering or who has never experienced any relapse, even if brief or minute, or any anticipatory dread of impending stuttering (internal stuttering), though this is not necessarily noticeable to others. (p. 183)*

This does not mean that adults who stutter are unlikely to benefit from therapy. However, they appear less likely to be "cured" than young children.

Level of Motivation

The more a client "invests" in therapy, the more likely he or she is to improve (Van Riper, 1973). Hence, the prognosis for significant improvement tends to be better for highly motivated clients than for less motivated ones.

Previous Therapy Experiences

The more the client regards previous therapy for the disorder as having been successful, the better the prognosis. As Sheehan (1970; quoted in Barbara, 1982) has indicated:

> *Being enrolled in therapy raises hopes and when nothing results, hopes are dashed, and future motivation is diminished. . . . Moreover, many stutterers acquire an attitude of hopelessness, give up the search, and deny themselves the possibility of future therapy that might really help them. (p. 74)*

If the client does not believe that it was helpful, he or she is likely to enter therapy hoping it will work, but not really expecting it to. Such an "expectation" can reduce the effectiveness of almost any intervention program.

Intervention Goals

The prognosis for modifying some of the behaviors in the set that defines a client's fluency disorder is likely to be better than that for modifying others. Hence, the prognosis for a particular client is a function, in part, of what the clinician hopes to accomplish.

Personality Attributes and Emotional Status

Aspects of a client's personality and emotional state can influence the likelihood that he or she will benefit from therapy (Van Riper, 1979). For example, a client who is extremely perfectionistic or chronically depressed probably is less likely to benefit than one who is not.

Attitudes of Family Members and Significant Others

The attitudes of family members and friends toward both the fluency disorder and the client can influence the prognosis. If their attitudes are such that they do not cause the disorder to become worse and they are supportive of the client's desire to seek therapy for it, the prognosis is likely to be better than if the opposite were true.

Presence of the Chronic Perseverative Stuttering Syndrome

Cooper (1993a) has suggested that for approximately one of every five individuals who stutter, "maintaining an acceptable level of fluency may require a *lifetime* [italics mine] of coping." He uses the label *chronic perseverative stuttering (CPS) syndrome* for their disorder. According to Cooper (1993a):

> *Because the CPS syndrome consists of multiple coexisting and interacting affective, behavioral, and cognitive components coalescing over a period of years, the hope for a complete cure or a total remission of symptoms appears remote. However, the outlook for these individuals is not bleak. With assistance, these individuals typically are able to develop and maintain a feeling of fluency control that enables them to communicate successfully in even the most challenging speech situations. The abundant number of professionally and personally successful individuals who are chronically disfluent testifies most tellingly to an optomistic outlook for those experiencing the CPS syndrome. (p. 13)*

As a person who has had this syndrome for more than 55 years and has treated persons who had it for more than 35 years, I can testify to both the reality of the syndrome and to an optomistic outlook for those who have it.

What information is needed to determine if a person has the CPS syndrome? This information can be gleaned from the items in the CPS Syndrome Checklist that Cooper developed as an aid for identifying such persons. The checklist is reproduced below (Cooper, 1993a):

- The individual's fluency disorder developed concomitantly with the development of language and speech.
- The individual's fluency disorder has persisted for 10 or more years.
- The individual's disfluencies are, or have been, accompanied by a fleeting but generalized feeling of loss of control.
- The individual has experienced periods of normal fluency accompanied by the feeling of control.
- The individual experiences a persistent fear of a catastrophic loss of fluency although, in fact, such occurrences occur rarely, if ever.
- The individual has identified one or more adjustments in speech production that generally, but not always, enhance fluency.
- Although capable of predicting the level of fluency to be experienced in most situations, the individual continues to experience unpredictable fluency failures.
- The individual has experienced fluent periods after a heightened or sustained period of psychic and physical concentration on attaining fluency, but has been unable to maintain that level of concentration or fluency.
- The individual's predominant self-perception is that of being a stutterer.
- The individual experiences periods of obsessive absorption in striving for normal fluency. (p. 13)

Not every stutterer who has the CPS syndrome will evince every characteristic in the checklist. However, the more of them a stutterer does evince, the more confident one can be that the diagnosis is correct.

A diagnosis of CPS syndrome does not necessarily mean that a speech-language pathologist can be of little help to the person. To the contrary, many can be helped by them to reduce both the severity of their stuttering and the extent to which it interferes with their life. In some cases, the diagnosis itself can be therapeutic. It can enable a stutterer to stop being obsessively absorbed with striving for normal fluency and to get on with his or her life.

COMMUNICATING QUESTIONS, ANSWERS, AND RECOMMENDATIONS

The final step in the evaluation process is communicating what was learned and what was decided. The persons to whom this may be communicated are the client, members of the client's family (such as his or her parents or spouse), and other professionals (including other speech-language pathologists). The clinician who did the evaluation may also be included because few clinicians can remember for more than a few weeks all that they learned during an evaluation.

Questions, answers, and recommendations usually are communicated both orally and in written form. They are likely to be communicated in an oral summary at the end of the evaluation. They also may be communicated face-to-face or over the telephone at some later time. In addition, they are likely to be communicated in a written report.

Most clinicians currently write evaluation reports using a microcomputer with word-processing software and in the future almost all are likely to do so. Preparing reports in this manner is more efficient than doing so with a typewriter. Changes can be made without having to retype the entire report, spelling errors and "typos" can be identified and corrected more easily, and sections can be written in the most convenient sequence and later rearranged (e.g., the "Recommendations" section can be written first and later inserted at the end of the report without having to retype it).

Another way that a microcomputer with word-processing software can facilitate report writing is to make it possible to use standard (boilerplate) sentences and paragraphs (see Appendix A). These may or may not require "blanks" to be filled in. Their use can facilitate the report-writing process by making it necessary for the clinician to create and "type" some sentences and paragraphs.

CONSIDERATIONS AND PROCEDURES FOR DETERMINING WHETHER A YOUNG CHILD IS BEGINNING TO STUTTER

Determining whether a young child—particularly a preschool-age one—is beginning to stutter may be very difficult. This is because the part-word and single-syllable word repetitions of children who are beginning to stutter (see the description of Bloodstein's Phase I stuttering in Chapter 4) are often quite similar to those of children who are not developing the disorder—particularly ones who are at the *upper end of normal limits* with regard to the amount of these disfluencies they produce.

When deciding whether a child is beginning to stutter you can make two kinds of errors. You can conclude that a child who is beginning to stutter is being normally disfluent. And you can conclude that a child who is being normally disfluent (perhaps at the upper end of normal limits) is beginning to stutter. While both kinds of errors are undesirable, one can have more serious consequences than the other. If you accept the diagnosogenic theory for the onset of stuttering (see Chapter 5), the second kind of error—diagnosing normal disfluency as being abnormal—would be more likely to have undesirable consequences than would the first.

The approach that I use is the following one. Because I accept the diagnosogenic theory as being the most likely explanation for most cases of stuttering, I try hard not to make the second kind of error. Consequently, I will only label a child's repetitions "abnormal" if there is considerable evidence to support such a diagnosis. I would not, however, label a child's repetitions as "normal" if they had the characteristics of Bloodstein's Phase II, III, or IV stuttering (see Chapter 4). Incidentally, labeling a child's repetitions as "normal" when they are really "beginning stuttering" could be therapeutic if it caused persons (especially the child's parents) to stop reacting to them in undesirable ways.

My decision about whether a child's disfluencies are abnormal is based both on information about them from informants (usually parents) and my observations of the child's speech. If the child has moments of stuttering while in therapy room, it is likely that he or she will have them elsewhere also. However, if he or she does not have them while in the therapy room, it is possible that he or she will in other environments. At the end of the diagnostic session, I ask the parents whether the child produced the disfluency behavior that concerned them during the session. If they indicate that they didn't hear any instances of the behavior, I ask them to tape-record the child's speech in situations in which he or she had exhibited it in the past and to make an appointment to see me when they have some instances of it on tape. During the session, we listen to the tape and I let them know whether the disfluencies they recorded suggest that their child has a disorder.

One factor that I consider when deciding whether a child's fluency level requires intervention is the child's awareness of and concern about his or her disfluencies. If a child is concerned about them, some intervention is likely to be needed regardless of whether they are normal or abnormal. Based on the diagnosogenic theory, such concern could precipitate stuttering if the disfluencies were normal or make the disorder more severe if they were abnormal (see Chapter 5).

One way to determine whether a child is concerned about being disfluent is to ask the parents whether he or she has ever said anything to them that would suggest such concern. Another way to determine it is to have the child do the three wishes task described previously.

ASSIGNMENTS

The three assignments at the end of Chapter 2 are also relevant for this chapter. Actually, they may be more relevant here than they are for the earlier one.

▶ 7

Intervention: Principles, Goals, and Strategies

After it has been established that a client has a fluency disorder and some of the behaviors in the set that defines it have been identified, intervention usually begins. This almost always includes an attempt *to assist the client and/or his or her parents and teachers* in either eliminating or modifying certain behaviors in this set. The italicized words appear in the preceding sentence because regardless of the intervention strategy used, the primary responsibility for implementing it is usually on the client, or in the case of a young child, on his or her parents and teachers (Starkweather, 1990). The role of the clinician is to be *helpful*—that is, to provide the client and/or his or her parents and teachers with at least some of the information and support needed to make the desired changes (Dopheide, 1987; Starkweather, Gottwald, & Halfond, 1990). This role could involve providing information about the disorder and techniques for modifying certain behaviors associated with it. It also could involve providing counseling for coping better with the disorder and offering the client support for attempting to change or for "accepting oneself and getting on with one's life." The clinical relationship can serve as a *catalyst* for change, but the client or parent (or possibly the classroom teacher) has to assume the primary responsibility for change outside of the therapy room (Starkweather, Gottwald, & Halfond, 1990; Van Riper, 1973).

Older children or adult clients should be informed at the beginning of the intervention process that they will have to function as their own therapist and that the clinician will do whatever he or she can to facilitate their doing so. They should also be told that the roles the clinician will assume in this process are those of consultant, teacher, and coach. Clients will be unlikely to improve if they do not assume this responsibility and will be unlikely to maintain any gains if they do not continue doing so (Adams, 1983; American Speech-Language-Hearing Association, 1995; Ingham, 1982; Johnson, 1987b; Kuhr & Rustin, 1985; Lay, 1982a, 1982b; Luterman, 1984; Maxwell, 1982; McDonough & Quesal, 1988; Williams, 1982). This appears to be why some persons who have fluency disorders—particularly those who stutter—relapse after therapy is terminated (Perkins, 1983b).

While clients have the primary responsibility for changing their behavior, it is not necessarily their fault if they are unsuccessful in doing so. They may have failed because the behavior they tried to eliminate could not, at that time, be eliminated (Cooper, 1987, 1993b; Freund, 1966) or the intervention that was used was inappropriate (Perkins, 1983b). According to Cooper (1986):

> *My research as well as my thirty years of experience with hundreds of stutterers of all ages convinces me that a significant number of disfluent stutterers will remain disfluent despite anything they might do or have done to them. Certainly, we all hope that the day will arrive when we have the ability to cure stuttering in everyone. Realistically, however, we know that such a time may never come. Until it does, I trust that our practitioners will communicate to those for whom normal fluency is an unrealistic goal the real sense of success that comes from being able to modify fluency. I have never known disfluent individuals unable to alter their fluency. (pp. 324–325)*

Cooper's final statement about "never having known disfluent individuals unable to alter their fluency" refers to stuttering—not the other fluency disorders (see Chapter 8).

The better able you are to understand the problems your clients will encounter as they try to change, the better able you will be to help them do so. One way to gain such understanding is to try to change an aspect of your own behavior (e.g., to exercise on a more regular basis, procrastinate less on keeping up with assignments, or reduce your intake of junk food). For a number of years I have required students in my fluency disorders course to do this. Judging by their comments, most have found the assignment to be a valuable—though not necessarily enjoyable—experience. If you decide to do it, you may find Lay's (1982b) suggestions helpful.

THE THERAPEUTIC RELATIONSHIP

The first step in the intervention process is to establish a good therapeutic relationship with the client and, possibly, some of his or her significant others (including parents, teachers, or spouse). The nature of this relationship can profoundly influence the effectiveness of any intervention strategy (Lay, 1982a; Peleman-Cappaert, 1994; Van Riper, 1979). A good one can enhance it and a poor one can practically guarantee its being ineffective.

What are the characteristics of a good therapeutic relationship? Some of those that are particularly important to consider when working with clients who have fluency disorders are listed below. For further information about these and others, see Chapter 11 in Silverman (1995), Van Riper (1979), and Lay (1982a).

The characteristics of a productive clinical relationship include the following:

- *Cultural Sensitivity.* The clinician is sensitive to the cultural values, practices, and beliefs of the client and his or her family when planning therapy and in interactions with them. These can make some intervention approaches less likely and others more likely to be effective than they would be in the clinician's own culture. For information about the types of cultural values, practices, and beliefs that can affect the clinical relationship, see Bebout & Arthur (1992), Cooper & Rustin (1985), Hammer (1994), Maestas & Erickson (1992), Matsuda (1989), and Shames (1989).
- *Mutual respect.* The client respects the clinician for his or her training, experience, and expertise. The clinician respects the client and manifests this respect by treating him or her as a person of worth, whom he or she wants to help.
- *Trust.* The client trusts the clinician to treat whatever he or she is told as confidential. Also, the client trusts the clinician not to recommend goals that are unattainable or intervention strategies that could be harmful or useless.
- *Honesty.* Both the client and clinician are honest with each other. They tell each other the truth, which may not be what the other wants to hear. For example, in a good relationship clients will not tell clinicians that they are improving or that they have done what was recommended when they have not. And clinicians will not tell clients that it's O.K. to avoid doing what they dislike doing if they know this is not true. Some of the assignments that clinicians give to clients who have fluency disorders (such as to bring their disorder out into the open) tend to make clients feel uncomfortable, and hence, they dislike doing them.
- *Empathy.* To be helpful to clients who have fluency disorders, clinicians need to have some insight into what they experience both while they are being abnormally disfluent and while they are trying to change. One strategy clinicians can use for developing such empathy is to perform the simulation assignment described in Chapter 1 and the behavior modification assignment described in an earlier section of this chapter.
- *Communication.* The client and clinician communicate reasonably well with each other in spite of the client's fluency disorder. Communication is the medium through which the clinician attempts to influence the client and the client attempts to make the clinician aware of his or her needs.
- *Hope.* The clinician continually offers hope to the client that he or she has the ability to improve. While the clinician cannot guarantee that the client will improve, he or she does offer hope to the client (and his or her significant others) that this can occur. The client's beliefs concerning his or her ability to change can significantly affect the outcome of therapy (Adams, 1983; Maxwell, 1982; McDonough & Quesal, 1988).

- *Success.* The clinician gives the client the opportunity to experience success whenever possible. "Nothing succeeds like success or fails like failure." Some clients who have fluency disorders enter therapy with the belief that they cannot be helped because of previous therapy experiences they regard as not having been successful. One way to help them cope with this belief is to give them the opportunity to experience success.
- *A contract.* The contract (which may be either written or oral) specifies what each promises to contribute to the relationship. The clinician usually promises to contribute his or her time and expertise and the client usually promises to follow through on the clinician's recommendations. A client who enters therapy without understanding the terms of the contract (what will be expected from him or her) will be less likely to meet the clinician's expectations than one who does. Also, such a client will be less likely to conclude, after a period of therapy, that he or she has benefited from it.
- *A "positive" placebo effect.* What clients believe about the efficacy of their treatment can influence the impact it is likely to have on them (Shapiro, 1964). If they do not expect it to be effective, it probably will be less likely to be so than otherwise ("negative" placebo effect). On the other hand, if they do expect it to be effective, it probably will be more likely to be so than otherwise ("positive" placebo effect).

How might clinicians behave in order to bring about a negative placebo effect? One way is to signal clients verbally or nonverbally that they do not have a high degree of confidence in the therapy they are using with them (Cooper & Cooper, 1985a). An example of this would be continually changing intervention strategies without giving the client a reasonable explanation for doing so. Such behavior is particularly likely to result in a negative placebo effect if intervention strategies tend to be changed whenever clients express concern about their progress.

Another behavior that could result in a negative placebo effect is to give clients a choice of intervention strategies, in particular, suggesting that if they have not tried a particular one yet, they may want to. This is unlikely to create a high degree of confidence in their clinicians' ability to help them. From the client's perspective, if the clinician knew which strategy is most likely to be effective, why would he or she be given a choice?

ESTABLISHING GOALS

One of the first tasks a clinician must accomplish when trying to be helpful to a client who has a fluency disorder is to establish goals and to communicate them *unambiguously* to him or her. If clients do not understand what their clinician wants them to accomplish, they obviously will be less likely than otherwise to succeed in doing so.

Therapy goals are derived from behaviors in the set that was identified during the evaluation as defining the client's fluency disorder. Achieving these goals eliminates or modifies these behaviors, thereby reducing—at least a little—the severity of the disorder.

Since there usually will be more than one possible goal, the clinician will have to decide which to work toward first. There are a number of factors that he or she should consider when doing so, including the following:

- The ease with which each can be achieved. It usually is desirable to select goals at the beginning of therapy that the client is likely to be able to achieve fairly quickly, particularly if he or she believes that previous therapy experiences were not successful. Having a client succeed in attaining a goal is probably the best way to convince him or her that change is possible.
- How interested the client is in achieving each. The client is likely to be more highly motivated to achieve some goals than to achieve others. If a client were highly motivated to achieve a particular goal, he or she probably would invest more to do so than otherwise. If there are several goals toward which a client could work, the amount of interest he or she would have in achieving each of them should be considered when deciding.
- The impact that achieving each goal would have on the severity of the client's disorder. Everything else being equal, the goals selected should be ones that if accomplished would significantly reduce its severity.
- The number of behaviors that are likely to be affected by achieving each. Accomplishing a goal may affect more than one behavior. For example, "bringing stuttering out into the open" can both make a client feel more comfortable (less anxious or embarrassed) and cause him or her to stutter less frequently (Van Riper, 1973).

Since in most cases it is desirable for a client to participate in the goal-setting process, how can this be accomplished? One way is to have him or her complete the *Stuttering Problem Profile* (Silverman, 1980b). This task (which is described in Chapter 6 and reproduced in Appendix C) enables clinicians to identify goals that clients are interested in achieving.

General Intervention Goals

What can a clinician attempt to accomplish that is likely to be helpful to a client who has a fluency disorder? Several general goals are discussed in this section that may or may not be appropriate for and achievable with a particular client.

To "Cure" the Client's Fluency Disorder

While this is the goal that both clinicians and clients regard as being the most desirable, it appears more likely to be attainable for young children than for adolescents and adults (Cooper, 1987; Freund, 1966; Wingate, 1976). For a client's fluency disorder to be regarded as "cured," it seems reasonable to require that the following conditions be satisfied:

- The amount of disfluency in the client's speech is within normal limits
- The client's fluency level has been within normal limits for at least five years
- The client no longer believes that he or she has a fluency disorder or will again develop one

The first of these conditions does not require the client to be almost completely fluent—it only requires that his or her disfluency level be somewhere in the normal range. The second is important because research indicates that a high percentage of those who are normally fluent at the termination of therapy relapse within five years (Boberg, 1981; Boberg et al., 1979; Conture & Guitar, 1993; Craig & Calver, 1991; Freund, 1966; Perkins, 1983b; Silverman, 1981). And the third is important if the disorder is stuttering because of evidence suggesting that fear of relapse can precipitate it (Bloodstein, 1987; Freund, 1966; Prins, 1993; Silverman, 1981, Van Riper, 1973).

Which clients who have fluency disorders will be most likely to attain this goal?—perhaps preschool-age children who are beginning to stutter. There are reports (such as Starkweather, Gottwald, & Halfond, 1990) that suggest that many such children recover completely. While there are reports in the literature of persons of all ages being cured of stuttering, the probability of this occurring appears to be negatively related to the length of time the person has had the disorder (Bloodstein, 1987; Cooper, 1987, 1993a; Freund, 1966).

To Reduce the Severity of the Client's Fluency Disorder

This goal should be attainable by almost any client who has a fluency disorder if:

- The client believes his or her severity can be reduced or, at least, has a "wait and see" attitude concerning this
- The client is sufficiently motivated to make the changes needed to do so
- The behaviors the clinician is encouraging the client to change are modifiable
- The intervention strategies used by the clinician are appropriate
- The client receives positive reinforcement from his or her significant others for changing

The first of these factors requires the client to not believe that therapy will fail. Unfortunately, as I indicated earlier in this chapter, clients who had therapy experiences they regarded as unsuccessful may have developed a "certainty" that they cannot be helped. This attitude, which has been referred to in the psychological literature as *learned helplessness* (Adams, 1983; Maier & Seligman, 1976; Seligman, 1975), needs to be changed—at least to one of "wait and see"—before such clients are likely to benefit from any attempt at intervention (Adams, 1983; Williams, 1982).

The second requires the client to assign a high priority to reducing the severity of the disorder. If the client does this, he or she should be more willing than otherwise to make the investments required to attain this goal.

The third requires that the client be capable of doing what he or she is being asked to do. Not all behaviors may be modifiable (Cooper, 1987) and not all clients may be capable of modifying those that are (Van Riper, 1979).

The fourth requires that the intervention strategies used be appropriate for the particular client being treated. Using ones that are appropriate for most clients but not for yours is one of the main reasons for intervention being unsuccessful (Adams, 1983).

The fifth requires most persons with whom the client interacts (particularly those whose opinions he or she values) to respond positively to his or her attempts to change. If they do not—or worse yet, respond negatively to these attempts—the client will be more likely than otherwise to stop trying to modify his or her behaviors (Adams, 1983; Boberg & Boberg, 1990; Daly, 1987).

Why might such persons respond negatively to a client's attempts to change? There could be several reasons. First, they may feel that the client's "new" way of talking calls more adverse attention to him or her than the "old" way. They could be right! For example, after stutterers were encouraged to pace their speech with a miniature metronome (Brady, 1968, 1971), it was discovered that doing this tended to make the speech of persons with relatively mild stuttering less acceptable to listeners than their "old" way of talking even though they stuttered less frequently while doing so (Silverman and Trotter, 1973).

A second reason why such persons may react negatively is that they have adapted to the clients "old" way of talking, but not yet to their "new" way. If persons who have fluency disorders are not constantly signaling listeners that they are embarrassed about it, listeners are likely to attend to, or abstract, their abnormal disfluency behavior less frequently than they did initially (Trotter & Kools, 1955). However, if clients change how they speak, listeners are again likely to attend to their disfluency and as a consequence may conclude that it has gotten worse. It is important that clients be made aware of this phenomenon at the beginning of therapy so that they will be less likely to become discouraged and stop trying to change if it occurs.

A third reason for negative reactions on the part of such persons is that the clients' attempt to change is adversely affecting their relationship with them because the clients are no longer willing to play their "old" roles. The clients may, for example, develop a better self-concept and, as a consequence, become less dependent and more assertive. While such changes are almost always desirable, they may be regarded as "threatening" by one or more of the client's significant others. For example, the client in his or her marriage may have played the submissive role and the spouse the dominant one. If the client becomes less willing to be dominated, the spouse may try to discourage him or her from changing further. If the clinician suspects that such a scenario is being acted out, both the client and those who are being threatened should be referred for counseling.

To Reduce the Extent to Which the Client is Handicapped by His or Her Fluency Disorder

The amount of abnormal disfluency in a client's speech does not necessarily determine how much he or she will be handicapped because of it. Some who have relatively little disfluency are more handicapped than some who have a great deal. The amount clients are handicapped is a function of how much the disfluency keeps them from doing what they want to do—how much it adversely affects their lives. One determiner of this is their attitude toward the disfluency. Consequently, for some clients with fluency disorders an appropriate goal is developing a less negative (or more objective) attitude toward the disorder, thereby reducing the amount it is handicapping to them. The goal is not to get clients to the point at which they do not care whether or not they have a fluency disorder. No sane person would want to have one, particularly considering the negative personality traits that tend to be projected on those who have such a disorder (see Doody, Kalinowski, Armson, & Stuart, 1993, and Ruscello, Lass, Schmitt, & Pannbacher, 1994, for discussions and bibliographies on this topic). Rather, the goal should be to persuade them to accept the fact they have the disorder and get on with their lives!

To Determine Whether It Is Possible to Reduce the Severity of the Client's Fluency Disorder

A clinician may not know at the beginning of therapy whether he or she can be helpful to a particular client. There can be a number of reasons—including uncertainty about the client's level of motivation to invest in therapy. An initial goal in such a case would be to assess his or her potential for improvement.

To Get the Client to Accept a Referral

Some clients who have fluency disorders need to be evaluated and possibly treated by professionals other than speech-language pathologists (Blaesing, 1982). The reason may or may not be directly related to their fluency disorder.

The most common type of referral that speech-language pathologists are likely to make for these clients is for psychotherapy. The practitioner to whom a client would be referred could be a psychiatrist, a clinical psychologist, or a psychiatric social worker. Among the reasons for making such a referral are chronic depression and poor social adjustment (Wakaba, 1983).

Clients and/or members of their families may regard a referral as threatening—particularly if it is to a psychotherapist—and, as a consequence, may not accept it. If you feel it is necessary or desirable for a client to be seen by another professional and the client (or a member of his or her family) refuses to accept the referral, one of your goals probably would be to persuade him or her to do so (Van Riper, 1979).

To Increase the Client's Motivation

Clients are unlikely to benefit from therapy if they are not sufficiently motivated to make the investments required. It is sometimes possible to increase their motivation for making these investments (Adams, 1983). If, for example, the reason for the lack of motivation was that the client did not expect therapy to be effective because of previous unsuccessful therapy experiences, proving that change is possible could result in an increase in his or her motivational level. An initial intervention goal for clients who believe this could be proving to them they can change by engineering it so that they do change some aspect(s) of their behavior.

Specific Intervention Goals

In the preceding section we considered some general intervention goals for clients who have a fluency disorder. We will consider some specific ones here.

What specific intervention goals might be established for a client who has a fluency disorder? This would be determined by the behaviors in the set that defines his or her problem. Those mentioned in this section are intended to illustrate both the types of goals one might have and how they are worded. The latter can influence how likely a client is to regard therapy as having been successful. Consider the following two wordings for a specific goal:

1. The client will no longer avoid contributing to class discussions.
2. The client will not avoid contributing to class discussions *as often as he or she did previously.*

A client would be more likely to feel that he or she had achieved the goal if it was worded like the second. If the first wording is used, even avoiding speaking in class once could cause a client to believe that he or she had "failed."

A clinician may find it advantageous to specify a specific minimum amount that a client should seek to change. The goal in the preceding paragraph, for example, could be rewritten as follows: "The client will reduce the amount he or she avoids contributing to class discussions *by about 10 percent.* This would permit him or her to do a lot of avoiding and still experience "success"!

One problem that a clinician may encounter when setting specific goals is that the client may have a *two-valued orientation* (Johnson, 1946). Persons who have such an orientation judge their performances as being either good or bad; successful or unsuccessful. For a performance to be regarded as a success, they must judge it to have been almost perfect—any significant deviation from perfection is likely to cause them to regard it as a failure.

How might having a two-valued orientation interfere with therapy? It could cause a client to fail more often than succeed. A client with such an orientation is likely to evaluate his or her performance in this manner regardless of how goals are worded. It is desirable, therefore, that the orientation be changed from two-valued to *multivalued*. With the latter there can be degrees of success and failure. While some clients will require psychotherapy to change their orientation, others will be able to do so by studying an appropriate self-help book, such as Wendell Johnson's *People in Quandaries*.

The following are examples of specific goals that might be established for a client who has a fluency disorder.

- The client will not avoid talking in specific situations as often as he or she did previously.
- The client will reduce the frequency of a specific behavior that occurs during moments of abnormal disfluency in a particular situation by 10 percent.
- The client will bring his or her fluency disorder "out into the open" (acknowledge it to listeners) more often than previously.
- The client will reduce his or her feelings of shame and embarrassment because of having the disorder.
- The client will judge his or her speech less often based on how fluent he or she was and more often based on how successfully he or she communicated.
- When angry, the client will communicate more often how he or she really feels (the client will reduce his or her tendency to be a "people pleaser").
- The client will develop a better self-concept.
- The client's knowledge about (understanding of) the disorder will increase.
- The client will become more confident that he or she can do something about the disorder and the impact that it is having on his or her life (that is, the client will not view himself or herself as frequently as "a giant in chains").

For further information about establishing goals for therapy, see Starkweather (1993).

SELECTING AND IMPLEMENTING INTERVENTION STRATEGIES

Factors Affecting the Choice of Strategy

After one or more goals have been formulated, the next step is selecting strategies for achieving them. A number of factors should be considered when doing so, including the following:

- The specific behaviors (including attitudes) that have to be modified
- The clinician's beliefs (hypotheses) about the causes of the behaviors
- The clinician's beliefs about how to modify behaviors having the hypothesized causes

- Economic and time constraints
- The client's therapy history
- The client's age and level of motivation to invest in therapy
- The clinician's faith in and competency with alternative strategies that could be used
- The attitudes of the client's significant others toward alternative strategies that could be used

Some possible impacts that each could have on the selection process are described in this section.

The intervention strategies a clinician selects obviously will be influenced both by what he or she is trying to accomplish and the specific behaviors that have to be modified. A single strategy may be appropriate for accomplishing more than one thing. For example, encouraging a client to bring his or her stuttering problem out into the open could accomplish several goals, including the following:

- Putting the client more at ease in speaking situations
- Putting those with whom the client communicates more at ease
- Reducing the severity of the client's stuttering
- Reducing the extent to which the client signals listeners that he or she is ashamed or embarrassed about stuttering
- Reducing the extent to which the client avoids speaking because of his or her stuttering

Another factor that is likely to influence the choice of intervention strategy is the clinician's beliefs (or hypotheses) about the cause(s) of the behaviors he or she seeks to modify. The program you develop for modifying a behavior should be based upon your "best guess" as to why the client is exhibiting it. If your hypothesis is correct, you are more likely to be successful than otherwise (Williams, 1968).

A clinician's beliefs about the best way to modify behaviors having a particular cause is also likely to influence his or her choice of intervention strategy. Authorities do not agree about what strategies are most likely to be successful for modifying some of the behaviors exhibited by persons who have fluency disorders, particularly the abnormal disfluency exhibited by stutterers. As a result, a relatively large number of strategies for reducing stuttering severity have been advocated and used by at least a few clinicians (see Ham, 1986, 1990b; Van Riper, 1973).

Two other factors that can influence the choice of intervention strategy are economic and time constraints. A clinician may reject a strategy that is likely to be effective because it is not practical for one or both of these reasons. It may require the client to invest more time in therapy sessions and/or daily practice than he or she is willing or able to. Or it may require the client to make a financial investment that he or she cannot afford.

A client's therapy history also can influence the choice of intervention strategy. If a client has tried a particular approach and has concluded rightly or wrongly that it was not effective, it may not be advisable to try that approach again, particularly if there is a viable alternative. The reason is that if you do so, the client is likely to expect it not to "work," which could reduce the likelihood of it being effective.

A client's age and level of motivation to invest in therapy can also influence the choice of intervention strategy. Some strategies that are appropriate for use with adults may not be appropriate for use with young children (Ham, 1990b). Also, some strategies that would be appropriate for clients who are highly motivated would not be so with others. Voluntary stuttering (Bryngelson, Chapman, & Hansen, 1955; Freund, 1966) is an example of such a strategy.

Thus far in this discussion of factors that influence the choice of intervention strategy the focus has been primarily on the client. A clinician's awareness of, confidence in, and competence to use alternative strategies can also influence this choice. Obviously, if a clinician is not aware of a particular strategy, it will not be considered. Also, the more confidence a clinician has in a particular strategy, the greater the likelihood that he or she will select it. Finally, a clinician is unlikely to select strategies that he or she does not feel reasonably competent to use, particularly if there are alternatives.

The choice of an intervention strategy may not only be influenced by factors pertaining to the client and clinician, but also by ones pertaining to persons with whom the client frequently interacts. The attitudes of a client's family, friends, teachers, employer, and others toward a strategy and the impact that it has on him or her can influence the choice, particularly if the client is a child. If a client does not receive positive reinforcement from these persons for trying to change in a particular way, he or she is less likely to succeed (Van Riper, 1973).

Strategies for Reducing Stuttering Severity

Most persons who stutter consult a speech-language pathologist because they either want to reduce the severity of their stuttering or to "cure" it. Many strategies have been recommended for achieving these goals during the past 2,000 years, and there is anecdotal evidence suggesting that most of them enabled at least one person to do so (Van Riper, 1973).

All of these strategies are not mentioned in this section. What is presented here is a scheme for conceptualizing their impacts on stuttering severity and brief descriptions of most of the ones that are currently being advocated and/or used in the context of this scheme. My intent is to provide you with the information needed to *select* a strategy—not that needed to use it. Providing such information in depth would have considerably increased the length (and cost) of this book. Furthermore, it is unnecessary to provide it here because in-depth information about each of these strategies is available from other sources. For some of them the information is in journal articles, for others it is in books, and for still others it is in both. Some sources of information about the strategies intended primarily for use with adults and older children are Blood (1993), Bloodstein (1987), Conture (1990b), Ham (1986, 1990b), Peters & Guitar (1990), Schwartz (1993), and Van Riper (1973). And some of those about the strategies intended primarily for use with young children are Conture (1990b), Conture & Guitar (1993), Culp (1984), Gregory & Hill (1984), Ham (1990b), Peters & Guitar (1990), Riley & Riley (1979), Shine (1984), Starkweather & Gottwald (1993), and Starkweather, Gottwald, & Halfond (1990). Several sources for information about a strategy should be consulted before attempting to use it. A single source is apt to be incomplete and/or reflect its author's biases.

The Interaction-Frame Model

This scheme (see Figure 7-1) was adapted from one proposed by Wendell Johnson (1946). Although it originally was promulgated in the context of a specific theory about the etiology of stuttering (in this case, the anticipatory-struggle hypothesis; see Chapter 5), it appears to be usable regardless of whether you believe the cause of this disorder is physiological, psychological, or some combination of the two. This is because it has been established unequivocally that the severity of a client's stuttering is likely to be influenced by both the reactions of persons in his or her environment and and his or her own reaction to it (see Chapter 2). There is no agreement, however, on the amount of influence that these are likely to exert on stuttering severity. Those who view stuttering, at least in part, as anticipatory-struggle behavior probably would ascribe a greater influence to the reactions than those who view its etiology as physiological (Quesal, 1989).

According to this scheme (see Figure 7-1), it is possible to reduce stuttering severity by targeting the behavior itself, the reactions of others to the behavior, and/or the client's own reactions to it. And by modifying one of these the other two are

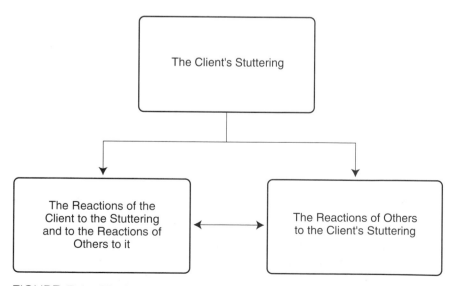

FIGURE 7-1 **The interaction-frame model.**

likely to be modified (which is the "interaction" aspect of the scheme). For example, by helping a client eliminate behaviors that occur during his or her moments of stuttering, you are likely to reduce negative reactions from listeners to the stuttering and, thereby, reduce the client's desire to avoid or conceal it. This, in turn, should result in a further reduction in stuttering severity (assuming that the desire to conceal stuttering tends to increase its severity) and a further reduction in negative reactions from listeners, and so forth. Consequently, this scheme indicates that we can reduce (not necessarily eliminate) undesirable reactions from listeners to a client's stuttering and undesirable reactions of a client to his or her own stuttering by focusing on modifying it, that is, by reducing its severity.

One important implication of the interaction-frame model is that it is possible to reduce a client's stuttering severity by modifying his or her attitude toward stuttering. Such modification may not only improve his or her self-concept and enable him or her to cope better with life, but may also reduce the amount that he or she stutters! The following are examples of attitudinal changes that, based on the model, would be likely to result in a reduced stuttering severity:

- Having less desire to avoid stuttering (Van Riper, 1982).
- Being more willing to bring the stuttering problem out into the open—that is, to openly acknowledge it (Silverman, 1988a).
- Judging performance in a speaking situation *less* on the basis of fluency level and *more* on that of success level in communicating (Yovetich, 1984).
- Developing a better self-concept through recognition by peers. Such recognition may be directly related to speaking—for example, a high school or college student may be regarded as a good debater in spite of the fact that he or she stutters (Silverman, 1960). An improved self-concept could also result from psychotherapy (Wakaba, 1983) or art therapy (Schmidt, 1994).
- Developing a stronger belief that he or she can cope with stuttering if it occurs and possibly desiring to have it occur in order to practice "controlling" it (Van Riper, 1973).
- Anticipating fluency more frequently than previously. Just as anticipation of stuttering is likely to lead to increased stuttering, anticipation of fluency is likely to lead to increased fluency (Van Riper, 1982).
- Becoming less embarrassed or ashamed about stuttering. This should result in a reduction in the desire to avoid it and, as a consequence, in a reduction in its severity (Bloodstein, 1987).
- Becoming less two-valued or less perfectionistic when evaluating one's performance and, as a consequence, experiencing "success" more often in speaking situations (Johnson, 1946).
- Feeling less of a need to overcome stuttering before going on with one's life. Gaining a greater realization that a person can succeed in life in spite of the fact that he or she stutters (Carlisle, 1985; Tillis & Wager, 1984). No longer feeling as much like "a giant in chains" (the "chains" being stuttering).

- Having more of a "what you see is what you get" attitude toward self and, consequently, feeling less of a need to impress people by being relatively fluent.
- Having more of a sense of humor about stuttering—perhaps even being able to laugh at "Porky Pig" cartoons (Johnson, 1987a; Manning & Beachy, 1994).
- Not being as likely to assume that people will think less of you if they know you stutter (Silverman, 1991).

There obviously is some overlap between these, and all are likely to lead to the same outcome: less desire to avoid stuttering. Such a reduction would be expected to result in increased fluency, at least temporarily (see Chapter 2).

Strategies for Modifying Moments of Stuttering Directly

Many strategies have been advocated and used during the past fifty years for *directly* modifying behavior that occurs during moments of stuttering. Judging by reports in the literature, most appear to have helped at least one stutterer, at least temporarily. One problem frequently encountered with all these strategies is clients being reluctant to practice and use them outside of the clinical environment (Starke, 1994). This may be partially due to the fact that they and their listeners tend to not regard the resultant "stutter-free" speech as sounding completely normal (Franken, Boves, Peters, & Webster, 1992).

The following are some intervention strategies that have been used alone or in combination during the past fifty years for reducing the frequency of moments of stuttering and/or for making them appear less abnormal. The order in which they are described is not intended to indicate their effectiveness. Nor are the books and articles cited necessarily the best or only ones for learning about them. They are, however, a good starting point.

Voluntary Stuttering.   Clients are told to speak disfluently on purpose (Bryngelson, Chapman, & Hansen, 1955). Specifically, they are told to do one of the following: imitate their own stuttering behavior, produce a relatively effortless repetition of the initial sounds of words (this has been referred to as the "bounce"), or simulate stuttering that is more severe than usual for them (Van Riper, 1973). Which approach to take would be determined by what the clinician hoped to accomplish. If, for example, the goal was to increase the client's awareness of behaviors that occur during moments of stuttering, they probably would be told to imitate their own stuttering behavior. On the other hand, if the goal was to desensitize them to their stuttering or to encourage them to bring their stuttering out into the open, any of the three could be used, though for desensitization the third might be most effective (Freund, 1966).

Clients usually are encouraged to try voluntary stuttering first in the clinic environment on a relatively small number of words. If this strategy were being used solely for increasing their awareness of what they do during moments of stuttering, they probably would not be encouraged to do it outside of the clinic environment. However, if it were being used (at least in part) for desensitizing them to their stuttering and/or for bringing their stuttering problem out into the open, they probably would be encouraged to do it on at least a few words outside of the clinic environment.

Most clients will find it difficult to do voluntary stuttering (particularly outside of the clinic environment) at least initially. For years their goal has been to stutter as little as possible. Now they are being told to do something that is likely to make their stuttering appear more severe than it would otherwise. In fact, if their stuttering is extremely mild, they probably are being asked to reveal their stuttering to at least a few persons who were not previously aware of it. They may benefit from doing so both because it could help to convince them that they can be accepted in spite of the fact that people are aware they stutter, and it could allow them to make use of at least some of the energy they usually devote to concealing their stuttering for more life-enhancing proposes. Clients who understand and accept their clinician's rationale for recommending voluntary stuttering probably will be more likely to try it than those who do not. There is a need, therefore, to make clients aware of this before encouraging them to try it.

One variation of voluntary stuttering, the *bounce* (Bryngelson, 1952; Johnson, 1946; Van Riper, 1973), has been used as a technique for reducing stuttering severity. Clients have been trained to repeat the initial syllables of words on which they do and do not expect to stutter in a relatively effortless manner. On those on which they expect to stutter, they are told to continue repeating the initial syllable until they either can say the word without stuttering or with only minimal stuttering. While this technique has been reported to be effective in reducing stuttering severity (Bryngelson, 1952), there is a potential "danger" associated with its use. Some who use it will develop the habit of repeating the initial syllables of words and will continue doing so even if the strategy is no longer effective for reducing the severity of their stuttering. This would tend to cause listeners to perceive their speech as being more abnormal than otherwise (Berlin & Berlin, 1964).

"Light" Consonant Contact.   This strategy—which has also been referred to as ventriloquism speech (Froeschels, 1950)—differs from the previous one in that the goal is to reduce voluntarily—rather than increase—stuttering severity. It is intended to provide clients with a tool for "breaking" (or reducing the tension in) blocks in which there are hard contacts involving one or more articulators (Ham, 1990b). During such a block, for example, there could be a hard, prolonged contact between the upper teeth and lower lip (if, e.g., the word contained an /f/ phoneme). Clients are taught both to produce consonant sounds on which they anticipate having a hard block with an extremely light contact and to try to change the strength of the contact between articulators to a light one while they are having such a block. While consonants that are produced in this manner may be perceived by listeners as distorted or even absent, such distortions and omissions are unlikely to seriously impede communication because of the redundancy present in language. Though it has been used mainly with older children and adults (Ham, 1990b; Ramig, 1984), a few attempts to use it with young children have been made (Ramig & Wallace, 1987). This strategy's ability to reduce stuttering severity may not be permanent (Ham, 1990b; Perkins, 1983b).

Another problem frequently encountered when using approaches such as this one in which clients are instructed to modify moments of stuttering while they occurring, is that they are of such short duration that doing so is extremely difficult, if not impossible. Zebrowski (1994), for example, found that for the stuttering children in her sample the duration of sound prolongations and sound/syllable repetitions was typically 750 milliseconds or less.

Cancellations, Pull-Outs, and Preparatory Sets.   These are a set of techniques, developed by Dr. Charles Van Riper of Western Michigan University, for enabling clients to reduce the severity of their moments of stuttering—for enabling them to stutter more fluently (Van Riper, 1973). While they can be used for the same purpose as the light-consonant-contact technique, they differ from it in several ways, including that the theoretical foundation on which they are based is stronger and a systematic program has been developed for teaching their use (see Van Riper, 1973).

The *cancellation technique* usually is taught first. After clients block on a word, they are supposed to (at least some of the time) pause briefly and think about what occurred during the block and then try to say the word again. The goal is not to say the word without stuttering, but to reduce, at least a little, the amount of abnormality that previously occurred while blocking on it.

There are several reasons why it seems reasonable to believe that the cancellation technique could contribute to reduced stuttering severity. First, it could help to convince clients that they can learn to reduce the severity of their moments of stuttering. Second, it can reduce their desire to avoid stuttering. To practice this technique it is necessary to stutter. A reduced desire to avoid stuttering is likely to result in reduced stuttering (see Chapter 2). And third, this technique can enable them to bring their stuttering problem out into the open. Listeners' curiosity about the cancellation technique would give them an opportunity to talk about or acknowledge their stuttering. Doing so should reduce its severity, at least a little (see Chapter 2).

The *pull-out technique* usually is taught after the client has made some progress mastering cancellation (Van Riper, 1973). It differs from cancellation in that it is used during a block, rather than after one has occurred. It is referred to in this way because it is a technique for "pulling out" of blocks. Clients are taught after they have begun blocking on a word to finish the word—terminate the block—with a relatively smooth, controlled prolongation of sounds. This is the aspect of the Van Riper approach that is most like the light-consonant-contact one (Ham, 1990b). Since much of the abnormality that occurs during moments of stuttering results from a frantic struggle to terminate blocks, terminating them in this manner would be expected to produce less abnormality and, hence, the blocks should be perceived as being less severe than they would have been otherwise.

The *preparatory-set technique* usually is taught after the client has made some progress in mastering the other two. It is intended to be used immediately *before* moments of stuttering. Van Riper (1973) based this technique on his observation that persons who stutter frequently exhibit certain abnormal behaviors—assume a particular kind of tense preparatory set—as they prepare themselves to begin saying words on which moments of stuttering occur. These abnormal behaviors include the following: tensing the musculature of the speech mechanism; saying the first sound of the word with a fixed position of the articulators rather than with a normal (coarticulatory) movement leading into the next sound; and initiating phonation before beginning to say the first sound of the word. He felt that this preparatory set was responsible for much of the abnormality that occurs during moments of stuttering (Van Riper, 1973). He recommended, therefore, that clients be taught to assume different—more relaxed—preparatory sets before beginning to say words on which they expect to stutter. Specifically, he recommended beginning with the articulators in a state of rest, saying the first sound as a movement leading into the next sound, and initiating air flow and phonation when beginning to say the first sound of the word (not before it).

After clients are proficient in all three techniques, they are told to use them in the reverse order in which they were learned (assuming that the order in which they were learned was the usual one). Before saying a word on which they expect to stutter, they should attempt to assume the "new" *preparatory set*. If they are not successful and begin to block with a great deal of abnormality, they should attempt to *pull out* of the block. And if they are not successful in pulling out of the block, they should use *cancellation* immediately after finishing the word to practice stuttering on it with less abnormality. For in-depth information about teaching these techniques, see Van Riper (1973).

Relaxation.   One fact about stuttering on which there is almost universal agreement is that those who have the disorder evince excessive muscle tension in their speech mechanism immediately before and during moments of stuttering. There is also almost universal agreement that this excessive tension is responsible for at least some of the abnormality present during moments of stuttering (Bloodstein, 1987). Hence, any intervention strategy that causes a client to be more relaxed while speaking should reduce his or her stuttering severity, at least a little (Wagaman, Miltenberger, & Arndorfer, 1993).

Two types of strategies for reducing tension when speaking have been used with persons who stutter: direct and indirect. Direct strategies are specifically intended either to cause clients to be more relaxed than usual when entering speaking situations or to train them to relax parts of their speech musculature when they feel tension in them. One such strategy that has been used with persons who stutter is progressive relaxation (Jacobson, 1938). Clients are taught to relax differentially various muscle groups, including those that make up the speech mechanism. Unfortunately, many have been unable to learn to use this technique well enough to reduce stuttering significantly in situations in which they tend to stutter a great deal (Bloodstein, 1987).

Another direct approach that has been utilized for this purpose involves the use of *suggestion* in either the waking or hypnotic state (Dempsey & Granich, 1978;

Francis, 1984; Ham, 1990b; Lockhart & Robertson, 1977; Macfarlane, 1990; McCord, 1955; Moore, 1946; Van Riper, 1973). Suggestion can be communicated by the clinician ("live" or on tape) or by the client to himself or herself—autosuggestion (see Boome & Richardson, 1931, for information about the use of autosuggestion in treating stuttering). A number of intervention strategies involving suggestion have been used with persons who stutter to bring about a more relaxed state while speaking (see Van Riper, 1973 for an in-depth discussion of these). Stutterers have, for example, been put into a relatively deep hypnotic state and given the posthypnotic suggestion that they will be relaxed when entering speaking situations and not stutter. Unfortunately, this type of posthypnotic suggestion, if effective, is usually so for only a short period of time (Gottlober, 1953; Ingham, 1984; Morley, 1957; McCord, 1955). While hypnosis by itself is regarded as being of questionable value in the treatment of stuttering (Ham, 1990b), it appears to have gained some acceptance when used to produce the relaxed state required for strategies such as systematic desensitization (Macfarlane, 1990; Wolpe, 1958).

A third direct approach uses electromyographic biofeedback instrumentation (Hasbrouck & Lowry, 1989; Ingham, 1993; Lanyon, 1977; Lanyon, Barrington, & Newman, 1976; Lanyon, Lanyon, & Goldsworthy, 1979). Surface electrodes are attached to the skin over a muscle that tends to tense during moments of stuttering (such as the masseter muscle), and the subject uses variations in the visual or auditory signal generated by the instrument both to monitor the level of tension in the muscle and to learn to relax it.

Indirect approaches that use suggestion for reducing tension while speaking usually do not involve the use of hypnosis. An example of such an approach would be the use of suggestion to modify aspects of clients' belief systems. One belief that clinicians may attempt to modify in their clients through the use of suggestion is that they cannot learn to reduce the severity of their stuttering. A client who regards previous therapy as having been unsuccessful is likely to have such a belief.

The suggestion that a client's severity of stuttering can be reduced would be communicated to him or her while in the "waking" state. However, the client may not be fully aware on a conscious level that the suggestion is being communicated because it may not be conveyed (or communicated completely) by what the clinician *says*. It may be communicated, in part, by the clinician behaving in a manner that *suggests* to the client that the prognosis for improvement is good. Or this idea may be communicated, in part, by the client meeting other stutterers who have improved—the fact that others have improved *suggests* to the client that he or she can also. The suggestion may also be communicated, in part, by the clinician having the client read research reports and other material that *suggest* persons who stutter can improve. Or, finally, it may be communicated, in part, by the client changing some aspect of his or her behavior that he or she did not believe could be changed (auto-suggestion).

This type of suggestion is responsible for the placebo effect (Shapiro, 1964). An intervention strategy can be effective, at least in part, because the client is led to believe through suggestion that it will be effective. Perhaps this is one reason why many seemingly different intervention strategies have been effective with persons who stutter.

Slow, Prolonged Speech.   Most persons who stutter do so less severely while speaking under the condition of delayed auditory feedback (DAF) in which there is a 250-millisecond delay (see Chapter 2). While doing so, their speaking rate tends to be slower than usual, and they tend to prolong sounds and syllables (Ryan & Ryan, 1995). Based on the assumption that it is these changes in speaking behavior rather than DAF, per se, that are responsible for the reduction in stuttering severity, a number of clinicians have attempted to teach delayed-auditory-feedback-type (slow, prolonged) speech to persons who stutter (Ingham, 1993; Martin, 1993; Ward, 1992). Some (Perkins, 1973; Robb, Lybolt, & Price, 1985; Shames & Florance, 1980) have recommended using a DAF unit, possibly a portable one (Craven & Ryan, 1984; Muellerleile, 1981), when teaching this form of speech—at least initially. Others (e.g., Ryan, 1971; Watts, 1971), however, have reported that it is not necessary to use such a device. They provide data that suggest that the *imitation* of speech produced under DAF is just as effective for reducing stuttering severity as is producing the altered speech pattern with a DAF unit. Those who do recommend using the device, however, gradually wean their clients from it. In some cases they do so by gradually increasing the interval of delay, thereby reducing the impact of the DAF unit on their clients' speech (Perkins, 1973). As this is being done, clients are encouraged to use the slow, prolonged DAF-type speech pattern voluntarily.

When clients use slow, prolonged speech, they are speaking in a nonhabitual manner. Speaking in such a manner tends to reduce stuttering severity (see Chapter 2). Hence, the reduction in stuttering that occurs while using slow, prolonged speech may result, at least in part, from speaking in a nonhabitual manner. If this is the case, then the effect of this strategy on stuttering may only be temporary.

There is an issue to consider before encouraging clients to speak in a manner, like the one just suggested, that listeners are likely to regard as abnormal. Will listeners tend to react more favorably to their "new" way of speaking than to their "old" way? There are data suggesting that listeners *may* react more favorably to a client's stuttering than to his or her "new" speech pattern if they regard it as sounding "unnatural" (see Berlin & Berlin, 1964; Franken et al., 1992; Kalinowski, Noble, Armson, & Stuart, 1994; Martin, Haroldson, & Triden, 1984; Onslow, et al., 1992; Perkins, 1983b; Silverman & Trotter, 1973c). According to Perkins (1983b, p. 157), "Unless use of fluency skills yields speech that sounds reasonably normal, stuttered speech is apt to seem preferable."

Rate Reduction.   Some persons who stutter become more fluent, at least temporarily, when they reduce their speaking rate (Ramig, 1984). This alone and in combination with other speech modification strategies has been used to reduce stuttering severity (Ham, 1988; Perkins, 1973; Ryan, 1974; Schwartz, 1976; Shames & Florance, 1980; Webster, 1980). It has been suggested, in fact, that this is an "active ingredient" in many of the strategies that have been used for this purpose (Ramig, 1984; Wingate, 1976).

Rhythmic (Metronome-Timed) Speech. Most persons who stutter become more fluent, at least temporarily, when they speak using an artificial rhythm—for example, when pacing their speech with the beats of a metronome (see Chapter 2). This phenomenon has been used clinically for several centuries (Eldridge, 1968). Two behavior-modification–based approaches that use rhythmic speech for reducing stuttering severity were developed during the past twenty-five years. With the first, metronome-timed speech (Brady, 1968, 1969, 1971; Meyer & Comley, 1969; Meyer & Mair, 1963; Silverman, 1971b, 1976; Trotter & Silverman, 1974), clients are encouraged to pace their speech with the beats of a miniature electronic metronome (one word or syllable per beat) that is worn like a behind-the-ear-type or eyeglass-type hearing aid (see Figure 2-1). With the second, syllable-timed speech (Andrew & Harris, 1964; Andrew & Ingham, 1972; Dalton & Hardcastle, 1977), clients are encouraged to speak rhythmically (one syllable at a time with even stress and timing) without using a device. Both have been reported to be effective in reducing the stuttering of some persons, at least temporarily (Andrews & Harris, 1964; Andrews & Ingham, 1972; Brady, 1968, 1969, 1971; Dalton & Hardcastle, 1977; Wingate, 1984c).

Clients using rhythmic speech—like those using slow, prolonged speech—are speaking in a nonhabitual manner. Doing so tends to result in reduced stuttering (see Chapter 2). Another factor that could partially explain this result is reduced fear of stuttering and desire to avoid it (see Silverman, 1971b).

Do listeners tend to react more favorably to clients' rhythmic speech than to their usual stuttering? There are data (Mallard & Meyer, 1979; Silverman & Trotter, 1973) suggesting that they may not, particularly if their usual stuttering tends to be relatively mild or if they pace their speech in a staccato, machine-like manner.

Speaking While Listening to Loud Masking Noise. Some persons who stutter become more fluent—at least temporarily—when they speak while listening to loud masking noise (see Chapter 2). Doing so interferes with their ability to monitor their speech auditorily and, as a consequence, there are changes in their speaking behavior—such as a tendency for their voices to grow louder. This phenomenon has been utilized clinically by having clients use portable masking-noise generators (e.g., Carlisle, 1985; Dewar et al., 1976; Ingham et al., 1981; Moore & Adams, 1985; Trotter & Lesch, 1967; Trotter & Silverman, 1973; Perkins & Curlee, 1969). These devices look like binaural body-type hearing aids. Some have a switch that clients can use to turn on the masking noise if they anticipate blocking or begin to block (Trotter & Lesch, 1967; Trotter & Silverman, 1973). Others, such as the Edinburgh Masker (Carlisle, 1985; Dewar et al., 1976; Ingham, 1993a; Ingham et al., 1981; Moore &

Adams, 1985), are voice actuated—that is, the masking noise is turned on when the person begins to phonate and turned off when phonation ceases. Some relatively severe stutterers have reported being helped by this type of device (Carlisle, 1985; Trotter & Lesch, 1967). The reduction in stuttering that occurs while using such a device may result, at least in part, from speaking in a nonhabitual manner.

Reducing Anomalies in Laryngeal Functioning.   Many persons who stutter have anomalies in laryngeal functioning during moments of stuttering (see Chapter 3). These include problems with initiating phonation and sustaining it in a relatively relaxed manner with adequate breath support. Several strategies have been proposed that require clients to monitor and attempt to modify one or both of these problems—that is, to have a gentle voice onset target (Miller, 1982; Stigora & DiSimoni, 1989). For example, Schwartz (1976) taught clients to monitor airflow and encouraged them to let some breath flow out passively before initiating phonation for each utterance. And Webster (1974, 1979, 1980, 1986), as a part of his Precision Fluency Shaping Program, taught clients to monitor onset of phonation (initially using a biofeedback device) and encouraged them to do it in a manner that is "gentle" (Mallard & Kelley, 1982; Pill, 1988). While many persons were reported to stutter less severely after learning to use these techniques, some were unable to maintain their posttherapy fluency level long term (Andrews & Tanner, 1982b; Pill, 1988).

The improvement in fluency reported by those who used these techniques may have resulted, in at least some cases, from speaking in a nonhabitual manner and/or from strong suggestion that the approach would be effective. With regard to the latter, Schwartz (1976) entitled his first book *Stuttering Solved* and his second (1986, with Carter) *Stop Stuttering*.

Reducing Abnormalities in Breathing.   Many stutterers exhibit abnormalities in respiratory functioning during moments of stuttering (see Chapter 2). Attempts have been made for hundreds of years to teach stutterers to breathe more normally (Van Riper, 1973). With one such contemporary approach—the regulated-breathing method (Andrews & Tanner, 1982a; Azrin & Nunn, 1974; Azrin, Nunn, & Frantz, 1979; Ingham, 1993a; Ladouceur, Caron, & Caron, 1989; Ladouceur, Coté, Leblond, & Bluchard, 1982; Waterloo & Gotestam, 1988)—clients are taught to

breathe in a smooth manner, to pause at natural juncturing points, to breathe deeply, to plan ahead for the content of speech, and to relax chest and neck muscles (Azrin et al., 1979).

While Azrin and his associates (1974, 1979) reported good results using it, Andrews & Tanner (1982a) and Ladouceur et al. (1982) were unable to replicate them. Hence, the usefulness of this technique for reducing stuttering is uncertain.

Another contemporary approach to treating stuttering by reducing breathing abnormalities is the perfectly mastered breathing (PMB) program (Tonev, 1994).

Punishing Stuttering and Positively Reinforcing Fluency. There have been attempts to reduce stuttering severity by using the operant conditioning methodology developed by B. F. Skinner and his followers (Curlee, 1993a; Gregory, 1968, 1969; Ingham, 1975, 1993a; Martin, 1993; Nittrouer & Cheney, 1984; Perkins, 1993; Siegel, 1993). If stuttering is the type of behavior that can be manipulated by response-contingent reinforcement, punishment should cause it to occur less frequently. And if speaking "fluently" is such a behavior, positive reinforcement should cause it to occur more frequently.

There have been a number of laboratory studies in which stuttering was reduced *temporarily* following response-contingent presentation of such stimuli as shock, noise, verbal disapproval, response cost, and time-out from speaking that probably would be interpreted by the recipient as punishment (see Chapter 2). A few attempts have been reported to use such reinforcement clinically with children who are thought to be beginning to stutter. For example, Martin, Juhl, and Haroldson (1972) reported on the use of a time-out procedure with two preschool children and Reed and Godden (1977) reported on the use of verbal disapproval (the words "slow down"), also with two preschool children. For all four children, a decrease in stuttering was reported following intervention. Onslow, Andrews, & Lincoln (1994) reported on its "successful" use with young children in a parent-administered program in which stutter-free utterances were rewarded with praise. In addition, Stocker and Gerstman (1983) have reported positive results from a strategy they refer to as the "probe technique" in which the therapist rewards the child for "reductions in dysfluencies with bits of candy or pennies" (p. 336).

Response-contingent punishment should be used with extreme caution with preschool children because there is reason to believe that it can precipitate stuttering. According to the diagnosogenic theory (see Chapter 5), communicating to children that their disfluencies (such as sound and syllable repetitions) are undesirable can precipitate the disorder. While the evidence certainly is not conclusive that doing so will always precipitate stuttering or that this is the only way stuttering can begin, it strongly suggests that it is *one* such way (Tudor, 1939; Silverman, 1988).

Concerns have been expressed about the reliability of perceptual judgments of moments of stuttering. Both interjudge and interclinic disagreements have be reported for relatively experienced judges (Ingham & Cordes, 1992). Consequently, it may not be possible to consistently punish moments of stuttering immediately after they occur.

Thus far response-contingent punishment of stuttering has been discussed. A second way that operant conditioning methodology has been used is reinforcement for periods of fluency. Moments of stuttering are ignored, and positive reinforcement is given for saying particular words or utterances fluently or for speaking fluently during a particular period of time. Leach (1969), for example, gave a twelve-year-old child one cent for each fifteen-second period of fluent speech, and Manning, Trutna, & Shaw (1976) gave three children—ages six, nine, and eleven—verbal rewards (such as "Good speech" and "You sounded real nice") for such performances. Some short-term improvement in fluency was reported in both studies.

Positive reinforcement for fluency may be interpreted by clients in the same manner as punishment for stuttering. By equating fluency with speaking well, you indirectly are equating being disfluent with speaking poorly.

Systematic Desensitization.   Stuttering severity varies on a situational basis (see Chapter 2). One reason a person stutters more than usual in some situations may be that a stimulus associated with them elicits higher than usual amounts of anxiety (Wolpe, 1958). If the reaction to this stimulus could be changed, there would likely be some reduction in stuttering severity (Brutten & Shoemaker, 1967). Systematic desensitization (which utilizes the reciprocal inhibition principle) has been used for this purpose (Wolpe, 1958; Brutten & Shoemaker, 1967; Walton & Mather, 1963).

The reciprocal inhibition principle, as formulated by Wolpe (1958), states that each time a person does not become highly anxious in the presence of a stimulus that ordinarily elicits a high level of anxiety, the link between that stimulus and the "old" response is weakened a little. How can it be arranged that a person will be unlikely to respond to such a stimulus with a high level of anxiety? One way is to produce in them an emotional state while they are in the presence of the stimulus that is not compatible with anxiety. One such state is deep relaxation (Wolpe, 1958). A person cannot be deeply relaxed and highly anxious simultaneously!

To desensitize a client to a stimulus using this principle, it is necessary to first get him or her deeply relaxed. A number of techniques can be used for this purpose (Jacobson, 1938; Wolpe, 1958). You would then present the stimulus a number of times in a way that should elicit a relatively low level of anxiety. If, for example, the act of talking on the telephone usually causes a client to become highly anxious, the stimulus could be presented to elicit a relatively low level by having the client repeatedly enter and leave a room in which there is a telephone, or imagine doing so. Imagining an act is reported to be as effective as actually doing it (Wolpe, 1958). When the client ceased responding to the stimulus with anxiety when presented in this manner, it would be presented in a way that would be expected to elicit a some-what higher level of anxiety. For example, the client would be required again and again to say something on the telephone (or to imagine doing so) to someone with whom he or she felt comfortable speaking. After the client ceased responding with anxiety to this version of the stimulus, it would be presented in a manner that would be expected to elicit a little more anxiety. This process would be repeated until the client ceased responding to the stimulus with a high level of anxiety when he or she encountered it in the "real world." Getting a client to this point can take many months (Wolpe, 1958).

The application of the reciprocal inhibition principle that was described in the preceding paragraph is highly structured. This principle also can be utilized in less formal ways. If, for example, a client were encouraged to discuss a situation that usually causes him or her to become highly anxious over and over again while he or she was fairly relaxed, this would tend to weaken the link between this situation and anxiety. This is one reason, incidentally, why psychotherapy in which clients "talk out their problems" is often beneficial (Wolpe, 1958). And this is also a reason why one may feel less anxious after talking with a friend about what is causing one's anxiety.

The reciprocal inhibition principle applied "informally" can be quite useful when working with persons who stutter. If, for example, the thought of bringing stuttering out into the open causes a client so much anxiety that he or she is unwilling to do it, having the client repeatedly talk about this with a person or group with whom he or she feels comfortable may reduce anxiety sufficiently to enable him or her to do it. This is one way, incidentally, that a support group, such as one sponsored by the National Stuttering Project (see Appendix B), can be helpful to persons who stutter.

Emotional Flooding (Implosive Therapy).   This, like systematic desensitization, is a behavior therapy method that involves having clients enter or imagine themselves in disturbing situations (Stampfl & Levis, 1967). While with systematic desensitization these situations are intended to be initially experienced by the client at a level that is only slightly disturbing, with emotional flooding they are intended to be experienced by him or her initially at a level that is highly disturbing—one that should produce an *emotional flood*. The theory is that repeatedly experiencing situations in this manner can cause the anxiety elicited by them to dissipate, or *implode* (Stampfl & Levis, 1967). Voluntary stuttering (Bryngelson et al., 1955; Van Riper, 1973), which is described elsewhere in this chapter, is an example of a technique that can produce such flooding. For further information about how this method has been used in the treatment of stuttering see Adams (1982) and Van Riper (1973).

Drugs.   There have been a number of attempts to use prescription drugs to reduce stuttering severity (Bloodstein, 1987; Brady, 1991; Ingham, 1984; Ludlow & Braun, 1993; Van Riper, 1973). Six that have been used with stutterers are bethanechol (Kampman & Brady, 1993); carbamazepine (Harvey et al., 1992); clomipramine (Stager et al., 1994); meprobamate (DiCarlo, Katz, & Batkin, 1959; Kent & Williams, 1959; Maxwell & Paterson, 1958), verapamil (Amster & Wark, 1994; Brady, 1994), and haloperidol (Andrews & Dozsa, 1977; Brady, 1994; Quinn & Peachey, 1975; Rosenberger, Wheelden, & Kalotkin, 1976). While these drugs appear to make some stutterers more fluent, most of those who become so eventually discontinue their use because of unacceptable side effects such as drowsiness and nausea (Bloodstein, 1987).

Acupuncture.   Acupuncture has been reported to be effective as a component of a therapy program for reducing stuttering severity (Brauneis, 1994). According to Brauneis (1994, p. 159), "Modern research has shown that acupuncture is able to influence neurophysiological and neurochemical (neurotransmitter) processes as well as relax the patient."

Strategies for Modifying Listeners'
Reactions to the Client's Speech Fluency

Most stutterers stutter more severely when talking to some persons than to others (see Chapter 2). Almost any older child or adult who has the disorder can name categories of people with whom he or she tends to stutter more severely than usual. An example of such a category for some stutterers is order takers in fast-food restaurants.

According to the interaction-frame model (see Figure 7-1) the reactions of listeners to stuttering can influence its severity. Stutterers tend to stutter more severely when with persons whom they expect to react negatively to their stuttering than when with those whom they do not expect to do so. This is because they tend to stutter most when they want to stutter least (Williams, 1982). Consequently, it may be possible to reduce the severity of a client's stuttering in some situations, at least a little, by changing the reactions of certain listeners to it.

We discussed, in the preceding section, how clinician-administered response-contingent punishment of stuttering and positive reinforcement of fluency can increase stuttering by increasing the desire to avoid it. A person who stutters is likely, at times, to receive both of types of feedback from listeners. One who laughs after the person stutters would be administering response-contingent punishment for stuttering. And one who compliments him or her for saying something fluently would be administering response-contingent reinforcement for fluency. Actually, anything a client interprets (rightly or wrongly) as being punishment for stuttering or positive reinforcement for fluency can have this effect.

Strategies for reducing the likelihood that particular listeners will unintentionally deliver response-contingent punishment for stuttering and/or response-contingent reinforcement for fluency are discussed in this section. These are of two types. With one the client attempts to modify these reactions, with the other, somebody else attempts to do so. The "somebody else" is most likely to be a clinician, a parent, or teacher.

Several strategies that a client could utilize for modifying these reactions are now considered. The first involves the use of response-contingent punishment. Immediately after the listener reacts to the client's stuttering or fluency in a way that he or she does not like, the client would do something that the listener would regard as adversive. One of my teenage clients solved the problem of being mocked frequently by a classmate for his stuttering by beating him up. And one of my adult clients, after being treated in a demeaning way by a store clerk because of his stuttering, asked to see the manager and complained. Both of these resulted in the client feeling more in control and less like a victim. Overtly expressing anger when it is appropriate to do so is also likely to benefit clients in other ways (Rubin, 1969).

Another strategy that a client could use for modifying such reactions is to bring his or her stuttering problem out into the open—to acknowledge it. Listeners are less likely to react to stuttering in ways that clients are likely to regard as objectionable if they do not have to play "The Emperor's New Clothes" game—make believe that they are not aware that the client's speech is abnormal. A client can acknowledge the problem verbally or through a printed message. He or she can do so, for example, by wearing a T-shirt on which is printed "I stutter. So what!" (Silverman, 1988; Silverman, Gazzolo, & Peterson, 1989). The findings of several studies (Silverman, 1988; Silverman, Gazzolo, & Peterson, 1989) suggest that listeners tend to react more positively to a stutterer who wears such a shirt than they would otherwise.

A third strategy that clients can use for this purpose is to present themselves as often as possible in a way that suggests they have a good self-concept (Cash & Pruzinsky, 1990). Doing so could involve being clean and well-groomed, being assertive, and not constantly signaling listeners that they are ashamed or embarrassed about stuttering. What clients perceive as reactions to their stuttering may actually be, at least in part, reactions to the feelings of shame and embarrassment about it that they are communicating to listeners. One way that they can do so is by having poor eye contact during moments of stuttering (see Chapter 3). Thus, encouraging clients to try to maintain normal eye contact at these times should help to reduce negative reactions to their disfluency. One strategy for helping clients learn to do this involves the use of response-contingent verbal reinforcement and successive approximations. The client initially would receive such reinforcement for even minimal attempts to improve eye contact during moments of stuttering. As his or her ability to approximate normal eye contact during them improved, he or she would cease receiving reinforcement for minimal attempts. Eventually, only those attempts that resulted in eye contact that was within normal limits would be reinforced.

A second strategy that may be usable for this purpose involves modifying clients' feelings of shame and embarrassment about stuttering. While it may not be possible to eliminate these totally, it should be possible to reduce them at least a little (Cash & Pruzinsky, 1990). These feelings are likely to have been caused, at least in part, by certain beliefs (or "certainties") that include the following:

- "I should be able to talk all the time without stuttering because I can do so some of the time."
- "If I had tried hard enough while in therapy, I would have learned to talk without stuttering."
- "I am weak. If I had been able to exercise a normal amount of self-control (will power), I would have been able to conquer my problem."
- "The cause of my stuttering is psychological (learned behavior) and, hence, I should have been able to conquer it."
- "People dislike listening to stuttering and, hence, I am making them feel uncomfortable."
- "Since stuttering reduces my speaking rate, I am taking more than my fair share of time while talking."

If it seems likely that a client's feelings of shame and embarrassment about stuttering arise, at least in part, from this source, the first step would be to identify the client's certainties and the second would be to reduce his or her confidence in their accuracy.

One way would be to present evidence that does not support them. The evidence could come from research data, the client's (or others) life experiences, and/or arguments developed by the clinician. The client initially is likely to reject such challenges to his or her belief system—or is likely to react in a manner that indicates he or she does not want to be "confused by facts." However, if the clinician is persistent, if the data are compelling, and if the arguments are cogent, the client's belief system is likely to be modified, at least a little. Techniques developed by the general semanticists for modifying erroneous beliefs can be useful here (see Johnson, 1946).

The focus so far has been on strategies that clients can use for modifying listener reactions to their disfluency. We will now consider ones that clinicians, parents, and teachers can use for doing so.

What strategies can clinicians use? In particular, how can they modify undesirable reactions of a child's parents to his or her disfluency when it appears to be "normal"? Since it seems likely that children can begin to stutter in the manner specified by the diagnosogenic theory (see Chapter 5), modifying parents' reactions may be necessary.

It may be possible to modify undesirable reactions of childrens' parents to their "normal" disfluency by doing one or more of the following:

- Providing parents with information about normal childhood disfluency.
- Providing them with information about how certain reactions to their child's disfluency could increase it. This can be done in a way that is unlikely to make parents feel guilty if they have already reacted inappropriately to it.
- Identifying undesirable reactions they are having to their child's disfluency and increasing their awareness of them.
- Teaching parents how to react appropriately to their child's speech disfluency.

Strategies to accomplish these are discussed below.

The first task in an intervention program for modifying parents' reactions to their child's disfluency is providing them with information about normal childhood disfluency (see Chapter 4). If their child's disfluency is found to be within normal limits, merely providing them with this information may be sufficient to eliminate undesirable reactions to it. That is, if they no longer regard the behavior as abnormal, they probably will cease reacting to it in undesirable ways, particularly if they are made aware that continuing to do so could cause it to become abnormal.

Several problems can be encountered when trying to convince parents that their child's fluency is within normal limits. The first is particularly likely to occur if a child's disfluency level is at the *upper end* of normal limits—that is, if he or she repeats sounds and syllables more often than most other children the same age. They may have a difficult time accepting that it is normal because they are aware of other children their child's age who are not as disfluent. It can be pointed out to them that there are *individual differences* in all aspects of childhood behavior, including disfluency, and that their child just tends to be more disfluent than many others of the same age.

Another problem that can be encountered when trying to convince parents that their child's fluency is within normal limits is their having a set to perceive their child's disfluency as stuttering because of a history of it in the family. They are particularly likely to have such a set if they remember a stutterer in the family being disfluent in a similar way during childhood. They can be made aware that most children born into families in which there is a history of stuttering do not stutter, even if one or both parents do so.

Parents probably should be given information about normal childhood disfluency even if their child exhibits abnormal disfluency behavior. There are at least two reasons. First, it is important for them to be aware that not all the disfluency in their child's speech is abnormal. Their child may not be stuttering, therefore, as severely as they think he or she is. And second, they have to learn to discriminate between normal disfluency and stuttering if they are being asked to inform the clinician about the child's stuttering at home.

After the child's parents have been given information about normal speech disfluency, the clinician's next task is to provide them with information about how certain reactions to their child's disfluency could increase it, in a way that is unlikely to make them feel guilty if they have already reacted to it in these ways. If this is not done, they are likely to interpret this information to mean that the reason for their child stuttering is poor parenting. This interpretation could cause them to feel guilty, to reject the clinician's recommendations, or both. To reduce the likelihood of such an interpretation, one or more of the following can be mentioned:

- They were reacting to the child's disfluencies in a way that would seem to be appropriate, based on "common sense." Unfortunately, this is one of those rare instances when common sense can lead you astray.
- They obviously reacted to their child's disfluency as they did because they loved and wanted to help him or her.
- Since there is a history of stuttering in their family and they heard that the disorder can be transmitted genetically, it is understandable why they perceived their child's repetitions as abnormal.
- Since the child's disfluency level appears to be at the upper end of normal limits, it is understandable why they perceived it as being abnormal.
- The fact that they brought their child in for an evaluation is evidence that they love their child and are willing to do whatever is necessary to help him or her.

After the parents appear to accept (perhaps with minor reservations) that certain of their reactions to their child's disfluency and/or demands they are placing on their child for fluency may be increasing his or her disfluency, the clinician should increase their awareness of them (Starkweather & Gottwald, 1990). There are two approaches that can be used, singly or in combination. The first is telling them, in a "face-saving" way, what they are doing that they need to change. The second is having them watch videotapes of the interaction between themselves and their child while the clinician points out both the desirable and undesirable ways they are reacting to his or her disfluency. Hopefully, there will be some of the former so that the experience will not be totally negative. Videotape the scene, if possible, so that they can see their child's face immediately after they react to the disfluency. This may help to increase their awareness of the effect their reactions are having on their child.

After the parents are made aware of what they are doing that needs to be changed, they are taught how to react appropriately to their child's disfluency. Doing so may involve training them to stop saying things that indicate to the child that he or she is doing something "bad" by being disfluent (such as "Take a deep breath before you talk.") and/or to stop doing the things (such as looking away) that communicate this message. This could involve teaching them *things to do* when their child is being disfluent such as listening to and concentrating on the "message" he or she is attempting to communicate and giving him or her positive reinforcement for communicating it successfully regardless of disfluency (Yovetich, 1984). It also could involve teaching them ways to manipulate unobtrusively their child's spontaneous communicative behavior that are likely to result in increased fluency (Langlois & Long, 1988; Starkweather & Gottwald, 1990). One approach that has been used for teaching parents how to react appropriately to their child's disfluency is having them watch videotapes of the clinician interacting with their child and then trying to imitate what they see (Daly, 1987).

Another group whose reactions may have to be changed is classroom teachers. How they react to a child's disfluency can strongly influence how his or her peers are likely to do so. If they react to it in undesirable ways, the child's classmates will be likely to also. An example of such a reaction would be refusing to allow the child to contribute to class discussions when he or she volunteers. Another example would be having the child give oral presentations to him or her privately, rather than to the class. The clinician, therefore, may have to counsel the child's classroom teacher in much the same way he or she would the child's parents. Such counseling, of course, should be done in a manner that is unlikely to make the teacher feel guilty or lose face. Otherwise, it could cause the situation in the classroom to deteriorate, rather than improve.

There is another reason why it may be desirable to work with the classroom teacher. He or she could provide the child an opportunity to bring the problem out into the open. The child could be encouraged to give an informal talk about it to classmates. The teacher may want to set the stage by providing information about stuttering (see FitzSimons, 1962), including the names of famous people who had the disorder, for example, Moses. The children probably should be given an opportunity to ask questions. It may be desirable for the child's speech-language pathologist to be present.

The approaches considered thus far for modifying parents' and teachers' reactions to children's speech disfluency attempt to do so directly—that is, by increasing their awareness of reactions that are desirable and undesirable. An indirect approach that may be usable for this purpose (alone or in combination with the others) is switching their attention and concern from fluency to another aspect of speech, language, and/or communication behavior and to treat it. Many young children who stutter or appear to be at risk for developing the disorder have articulation, auditory processing, language formulation, and/or oral motor problems (Riley & Riley, 1979). Riley & Riley (1979) have described a program for treating young children who stutter that has this as a component.

Strategies to Modify Clients' Reactions to Their Stuttering and the Reactions of Others to It

The more clients are disturbed by their stuttering and others' reactions to it, the stronger will probably be their desire to avoid stuttering and, hence, the more severely they are apt to stutter (see Figure 7-1). Remember that stutterers tend to stutter most when they want to stutter least (Williams, 1982)!

This section focuses on strategies for modifying the reactions of clients to their stuttering and the reactions of others to it or for *desensitizing* them to these reactions. The reciprocal inhibition principle (Wolpe, 1958) can be used to explain how such strategies work. This principle, which was discussed earlier in this chapter, states that each time a person does not experience anxiety (or as much anxiety as usual) while in the presence of a stimulus that usually elicits it, the link between that stimulus and the old, anxiety-type response is weakened. Hence, if clients can be kept a number of times from reacting to their stuttering and to their anticipation of it with the usual amount of anxiety, there should be a reduction in the amount of anxiety these stimuli tend to elicit. Consequently, there should be some reduction in the severity of their stuttering. The same should be true for anticipated undesired listener reactions to their stuttering.

Is it possible completely or almost completely to desensitize clients to their stuttering and negative reactions of listeners to it? While clinical experience suggests that this is not an attainable goal for many clients, *reducing* the amount of anxiety with which they tend to react to these occurrences should be an attainable goal for almost all of them (Wolpe, 1958). Even if this amount were only reduced 15 or 20 percent, it would contribute to the overall goal of reducing stuttering severity.

While any strategy that can cause clients to respond to stuttering or negative listener reactions to it with less than the usual amount of anxiety is worth considering, some are less acceptable and/or practical than others. For example, voluntary stuttering outside of the clinic environment (Bryngelson, 1952; Bryngelson et al., 1955) can be effective, but many stutterers are unwilling to do it. And using systematic desensitization with hypnotic relaxation (Wolpe, 1958) can be effective, but very few speech-language pathologists have been trained to use hypnosis.

The following strategies can be used (singly or in combination) for desensitizing clients to their stuttering or negative reactions to it.

Voluntary Stuttering.   Voluntary stuttering (Bryngelson, 1952; Bryngelson et al., 1955), which is described in this chapter, can be an effective strategy for desensitizing clients if they are willing to do it and can remain relatively relaxed while doing so.

This strategy can be used in several ways. One is for the client to voluntarily stutter for a period of time in all (or almost all) situations. Another is for the client to use it as a tool to temporarily reduce his or her anxiety in specific situations. A client who is experiencing a great deal of anxiety about the possibility of stuttering—or stuttering severely—in a particular situation, may be able to reduce it by voluntarily stuttering. The second of these is likely to be more acceptable to clients than the first because it does not require them to do as much voluntary stuttering and it gives them *control* over when they will do it. The act of feeling in control, by itself, may reduce a client's anxiety level (Van Riper, 1973).

Systematic Desensitization.   Systematic desensitization (Wolpe, 1958), which is described in this chapter, also can be used for this purpose. After a client is relaxed, he or she is either made to experience a stimulus that is related to stuttering or others' reactions to it or is asked to imagine doing so a number of times. An example of such a stimulus would be stuttering while talking on the telephone. If the client can remain fairly relaxed while doing this, the strength of the link between this stimulus and anxiety should be reduced, at least a little.

Paradoxical Intention.   Paradoxical intention (Frankl, 1939, 1985) is a technique in which the client is encouraged to *intend,* or wish, something to occur that he or she fears. According to Frankl (1985, p. 147): "This procedure consists of a reversal of the patient's attitude, inasmuch as his fear is replaced by a paradoxical wish. By the treatment the wind is taken out of the sails of the anxiety." Paradoxical intention has been used for treating a number of conditions in which there is anticipatory anxiety (Frankl, 1985; Freund, 1966).

How might paradoxical intention be used for desensitizing clients to their stuttering? They could be told that when they anticipate stuttering or begin to stutter they should resolve deliberately to show people how severely they can do so. That is, rather than desiring to avoid stuttering, they should have the paradoxical intention: desiring to stutter as much as possible. If they are successful in doing this for a period of time, the amount of anxiety that the anticipation of stuttering tends to elicit should be reduced.

The effect of paradoxical intention on anxiety can be explained by the reciprocal inhibition principle (Wolpe, 1958). By desiring to stutter, clients experience less anxiety than usual when they do stutter or anticipate doing so. Consequently, there is a weakening in the link between stuttering and anxiety.

Training Clients to *Control* (Modify) Their Moments of Stuttering.   To learn to do this clients have to practice, and they cannot practice if they do not stutter. Hence, stuttering becomes desirable behavior and, consequently, less likely than before to elicit high levels of anxiety.

This strategy may be usable for encouraging clients to adopt the mind-set required for using paradoxical intention (the strategy that is discussed before this one). It would be easier for some to adopt this mind-set (decide that they want to stutter) if they were doing it for a purpose.

Assertiveness Training. Assertiveness training (Cohen, Thompson, Ruppel, & Flaherty, 1975; Schloss, Espin, Smith, & Suffolk, 1987; Schloss, Freeman, Smith, & Espin, 1987; Wolpe, 1969; Wolpe & Lazarus, 1966), a technique for enhancing interpersonal skills, can facilitate the development of a state which, like relaxation, is not compatible with anxiety (Wolpe, 1969). Hence, if stutterers behave in an assertive manner in situations in which they usually tend to stutter relatively severely, they are likely to become less anxious in them than usual and, consequently, are likely to stutter less severely than they usually do (Schloss et al., 1987). Based on the reciprocal inhibition principle (Wolpe, 1958), being assertive in the presence of stimuli that ordinarily elicit relatively high levels of anxiety should cause them to elicit less of it, thereby weakening the link, at least a little, between these stimuli and anxiety.

Talking with Clinician or Support Group. Having clients talk with a clinician or a support group about their stuttering and their reactions to it can reduce the anxiety these usually elicit, provided that the clients are not highly anxious while doing so (Moore & Rigo, 1983). Here, again, the mechanism can be regarded as being the reciprocal inhibition principle (Wolpe, 1958). Because clients are talking about these problems without becoming as upset as they usually do, the strength of the link between them and anxiety is weakened a little.

The ameliorating effect of such talking explains, in part, why some stutterers benefit from attending meetings of a support group, such as ones sponsored by the National Counsel on Stuttering and the National Stuttering Project (Diggs, 1990; Paul-Brown, 1990). Most persons who participate in them on a regular basis probably enjoy doing so (experience "positive" emotion). Hence, when they talk with group members about their stuttering and negative reactions to it, they are unlikely to become as upset about them as they usually do.

While these are not the only strategies that have been used for desensitizing clients to their stuttering and reactions to it, they include the ones that have been utilized most often for this purpose. For further information both about them and the other strategies see American Speech-Language-Hearing Association, 1995; Bloodstein (1987), Curlee (1993b), Ham (1986, 1990b), Kelly (1955), Van Riper (1973), and Wolpe (1969).

Our focus thus far in this section has been on strategies for reducing clients' desire to avoid stuttering by desensitizing them to it. There is a second approach that can be used for this purpose: reducing their tendency to use fluency as the primary measure of how well they speak. Many clients tend to overvalue fluency (Perkins, 1983b). This approach can be implemented by encouraging them to redirect their attention from how they are speaking to what they are saying (Gerstman, 1983;

Yovetich, 1984). The less frequently they judge how well they speak by how much they stutter rather than by how well they communicate, the weaker should be their desire to avoid stuttering. Yovetich (1984) has described a strategy, which he refers to as message therapy, for doing this with children. Shklovskii, Krol, & Mikhailova (1988) have described a group psychotherapy program for adults that attempts, in part, to make participants more aware of verbal and nonverbal aspects of their communication and to try to "normalize" these. If the program is successful, the result should be their considering these more and stuttering less when judging how well they spoke in a particular situation.

Maintenance of Fluency Following Treatment

Fewer than 50 percent of older children and adults who acquire more normal fluency during treatment are able to maintain it permanently (Bloodstein, 1987; Ingham, 1993a; Kamhi, 1982; Perkins, 1981; Starkweather, 1990). According to Perkins (1983b):

> *Judging from published and unpublished reports of fluency shaping programs, reports that accord with our experiences, the most predictable outcome is relapse of varying amounts and durations. Not that all progress is lost or that other forms of treatment yield better or more permanent results. Quite the contrary. But the expectation of permanent fluency is an expectation rarely realized. (p. 158)*

The relapse rates that have been reported for young children, particularly preschool-age ones, are considerably less (Starkweather, 1990; Starkweather, Gottwald, & Halford, 1990).

A program for posttreatment maintenance of fluency can minimize, or even prevent, relapse (Boberg, 1981; Boberg et al., 1979; Boberg & Sawyer, 1977; Hanna & Owen, 1977; Howie, Tanner, & Andrews, 1981; Ingham, 1993b; Johnson, 1987b; Kuhr & Rustin, 1985; Pill, 1988; Schwartz, 1994; Shenker & Finn, 1985). It could include periodic clinic contacts to check on status and/or periodic participation in refresher programs (Boberg, 1981) or self-help groups for former clients (Howie et al., 1981). For children it could include training parents to administer a fluency maintenance program (Schwartz, 1994). It may be desirable to encourage clients to participate in such programs regardless of whether they appear to be experiencing relapse. And it is quite possible that to maintain treatment gains they will have to continue to work on their speech for the rest of their life (Ingham, 1993b).

There are several things that can be done while clients are in treatment that have been reported to reduce the likelihood of their relapsing following it, permanently or for a relatively long period. One is communicating the importance of and training them to be their own clinician—to do self-therapy (Boberg, 1976; Costello, 1975; Hanna & Owen, 1977; Kuhr & Rustin, 1985; Martin & Haroldson, 1982; Ryan & Van Kirk, 1974). Another is modifying their self-concepts and attitudes toward speaking (Guitar, 1976; Guitar & Bass, 1978; Kuhr & Rustin, 1985). The goal is to make both more similar to those of "normal speakers." A third is to "normalize" fully their speech fluency before permanently terminating therapy (Adams & Runyan, 1981; Andrews & Craig, 1988; Runyan & Adams, 1978, 1979). If this is done while they exhibit "tenuous fluency" (Adams & Runyan, 1981)—while they continue to exhibit behaviors in rate, rhythm, or vocal characteristics that would enable listeners to differentiate their speech from that of normal speakers—they may have a greater potential for relapse (Shenker & Finn, 1985). The fluent speech of some stutterers who were regarded by their clinicians as having been "successfully therapeutized" has been shown to be perceptually different from that of normal speakers (Ingham, Gow, & Costello, 1985; Onslow, Hayes, Hutchins, & Newman, 1992; Onslow & Ingham, 1987; Runyan & Adams, 1978, 1979). However, there is a little evidence that providing clients with feedback about this can enable them to make their speech sound more normal (Ingham, Martin, Haroldson, Onslow, & Leney, 1985). A fourth is to prepare them for and train them to cope with relapse, to "cease pretending that the majority of stutterers will be able to maintain fluent or stutter-free speech on a long-term basis" (Kamhi, 1982, p. 460). And a fifth is to desensitize them to feeling pressured to speak faster if the strategy they are using to reduce stuttering severity results in a reduction in speaking rate (Craig & Calver, 1991).

One issue relevant to maintaining fluency is assessing whether a relapse is occurring. Ordinarily, the sooner it can be detected, the better the prognosis for the client successfully coping with it (Hillis, 1993). While casual observation often is adequate for detecting a relapse—particularly one of relatively large magnitude—after it has occurred, it may not be adequate for detecting its beginning stages. Clinicians have used both overt and covert procedures for observing their clients' fluency posttherapy, and there is some data suggesting that, for individuals (as opposed to groups), some overt ones may lead to underestimates of amount of disfluency (Andrews & Craig, 1982; Howie, Woods, & Andrews, 1982; Ingham, 1990b).

Strategies for Reducing the Amount Clients Are Handicapped by Stuttering

Our primary focus thus far has been on reducing stuttering severity. For most adults who stutter, this is unlikely to be the only important goal. The set of behaviors that defines their stuttering problem will include ones that are not aspects of speaking behavior. They result from living with the disorder and can contribute significantly to the amount that clients are handicapped.

The amount clients are handicapped by stuttering (or another fluency disorder) is determined by how much it keeps them from doing what they want to do. The severity of the handicap is not necessarily related to the amount of disfluency. Some persons who stutter very little are more handicapped because of their attitude toward it than some who do so a great deal.

The amount that they are handicapped is determined, in part, by their beliefs about the impact the disorder has on them. Some such beliefs, or *certainties,* can cause them to limit their activities and, thereby, increase the amount they are handicapped. One or more of their certainties may not be true. Modifying these should cause them to place fewer limitations on themselves and, as a consequence, be less handicapped than previously. Strategies for working toward this goal are discussed next.

The following are examples of certainties that can cause clients to limit their activities:

- "A person who stutters cannot be successful in a field that requires a great deal of talking, such as teaching, acting, law, politics, public relations, the clergy, sales, speech-language pathology, and medicine." While a person who stutters may have difficulty getting hired in such a field (Silverman & Paynter, 1990), the fact is that persons who stutter have been successful in all of them. The memberships of the National Stuttering Project and the National Council on Stuttering, for example, have included persons who were employed in these fields for a number of years.

- "A person who stutters must conquer the disorder before getting on with his or her life." Persons who have this belief tend to put their life "on hold." While clients certainly should be encouraged to try to reduce the severity of their stuttering (assuming that this, for them, would be an attainable goal), it probably is unnecessary for them to put their life on hold until they do so. Many persons who stutter relatively severely appear to have had satisfying lives, professionally and otherwise.

- "A person who stutters in unworthy." Persons who have this belief tend to withdraw from people—they may almost become hermits. An extreme example would be an attorney with whom I worked briefly who stuttered. He lived for a number of years on a small island in the Pacific because he did not feel he was sufficiently worthy to live on the mainland. Those who view themselves in this way obviously have a poor self-concept and may benefit from psychotherapy.

- "A person who has normal speech will not want to date someone who stutters." Clients who have this belief will rarely, if ever, try to get a date because they anticipate rejection. While there probably are such persons who would refuse to date someone for this reason, the fact that many persons who stutter are married to non-stutterers suggests that this in not true in general. While a person who stutters may attribute his or her lack of success in dating to stuttering, the real reason may be a poor self-concept. He or she may not dress attractively, be well-groomed, have a good sense of humor, and/or in other ways be the kind of positive person with whom people enjoy spending time.

- "If I talk in a particular situation, people will react to my stuttering in ways I'll find upsetting." Clients are likely to avoid talking in certain situations at least some of the time because of bad experiences they have had in the past. For example, a child may avoid asking questions in class or contributing to class discussions because classmates have laughed at his stuttering. Clients assume that because their stuttering was reacted to negatively in the past, it is likely to be treated this way in the future. This may or may not be true. If it is not true, then they are unnecessarily handicapping themselves by not talking. And if it is true, they may be losing more than they gain by doing so. For example, while children can reduce negative reactions to their stuttering by not participating in class discussions, doing so can also contribute to their doing less well academically than they would have otherwise (Williams, Melrose, & Woods, 1969).

• "Because I stutter I can't participate in a particular activity I think I'd enjoy." Over the years I have met persons who stutter who have participated in a wide variety of activities, many of which involve speaking. They have been debaters, actors, singers, telephone answerers on suicide "hot lines," members of volunteer fire departments, leaders of religious services, and advocates for political candidates and causes. They have even run for and been elected to political office. Hence, clients who have this certainty may be handicapping themselves unnecessarily.

Persons who have other fluency disorders can also be handicapped by these certainties.

Intervention for reducing the amount clients are handicapped by their beliefs is a two-step process (Johnson, 1946). The first, which is identifying them, involves questioning clients in a way that will reveal the limitations they are placing on themselves. Answers to the following questions can provide useful information: "If your stuttering were to disappear tomorrow, what effects would it have on your life? What would you do that you do not do now? Would you change jobs? If you think that you might do so, what field would you enter? Do you think you would do better in school? Why? Are there activities you would engage in that you do not engage in now? With what people, if any, would you talk more often? Would you date more often? Would you feel better about yourself—more 'worthy?' Would you further your education? Would you have more friends?"

After at least some of a client's certainties have been identified, an attempt can be made to modify them. Doing so usually involves providing the client with information and/or experiences that hopefully will cause him or her to question their accuracy. Such information can be provided in several ways. First, the clinician can do so orally. Second, the clinician can encourage the client to read material that provides it. And third, the clinician can encourage the client to talk to stutterers who do not have these certainties.

The process used for encouraging clients to modify their certainties is similar to hypothesis testing in research (Silverman, 1993). Certainties can be looked upon as hypotheses that may or may not be valid. To assess their validity, clients would be encouraged to make the observations necessary to "test" them as objectively as they can. If, for example, one of a client's certainties pertains to how specific listeners will react to his or her stuttering (e.g., how classmates will react if he or she stutters while asking questions in class), the client would be encouraged to stutter while talking to them and observe how they react. If they do react negatively, this would suggest that the certainty is accurate. On the other hand, if they do not do so, this should make the client at least a little less confident in its accuracy. Since a single observation is not adequate for testing any hypothesis, clients should be encouraged to test their certainties more than once.

What if this process indicates that such a certainty probably is accurate—that, for example, stuttering decreases employability in some occupations even if it does not interfere with job performance (Hurst & Cooper, 1983a, 1983b)? Should the client be encouraged to accept the limitations it imposes? If these are ones that the client is highly unlikely to be able to overcome, it probably would be best for his or her mental health that they be accepted. On the other hand, if there is a good chance they can be overcome and the client is willing "to pay a price" for trying, whether he or she should be encouraged to do so would depend on whether the potential benefits from trying exceeded the potential losses from doing so.

Counseling the Client's Family

There may be a need to counsel members of the client's family for reasons other than having them do things to facilitate his or her therapy. They may need help in coping with situations they themselves encounter because they live with a person who has a fluency disorder. Perhaps the persons who are most likely to be in need of such help are the parents of children and the spouses of adults who have such a disorder. For descriptions of coping strategies for parents, see Conture & Fraser (1989) and Zebrowski & Schum (1993), and for spouses, see Boberg & Boberg (1990).

Prevention of Stuttering

The best way to "cure" stuttering would be to prevent it from occurring. Just as there is controversy about the cause of stuttering, there is controversy about whether it can be prevented (see the papers in the first issue of the *Journal of Fluency Disorders* for 1992). Whether one is an optimist or pessimist is largely a function of what one believes to be the etiology of the disorder. Those who believe that it is mostly organic (e. g., genetic) tend to be pessimistic (see Hamre, 1992a, 1992b) and those who believe that it is mainly psychological—particularly those who accept the diagnosogenic theory—tend to be the opposite (see Crowe & Robinson, Jr., 1993). I am firmly convinced (perhaps deluded) that during my thirty-five years of clinical practice the counseling I gave (based on the diagnosogenic theory) to the parents of a number of young children who appeared to be at risk for developing the disorder because of a history of stuttering in the family kept at least a few from developing it.

SELF-HELP FOR STUTTERING

The self-help movement has come a long way since its beginnings in 1935 with the founding of Alcoholics Anonymous. Today an estimated 12,000,000 people "get help from helping" in approximately 500,000 such groups (Diggs, 1990).

There are local self-help groups for persons who stutter, some of which are affiliated with national organizations (see Appendix B). Those who participate in them may or may not be receiving therapy concurrently. In some a speech-language pathologist attends meetings on a regular basis.

Through participating in meetings sponsored by local and national groups and reading their newsletters, stutterers are likely to become more aware that the problems they encounter in living with the disorder are not unique and can be coped with. They also may benefit from learning about the experiences others have had with particular approaches to therapy, about speech-language pathologists in their community who are experienced working with persons who have the disorder, and about books that may help them better to understand and cope with stuttering (e. g., Carlisle, 1985; Fraser, 1972). According to Diggs (1990):

> *Many self-help organizations encourage discussing how members cope with upsetting events. Problems are shared with other people who care. As one consumer said, "I'm not singled out. Somebody else is in the same boat." Members listen without judgment and learn together, recognizing others rights to their own beliefs.*
>
> *Through such experiences, many self-helpers decide for the first time that they don't have to hide their problem. A sense of normalization grows from being with people who share a problem, and often a social support system emerges. This socialization process seems to be quite important in the generic self-help movement, but may be even more critical to people with communication disorders where often the problems themselves promote social isolation. (p. 33)*

Speech-language pathologists should refer clients to such groups if they feel they could benefit from participating in them. Those who have the chronic perseverative stuttering syndrome are particularly likely to do so (Cooper, 1993a). Some speech-language pathologists resist making such referrals (Pill & St. Louis, 1994). According to Cooper (1986):

> *Many factors might be cited to explain the typical professional's lack of enthusiasm for self-help groups. I suspect that one of those factors is the professional's failure to accept the fact . . . that some individuals will continue to stutter no matter what they may do or have done to them and that even some successfully controlled stutterers need such continuing support to maintain their control. Clinicians may be uncomfortable with the existence of groups of individuals who may or may not continue to experience disfluencies but appear to benefit from the association with others with similar experiences. Perhaps professionals experience discomfort believing that they or their colleagues have failed if former clients seek such support. (p. 325)*

Such resistance also can result from misconceptions clinicians have about these groups. They may think, for example, that group members just talk about depressing experiences and feel sorry for themselves. In conclusion, I agree with Diggs (1990, p. 33) that "Consumers are becoming more interested in taking charge of their own lives. Professionals need to recognize this trend and acknowledge the potential benefits of self-help."

The families of persons who stutter—particularly the parents of young children who do so—may also benefit from participating in self-help groups (Aguirrebengoa, 1994).

Self-help groups for persons who stutter or have another fluency disorder exist in many countries. Information about them can be obtained from the European League of Stuttering Associations (ELSA) and the International Stuttering Association (ISA), a worldwide network of national self-help organizations (Pill, 1994). According to Pill (1994):

> *Around the world, support groups are variously termed self-help groups, therapy groups, and maintenance groups among other labels. Some groups dissociate themselves from speech professionals, some are autonomous organizations which communicate and closely cooperate with clinicians, and others function primarily as proponents of particular treatment methods or programs. (p. 201)*

For further information about self-help groups for persons who stutter and their families, see Aguirrebengoa (1994), Alm (1994), Carlisle (1987), Köpf & Christmann (1994), Krauss-Lehrman & Reeves (1989), and Ramig (1993).

While members of self-help groups usually interact face-to-face, other options are possible. Starkweather (1994), for example, has reported on an electronic self-help group in which stutterers interact through e-mail.

In addition to there being self-help groups for persons who stutter and their families, there are self-help books. The Speech Foundation of America has published some that are coauthored by speech-language pathologists regarded as authorities on stuttering (see the books edited by M. Fraser and J. Fraser & Perkins in the reference list). These books are usable for parent counseling and for communicating to teenage and adult clients that their experiences with and feelings about stuttering are not unique and that the disorder can be coped with.

ASSESSING/DOCUMENTING THERAPY OUTCOME

The philosophy of management throughout this chapter (and, indeed, throughout this book) is based on the assumption that management of stuttering usually has two aspects: reduction (or elimination) of abnormal disfluency and reduction of the extent to which the disorder (assuming that it is not cured) interferes with the client's life. Consequently, when assessing/documenting therapy outcome, both aspects should be considered.

What strategies are likely to yield data possessing adequate levels of validity, reliability, and generality for this purpose? Pros and cons of a number of them are discussed in the *Proceedings of the NIDCD Workshop on Treatment Efficacy Research in Stuttering,* which was published in 1993 in the *Journal of Fluency Disorders* (pp. 121–361), and in papers by Hillis (1993) and Franken, Boves, Peters, & Webster (1995).

In my own clinical practice, the strategy I have found most useful for gathering such data is questioning the client and possibly members of his or her family as well as others (such as teachers) who spend a significant amount of time with the client. I ask if aspects of the client's stuttering problem have changed and, if so, how. For gathering such data from the client, the *Stuttering Problem Profile* (see Appendix C) can be helpful: The client is asked for each statement circled whether he or she is any closer to being able to make it than previously.

My decision to evaluate therapy outcome *clinically,* primarily by questioning clients and those with whom they interact, was based on the results of a large-scale study of approaches for evaluating stuttering therapy that was summarized in a report by Drs. Wendell Johnson and William Trotter of the University of Iowa to the federal agency that funded it. The study was done in the late forties or early fifties and, to my knowledge, was never published. One conclusion was that questioning a client about how he or she has changed yields data that are as valid and reliable as those yielded by the twenty or more "objective" measures they evaluated. If a client has changed in any meaningful ways outside of the therapy room, the client and/or members of his or her family are likely to be aware of them. The findings of a recent study by Finn & Ingham (1994), incidentally, in which stutterers were shown to be able to reliably rate an attribute of their "speech quality" tends to support this conclusion.

ASSIGNMENTS

Behavior Modification

Select an aspect of your behavior that you would like to modify and attempt to do so for a period of at least two months. Changes that my students have attempted to make include exercising more frequently, studying on a more regular schedule, losing weight, eating less junk food, keeping their apartments cleaner, biting their fingernails less frequently, being on time more often, watching less TV, and being less "negative" when talking with people. Keep a weekly journal in which you describe your successes and failures as honestly and objectively as you can. What problems did you encounter while doing this assignment? How did your motivation level vary during the months you were "in therapy"? What insights did you gain that hopefully will result in your functioning as a more effective clinician? This assignment is quite similar to one used by Leahy (1994).

Fluency Facilitating Speech Strategy

A number of fluency facilitating speech strategies are described in this chapter. Use one in all communication situations for at least a day. An example you could use for this assignment is "a lengthening of vowels beyond that perceived...[by you] as being normal, short utterance lengths, and the use of frequent pauses" (McKeehan, 1994, p. 114). How did people react while you were using the strategy? How did their reactions affect you? What did you learn while doing this assignment that will affect your use of such strategies with clients? [This assignment is based on one described by McKeehan in her 1994 paper.]

Badge Wearing

One strategy for bringing stuttering out into the open is wearing a badge or a shirt on which a message is printed acknowledging the disorder. There is a store or cart in some shopping malls at which you can have such a badge printed. Have one made that says "I stutter. So what!" and wear it for a day. Did you feel self-conscious at first while wearing it? It you did, were you less self-conscious at the end of the day than you were at the beginning? What reactions, if any, did you get while wearing it? In what situations do you think a stutterer might benefit from doing so?

Certainty Testing

We discussed in this chapter how people are handicapped by their "certainties." Identify one certainty you have that may be handicapping you. If possible, test it and describe what happened when you did so.

Support Group

There are support/self-help groups for persons who stutter in many communities. If there is one in your community, attend a meeting. In what ways did the participants appear likely to benefit from participating in the group? Should speech-language pathologists refer clients to them? Why?

Telecommunication Relay Service

Telecommunication relay services (TRSs) enable a speech-impaired person to communicate by telephone without having to speak. They do so by typing what they want to "say," using either a microcomputer with a modem attached or a telecommunication device for the deaf (TDD). For many stutterers, the telephone situation is one in which they stutter very severely (see Chapter 2). Make at least two calls using your state's TRS. Under what circumstances might a stutterer benefit from using one?

▶ 8

Other Fluency Disorders

Our focus in previous chapters has been on the most frequently occurring and most thoroughly researched disorder of fluency—stuttering. Here it will be on the symptomatology, phenomenology, etiology, and management of five other fluency disorders—cluttering, neurogenic acquired stuttering, psychogenic acquired stuttering (hysterical stuttering), acquired stuttering following laryngectomy, and spastic dysphonia. While the latter—spastic dysphonia—usually is not classified as a fluency disorder, there is reason to believe that at least some cases should be (Salamy & Sessions, 1980; Silverman & Hummer, 1989). We also will briefly consider stutter-like disfluencies in manual communication, stuttering-like behavior during the playing of wind instruments, and malingering. The chapter ends with a description of the differential diagnostic procedure used to distinguish stuttering from cluttering, neurogenic acquired stuttering, and psychogenic acquired stuttering.

Much of the information about management presented in Chapters 6 and 7 is relevant to these disorders. The problems with which a client who has them must cope can be conceptualized as consisting of a set of behaviors, some of which also are found in the sets of persons who stutter. This is particularly likely to be true for behaviors that can cause clients to limit their activities, that is, be handicapped. The stuttering simulation assignment at the end of Chapter 1, incidentally, also provides insights into how listeners tend to react to persons who have one of these fluency disorders.

CLUTTERING (TACHYPHEMIA)

Cluttering, or tachyphemia, is a disorder that begins during childhood and is thought by some to have a genetic basis (Arnold, 1965; Myers & St. Louis, 1992). It is reported to have been first differentiated from stuttering in 1830 by Colombat (Weiss, 1964). The disorder has received considerably more attention in the European literature than in American (St. Louis & Rustin, 1992). In fact, until recently most of those who wrote about it in the American literature were Europeans. According to Daly (1986):

> *American speech-language pathologists have not, by and large, accepted cluttering as a clinical entity, nor have they incorporated information about cluttering into their clinical decision-making processes. Although considerable literature on cluttering exists, American authors treat the problem of cluttering in a most cursory manner. Typically, only a paragraph or two are devoted to this ill-understood disorder. Many authors omit any mention of cluttering. (p. 156)*

During the past decade it received more attention in the English-language literature than it had previously (e.g., Daly, 1986, 1993a, 1993b; Diedrich, 1984; Myers & St. Louis, 1992; St. Louis, 1993; St. Louis & Hinzman, 1986; St. Louis, Hinzman, & Hull, 1985; Tiger, Irvine, & Reis, 1980).

Unfortunately, like stuttering, there is no universally agreed-upon definition for this disorder. One of the most accepted (judging by the frequency with which it has been referred to in papers on cluttering) appears to be that of Weiss (1964):

> *Cluttering is a speech disorder characterized by the clutterer's unawareness of his disorder, by a short attention span, by disturbances in perception, articulation and formulation of speech, and often by excessive speed of delivery. It is a disorder of the thought processes preparatory to speech and based on a hereditary disposition. Cluttering is a verbal manifestation of Central Language Imbalance, which affects all channels of communication (e.g., reading, writing, rhythm, and musicality) and behavior in general. (p. 1)*

Weiss, then, views cluttering as one manifestation (symptom) of a generalized disturbance in language functioning—one "tip" of a submerged iceberg (see Figure 8-1).

Daly's definition of cluttering (1993b) describes the speech and language processing disturbances of persons who have the disorder in more detail:

> *Cluttering is a disorder of both speech and language processing that frequently results in rapid, disrhythmic, sporadic, unorganized, and often unintelligible speech. Accelerated speech (or tachylalia) is not always present, but impairments in formulating language almost always are.... Those who clutter confuse their listeners with incomplete and awkward sentences, false starts, sound sequencing errors, and word-retrieval prob-*

FIGURE 8-1 **Cluttering viewed as one symptom of a generalized central language imbalance. (*Source:* From Weiss, 1964.)**

lems. Their garbled speech is confounded by a lack of clarity of inner language formulation. Equally frustrating for clinicians are the absence of self-awareness and unconcerned attitude of many clients who clutter. Their self-monitoring skills for speech and social situations are deficient. (p. 7)

What specific symptoms (speech, language, and behavioral) and other characteristics *may* be exhibited or shared by persons who have this disorder? St. Louis & Hinzman (1986) compiled the list in Table 8-1 from six publications dealing with the symptomatology and etiology of cluttering. Few persons who clutter are likely to exhibit all of them. However, judging by the data presented in this table and other literature on cluttering (including the study by St. Louis, Hinzman, & Hull, 1985), there are certain symptoms that tend to be manifested by most persons who have the disorder. These include a rapid speaking rate, speech disfluencies (particularly repetitions), a lack of awareness of the disorder (including the disfluencies and the rapid speaking rate), and articulation and language problems. St. Louis & Hinzman (1986) synthesized the following description of persons who have this disorder from the data they distilled from the literature (see Table 8-1):

Their speech is noticeable because it usually sounds "cluttered" as though they are talking without a clear idea of what they want to say. Their conversation is hard to follow because they seem to talk too fast, in a jerky fashion, and seem to run words and sentences together. Clutterers may also repeat sounds, syllables, or phrases excessively. Despite these characteristics, they are typically unaware of any difficulty and may be talkative and outgoing.

TABLE 8-1 **A sampling of symptoms and other characteristics that the literature associates with cluttering.**

Symptom
Fast speech rate
Run-on sentences
Disorganized thinking
Irregular speech rate
Unawareness of the problem
Word repetitions
Sound/syllable repetitions
Phrase repetitions
Inability to get to the point
Reduced attention span
Revisions
Academic achievement difficulties
Misarticulations
Poor syntax
Circumlocutions
Interjection overuse
Motor coordination problems
Language delay
Learning disabilities
Struggle during speech
Neurological impairment
Tension during speech
Prolongations
Handwriting difficulties
Family history of cluttering
Monotone speech
Social maladjustment
Secondary behaviors
Poor music abilities

Source: From St. Louis & Hinzman, 1986.

Clutterers may also have academic problems in various subjects, yet they may or may not be severe enough to require specialized educational placement. In fact, some clutterers may excel in certain areas, such as in mathematics.

Overall, clutterers seem disorganized, always in a hurry, and unable to concentrate, perhaps due to a poorly developed attention span. In many things a clutterer does—speaking, writing, reading or working at specific activities—there is a curious tendency to function in constant disarray. (pp. 134–135)

The speech disfluency of clutterers has been reported to differ from that of stutterers in several ways (see Table 8-2). The first concerns level of awareness of it. Stutterers tend to be aware of their disfluencies, but clutterers do not.

Clutterers, like stutterers, tend to be more fluent in some situations than in others. However, the impacts of some situations on their fluency levels is quite different (see Table 8-2). While stutterers tend to be *less* fluent when they feel it is important to be fluent, clutterers tend to be *more* fluent in this circumstance. Thus, stutterers tend to be less fluent with authority figures than with young children, and clutterers tend to be less fluent with young children than with authority figures.

Asking clutterers to pay attention to their speech usually results in less disfluency—at least for a few minutes after they are told to do so (see Table 8-2). Asking stutterers to attend more to their speech usually results in increased disfluency.

Some children seem more likely than others to develop cluttering. Like stuttering, more males than females develop the disorder (Myers & St. Louis, 1992). And,

TABLE 8-2   **Differences between stuttering and cluttering.**

	Cluttering	**Stuttering**
Awareness of disorder	Absent	Present
Speaking under stress	Better	Worse
Speaking in relaxed situation	Worse	Better
Calling attention to speech	Better	Worse
Speaking after interruption	Better	Worse
Short answers	Better	Worse
Foreign language	Better	Worse
Reading a well known text	Worse	Better
Reading an unknown text	Better	Worse
Handwriting	Hasty, repetitious, uninhibited	Contracted, forced, inhibited
Attitude toward own speech	Careless	Fearful
Psychological attitude	Outgoing	Rather withdrawn
Aptitude (academic)	Underachiever	Good to superior
EEG	Often diffuse dysrhythmia	Usually normal
Goal of therapy	Directing attention to speech details	Diverting attention from speech details

Source: From Weiss, 1967.

also like stuttering, it is more likely to occur in families in which there is a history of the disorder than in those in which there is no such history (Myers & St. Louis, 1992).

As Weiss (1964) and others have noted, clutterers appear to have a language disorder in addition to a fluency one. Children who have this disorder are more likely to be delayed in language development than are their peers (Daly, 1992).

While stuttering and cluttering are separate disorders, a person can have both (Arnold, 1965; Daly, 1986, 1993b; Freund, 1966; Grewel, 1970; Preus, 1987, 1992; Weiss, 1964; Winkelman, 1994). Daly (1993b), based on a review of the literature, has estimated that between one-third and two-thirds of stutterers exhibit some symptoms associated with cluttering. According to Freund (1966):

> In a typical case of cluttering-stuttering, the expectancy of difficult speech sounds, tonic efforts, postponements and avoidance devices, etc., are much less marked than in typical cases of common ... stuttering. In the former, the stutter symptoms, consisting usually of quick reiterations often of vowels within or between syllables with not too much effort combined, vary in direct proportion to the severity of the underlying "cluttering." The latter can be clinically defined as an overly hasty and poorly organized speech. (pp. 140–141)

Treatment Strategies

There appears to be good agreement among authorities that persons who have this disorder are abnormally disfluent because they do not monitor their speech adequately (e.g., Daly, 1986, 1993b; Luchinger & Arnold, 1965; Weiss, 1964). This may also be the reason for their language and articulation disorders (Myers, 1992). Consequently, they usually aren't aware of their disfluency and other speech-language disorders (Daly, 1986). Although they usually do not monitor their speech adequately, they apparently can do so judging by the fact that they tend to be more fluent when performing a task that requires them to pay attention to how they talk—as in reading unfamiliar material or speaking a foreign language (see Table 8-2). Therefore, to reduce their disfluency, it is necessary to get them to monitor their speech more carefully.

Their lack of self-monitoring affects aspects of their speaking behavior other than fluency. Their rate of speaking tends to be excessive, and they make frequent errors related to language formulation and expression (Luchinger & Arnold, 1965). The general disturbance in speech-language functioning of many persons who have this disorder caused Weiss (1964) to hypothesize that cluttering is one manifestation (symptom) of a central language imbalance in the area of verbal utterances (see Figure 8-1). This underlying condition (portion of the "iceberg below the surface"), according to Weiss (1964), also produces disorders that are not directly related to speech and language functioning (see Figure 8-1). Clients who have this disorder, therefore, are also likely to have others that require treatment.

One problem likely to be encountered (at least at first) when working with clients who clutter is lack of motivation. Most are seen by speech-language pathologists because they are told by someone (usually a parent, teacher, or employer) that they need therapy. Their attitude upon being told so is likely to be negative. According to Daly (1986):

> *cluttering children are frequently confused by a listener's inability to understand their speech. Clutterers accept no blame for the communication breakdown, thinking instead that the listener should pay closer attention. Adolescent and adult clutterers are annoyed and often angered by the persistent attempts of teachers or speech-language pathologists to find a problem, when in the clutterers' minds none exists. (The author has treated a number of salesmen who clutter. Their sales managers insisted that treatment be obtained because customers had complained that the salesmen were difficult to understand. Even when therapy was mandatory to maintain employment, some adult clutterers would not take their speech treatment seriously. They preferred to believe that their boss was being "hard-nosed" or unreasonable.) (pp. 159–160)*

It may be possible to motivate clutterers to invest in therapy by making them more aware of the effect that improved self-monitoring has on their speech and by having them receive positive reinforcement for attempting to improve it, particularly from those who previously complained about it. The first can be accomplished by having them listen to tape-recordings of their speech, *both* while they are and are not adequately monitoring it (Daly, 1987). And the second can be done by making persons who are concerned about their speech aware of the importance of providing such reinforcement (Daly, 1986).

Lack of motivation isn't the only problem encountered when working with clutterers. Because their fluency tends to increase significantly when they speak at a rate slower than their usual one, usually one goal of therapy is to encourage them to do so. However, many clutterers cannot tolerate speaking at such a rate unless they are desensitized to doing so. Van Riper (1992) has suggested several strategies for desensitizing a clutterer to a slower speaking rate:

> *At first don't ask him to speak slowly even though, when he does so, his communication will markedly improve. You'll find that he cannot tolerate the slower rate. Instead, find other ways of slowing him down until that tolerance is increased. Try reading in unison and begin by using a very fast rate yourself, then gradually returning to a more normal rate. Have him learn to shadow your speech and then the speech of others. Have him repeat phrases and sentences that you utter with different tempos. Have him write down the words he wants to say before saying them. Have him tap the words of his forthcoming utterance before he speaks them or hums them.*

Record samples of his rapid, confused speech, desensitize him to them, then have him translate. Have him teach you how to speak clutteringly. Using recorded speech samples, jointly analyze the omissions, repetitions, slurrings, and other cluttering features. With prepared written material teach him how to clutter on purpose before trying to say it better. Have him echo both your deliberately cluttered speech and then your normal version. Using more prepared sentences, have him read them faster and faster until complete breakdown occurs, then listen to the recording.

A most valuable technique is to teach him to pause and to tolerate that pause for increasing lengths of time. For this you will have to use modeling and various signals to indicate when to stop and when to get going again. Adequate pausing will slow down his speech more than any amount of exhortation to talk slowly. The clutterer's speech is highly disorganized and he needs some training in this area. . . . Have him paraphrase things he reads or what you tell him. . . . Do some role playing of situations in which he must speak coherently such as applying for a job or asking for a date or giving directions to a stranger hunting for a store. (p. viii)

Other authors also have suggested strategies for encouraging clutterers to monitor their speech more closely and to develop tolerance for a slower speaking rate. They include the following:

- Having clients use a miniature masking noise generator, such as the Edinburgh Masker, while speaking (Dewar, Dewar, & Anthony, 1976). The resulting disturbance in auditory feedback causes them to concentrate more than usual on how they are speaking.
- Having clients pace their speech with a metronome (Tiger, Irvine, & Reis, 1980). Doing so would cause them to concentrate more on how they are speaking and thus reduce their speaking rate.
- Using a delayed auditory feedback (DAF) device to desensitize clients to slower speech (Daly, 1992). If they can learn to tolerate slow, distorted DAF speech, they will almost certainly be better able to tolerate a slower speaking rate.
- Telling clients to pronounce each syllable slowly, giving each syllable equal stress (Weiss, 1964). The resultant speech sounds similar to the one produced by a DAF machine. This exercise tends to heighten their awareness of tactile and kinesthetic feedback (Daly, 1986).
- Having the client practice reading material aloud, the words in which are exposed one at a time through a hole, a "window," in a sheet of paper at a relatively slow rate. This exercise can be used to desensitize a client to slower speech. (See Daly, 1988, for structured therapy materials and evaluation forms for this task.)
- Having clients count backward by a specific amount (ones, twos, threes, or fours) to increase their concentration (Weiss, 1964).

- Having clients speak in unison with or "shadow" (see Chapter 2) tape-recordings made by the clinician in the which the rate/prosody are appropriate. Ham (1988) has described in detail a program that can be used for this purpose.
- Having clients visualize themselves speaking fluently in as many situations and with as many people as possible, including those who have reacted negatively to their speech (Daly, 1988; Daly, Thompson, & Simon, 1985).
- Encouraging clients to watch videotapes of themselves both while they are and are not adequately monitoring their speech (see Daly, 1987).
- Using Shames & Florance's (1980) Stutter-Free Speech Program. Daly (1986) has reported some success using a modified version of the program with clutterers. He concluded that this program was beneficial because "Their emphasis on slow, smooth speech initiations and continuous phonation, first with delayed feedback and later without it, provides the clutterer with concrete, verifiable components of the speech act that can also be monitored" (Daly, 1986, p. 181).

How likely is a person who has this disorder to be completely cured? The prognosis for a cure is poor, but better for children than for adults (Daly, 1986, 1993b; Luchinger & Arnold, 1965; Myers & St. Louis, 1992; Weiss, 1964).

For further information about the symptomatology, etiology, and management of cluttering, see Arnold (1965), Bradford (1963), Dalton & Hardcastle (1977), Daly (1986, 1992, 1993b), Freund, (1966), Luchinger & Arnold (1965), Myers & St. Louis (1992), St. Louis & Hinzman (1986), St. Louis, Hinzman, & Hull (1985), *Studies in Tachyphemia* (undated), Tiger, Irvine, & Reis (1980), and Weiss (1964).

NEUROGENIC-ACQUIRED STUTTERING

A number of case descriptions of stuttering acquired during childhood (see Aram, Meyers, & Ekelman, 1990; Meyers, Hall, & Aram, 1990; Nass, Schreter, & Heier, 1994) and adulthood (see Abe, Yokoyama, & Yorifuji, 1992, 1993; Andy & Bhatnagar, 1991, 1992; Ardila & Lopez, 1986; Balasubramanian & Hayden, 1994; Bhatnagar & Andy, 1989; Byrne, Byrne, & Zibin, 1993; Canter, 1971; Chen & Peng, 1993; Culatta & Leeper, 1988; Davis, 1993; Fleet & Heilman, 1985; Freeman, 1982; Helm, Butler, & Benson, 1978; Helm, Butler, & Canter, 1980; Helm-Estabrooks, 1986, 1993; Hertrich & Ackermann, 1994; Horner & Massey, 1983; Lebrun & Leleux, 1985; Lebrun, Leleux, Rousseau, & Devreux, 1983; Ludlow, Rosenberg, Salazar, Grafman, & Smutok, 1987; Market, Montague, Buffalo, & Drummond, 1990; Mavlov, 1994; Mazzucchi, Moretti, Carpeggiani, Parma, & Paini, 1981; McClean & McLean, 1985; Nagafuchi, 1994; Nass, Schreter, & Heier, 1994; Nowack & Stone, 1987; Quinn & Andrews, 1977; Rao, 1991; Rosenbek, Messert, Collins, & Wertz, 1978; Sakai, Miyamura, & Kuzuhara, 1992; Stewart & Grantham, 1993; Weiner, 1981) following damage to the central nervous system have appeared in the literature. Most of these pertain to persons who had no history of stuttering, and whose onset of the disorder (which was usually sudden) was associated with a neurological event. A few of them pertain to persons who experienced a recurrence or worsening of childhood stuttering following brain damage. The neurological events with which the onset of their stuttering was associated included strokes, head trauma, extrapyramidal diseases, tumors, dementia, drug usage, anoxia, and cryosurgery (Helm-Estabrooks, 1986). Their disorder was referred to as neurogenic-acquired stuttering, stuttering associated with acquired neurological disorders (SAAND), neurogenic stuttering, acquired stuttering, neurological stuttering, neurological disfluency, cortical stuttering, or stuttering of sudden onset.

The types of abnormal disfluency behaviors observed in the speech of persons who have this disorder include repetitions and/or dysrhythmic phonations. The specific symptomatology is determined, in part, by the neurological condition (site of lesion) with which the disorder is associated. The following three descriptions from published case reports are representative:

1. *A 62-year-old man who had a stroke:* Conversational speech was characterized chiefly by repetitions of syllables and short words and by sound prolongations, for example, "be-be-because," "until-til," and "I was, I was, I was..." Repetitions were dysrhythmic and both clonic and tonic in nature. He frequently attempted to avoid disfluencies by pausing and restarting phrases. (Helm-Estabrooks, 1986, p. 196)

2. *A 22-year-old woman who had an episode diagnosed as viral meningitis:* She stuttered on 95 percent of the words she spoke, repeating initial consonants four to six times and medial consonants three to four times. The stuttering was not specific to any phoneme or group of phonemes. There was no adaptation effect. Whispering made no difference. She demonstrated marked effort in the production of speech but not poor eye contact, distracting sounds, or excessive body movement. (Nowack & Stone, 1987, pp. 142–143)

3. *A 62-year-old man with right cerebral damage:* Disfluency was characterized by sound, syllable, word, and phrase reiterations. Word and phrase repetitions were more frequent than sound and part-word repetitions. The latter occurred primarily in initial position, while word and phrase iterations could occur anywhere in the sentence, including at the end.... On one occasion, the target sentence *I can't walk* was actualized as "can't-can't-can't-can't walk-can't-can't-can't walk-can't-can't-walk." Having been asked what a robin was, the patient answered, "A bird-a bird-a-a-a bird-bird-bird-bird, a robin-robin is a bird b-b-b-b-b-bird." Dysfluencies were more numerous in spontaneous speech than in repetition and in oral reading. Few iterations occurred in recitation and none could be observed in singing. (Lebrun & Leleux, 1985, p. 138)

While the symptomatology of this disorder appears to vary, in part, depending on the neurological condition with which it is associated, are there characteristics other than time and nature of onset that tend to differentiate it from stuttering? Canter (1971) has suggested seven such characteristics, all of which he cautions are *unlikely* to apply to any one client:

1. Repetitions and prolongations are not restricted to initial syllables.
2. The phonemic foci of the dysfluencies may differ from developmental stuttering, that is, the /r/, /l/, /h/ sounds may be targets for dysfluency.
3. There is no particular relationship between dysfluency and the grammatical function of words, so that small function words may be as troublesome as substantives.
4. Dysfluency is not necessarily in direct relationship to propositionality, so that self-formulated speech may be easier than more automatic speech tasks such as the Lord's Prayer.
5. There is no observed adaptation effect, that is, improved fluency with repeated readings of a passage.
6. The speaker may be annoyed, but not necessarily anxious, about his stuttering.
7. There may be no secondary symptomatology such as facial grimacing or fist clenching.

While Lebrun et al. (1983) have raised questions concerning whether these are characteristics of the speech of most adults with the disorder, Market et al. (1990) have reported data that provide some support for their being so, particularly for the first, second, sixth, and seventh characteristics.

Treatment Strategies

Several strategies that have been suggested for reducing the abnormal disfluency associated with this disorder are described here.

Word-retrieval deficits appear to be at least partially responsible for the abnormal disfluency exhibited by some persons who have this disorder (Brown & Cullinan, 1981; Meyers et al., 1990). It has been suggested that teaching a delay strategy to provide more time for word retrieval may be one way to reduce such disfluency (Linebaugh, 1984). One such strategy is self-monitoring.

Whitney and Goldstein (1989) described a self-monitoring program they found successful in reducing the disfluency of three mild aphasics. Three disfluency types were used as target behaviors: repetition (part-word, word, and phrase), interjection, and revision (see Chapter 1). Target behaviors are treated one at a time. The program consists of the following four steps:

Step 1. Clients listen to tape-recordings of their speech while their clinician points out instances of the target behavior to them. The purpose is to begin to make them aware of the behavior they are to self-monitor.

Step 2. Clients listen to other tape-recordings of their speech and signal (e.g., activate a counter) each time they hear the target behavior. If they do not signal an instance within three seconds after it occurs, the clinician stops the tape and points it out to them. If they accurately identify most instances, this would suggest that they understand what their clinician wants them to self-monitor.

Step 3. Clients self-monitor while performing a speaking task (such as describing a picture). They are told to signal each time they produce the target behavior, in the same way they did in Step 2. If they do not signal an instance within three seconds, the clinician stops them and points out the target behavior, using a recording.

Step 4. Clients self-monitor while performing the speaking task used in Step 3 without the clinician providing feedback and reinforcement. Their performance is recorded and the amount of the target behavior they evince is compared to that in a recording they made before beginning the training program. If there is less of the target behavior in the post- than in the preintervention recording, this would suggest that self-monitoring could be helpful for decreasing their disfluency. They would then be encouraged and trained to use it outside the clinic environment.

Whitney & Goldstein (1989) used this program for more than ten sessions with each client. It probably would take considerable practice before most clients would be able to self-monitor successfully during nonstructured conversational speech.

This strategy may also be worth trying with clients who are excessively disfluent for other reasons—such as a relatively mild dysarthria—because it reduces their speaking rate. To determine whether a client would be likely to benefit from the use of this strategy, have him or her speak at a very slow rate. If doing so results in increased fluency, it is likely that he or she would be helped by self-monitoring.

Several other strategies have been suggested for reducing the speaking rates of clients who exhibit this type of disfluency. These include having them pace their speech in a syllable-by-syllable manner auditorily with the beats of a metronome or tactilely with a pacing board (Helm-Estabrooks, 1986). With the latter, the client taps his or her finger from square to square while speaking in this manner (see Helm-Estabrooks, 1986, for a drawing of this board and further information about tactile pacing). Other strategies that have been suggested for this purpose include speaking under the condition of delayed auditory feedback (Helm-Estabrooks, 1986).

Fluency-enhancing strategies used for treating stuttering—including utilizing a slow rate, learning to initiate phonation with an easy onset, and systematic desensitization—have also been used with such clients (Market et al., 1990; Meyers et al., 1990; Rousey, Arjunan, & Rousey, 1986).

Thus far, the discussion has been on treating clients with neurogenic-acquired stuttering by encouraging them to speak in a manner that will cause the abnormal disfluency to occur less frequently. Since the disorder results from the abnormal functioning of one or more structures in the central nervous system (Lebrun, Leleux, & Retif, 1987; Ludlow et al., 1987), if it were possible to reduce the extent to which they malfunction, it also would be possible to reduce the disfluency that results from that malfunction. There is some evidence that it may be possible to treat the disorder in this manner. Bhatnagar and Andy (1989), for example, have described a person with this disorder who had a thalamic stimulation electrode implanted because of chronic pain. Within the first three weeks of daily self-stimulation, a noticeable reduction was reported in the client's disfluency. After two months, the client was reported to have become almost normally fluent. A two-and-a-half-year posttherapy followup indicated that he had not relapsed. (In another paper [Andy & Bhatnagar, 1991], incidentally, they reported that electrical stimulation at the same thalamic site in a normal speaker during surgery resulted in abnormal disfluency.) Also, Manders & Bastijns (1988) described a child with this disorder who recovered after an epileptic attack—a condition that by causing further damage that may have normalized the functioning of some structure in the central nervous system. Others (Helm, Yeo, Geschwind, Freedman, & Wenstein, 1986; Jones, 1966; Van Riper, 1982) have reported similar outcomes. Perhaps, sometime in the future, it will be possible to normalize the functioning of such structures through the use of pharmacological agents (Helm-Estabrooks, 1986).

For further information about this disorder, see Freeman (1982), Helm et al. (1980), Helm-Estabrooks (1986, 1993), and Lebrun et al. (1983).

PSYCHOGENIC-ACQUIRED STUTTERING (HYSTERICAL STUTTERING)

A number of reports of stuttering acquired during adulthood at least partially as a reaction to acute or chronic psychological disturbances have appeared in the literature (e.g., Attanasio, 1987a; Bluemel, 1935, 1957; Breuer & Freud, 1936; Deal, 1982; Deal & Doro, 1987; Dempsey & Granich, 1978; Freund, 1966; Luchinger & Arnold, 1965; Mahr & Leith, 1992; Preacher & Harris, 1946; Roth et al., 1989; Wallen, 1961). These are reports of persons who did not appear to have a childhood history of stuttering and the onset of their disorder—which was usually sudden and could not be accounted for solely on the basis of central nervous system damage—appeared to be associated with some form of psychological stress (Roth et al., 1989). One young man, for example, suddenly began to stutter after his ship received a direct missile hit during the Korean conflict (Dempsey & Granich, 1978). Another suddenly began doing so during an acute anxiety attack (Wallen, 1961). And a third is reported to have started stuttering when his marriage began to experience difficulty (Attanasio, 1987a). In some cases, the presence of psychopathology was established through performance on the Minnesota Multiphasic Personality Inventory (MMPI) (Roth et al., 1989).

What behaviors are exhibited by persons who have this disorder and how does it develop? The following list of symptoms and onset characteristics that *may* at least partially define this disorder was adapted from one developed by Deal (1982, p. 304):

1. The onset is sudden.
2. The onset is related to a significant event that could have resulted in extreme psychological stress.

3. The abnormal disfluency behavior consists primarily of repetition of initial or stressed syllables.

4. This disfluency behavior is affected little by choral reading, white noise, delayed auditory feedback, singing, or other conditions that have been reported to influence the disfluency behavior of "ordinary" stutterers (Starkweather, 1987).

5. There may be no conditions under which a person who has this disorder is completely fluent.

6. The person may appear to have an indifferent attitude toward the disorder. "He seems to feel no responsibility for what he does. He is relatively detached from the symptom" (Freund, 1966, p. 139). This phenomenon has been referred to in the psychiatric literature as *la belle indifférence* (Roth et al., 1989).

7. The person does not exhibit secondary symptoms. He or she does not appear to avoid sounds, words, or speaking situations.

8. The person maintains normal eye contact (Freund, 1966; Deal & Doro, 1987).

9. The person may evidence the same pattern of repetitions during mimed reading aloud. This phenomenon also was reported by Deal & Doro (1987). "The continuation of stuttering-like behaviors during miming may be analogous to Hoover's sign, which is observed in some hysterias. When a supine patient is asked to lift one leg, the other leg also tends to lift; however, this action is absent in patients presenting hysterical paralysis of one leg. It is as if the patient's mind is unaware of body mechanics. By analogy [the patient with this disorder may be unaware] that stuttering-like movements rarely occur when miming words." (Deal, 1982, p. 304)

Hence, a typical patient who has this disorder is an adult, with no previous history of stuttering, who suddenly begins to stutter after (or while) experiencing a great deal of psychological stress and who has no neurological condition that could account for the behavior. Furthermore, the patient's disfluency may not vary on a situational basis and he or she may not exhibit any behavior that indicates a desire to avoid it.

Treatment Strategies

The treatment of clients who have this disorder may require a combination of psychotherapy and speech therapy (Roth et al., 1989). With regard to the speech therapy component of management, they are,

> *as a group, receptive and responsive to speech therapy, if the same techniques used in the treatment of adult stuttering that originates in childhood are applied.... When patients are persuaded that they have greater-than-expected capacity for fluent speech and are shown how to decrease the severity of stuttering blocks through the use of such traditional techniques as easy onset of voicing, light touch, or bounce during phonatory or articulatory blocking or struggle, their stuttering can diminish or disappear. A*

> *strong attitude of clinician encouragement and optimism seemed to be an*
> *indispensable component of such therapy. (Roth et al., 1989, p. 64).*

If there is any doubt about the client's emotional health, he or she should be referred
to a psychologist or psychiatrist for evaluation (Roth et al., 1989).

For further information about this disorder, see Arnold (1965, pp. 781–782),
Deal (1982), Freund (1966, pp. 139–140), Mahr & Leith (1992), and Roth et al.
(1989).

SPASTIC DYSPHONIA (SPASMODIC DYSPHONIA)

The focus in this chapter has been on disorders that are usually labeled as fluency ones.
Might there be others that are not usually labeled as such? A number of comments in
the literature (see Aronson, 1990; Arnold, 1959; Boone, 1987; Cannito, Vogel, Deal,
& Watson, 1995; Luchinger & Arnold, 1965; Salamy & Sessions, 1980; Silverman &
Hummer, 1989) suggest that there is such as disorder—spastic dysphonia.

Spastic dysphonia has been referred to by clinicians as "stammering of the vocal
cords and laryngeal stuttering" (Aronson, 1973) and the resultant speech has been
labeled "disfluent" by listeners (Silverman & Hummer, 1989). Persons who have
spastic dysphonia (specifically, adductor spastic dysphonia) evince "a repeated
blockage of phonation by spasms of the adductor muscles of the larynx, resulting in
an intermittently strangled, choked utterance" (Bloodstein, 1984, p. 204). The severity of their problem appears to vary on a situational basis. According to Boone
(1987):

> *The patient may experience a normal voice in some situations, such as talk-*
> *ing to a cat, repeating a memorized verse, or singing. It is no wonder that*
> *spastic dysphonia has been described as "laryngeal stutter"...with the*
> *faulty voice varying in severity according to how the speaker views the lis-*
> *tener. The more critical the communicative act, such as giving one's name*
> *to a ticket seller on the telephone, the more likely it is that the laryngeal*
> *tightness will occur and the voice will be shut off. (p. 285)*

Persons with this disorder also have been reported to speak normally when reading
in chorus, speaking to children, and speaking when no listener is present (Arnold,
1959) and to demonstrate the adaptation effect—that is, the number of strain-stran-
gle syllables decreases significantly during successive readings of a passage (Salamy
& Sessions, 1980).

The symptomatology and phenomenology of stuttering and spastic dysphonia
seem similar. Both disorders are characterized by intermittent disturbances in the
ability to control the musculature of the speech mechanism (particularly that of the
larynx) in the manner necessary to produce fluent speech. Also, the severity of both

disorders varies on a situational basis. In fact, both stuttering and spastic dysphonia appear to increase and decrease in severity under the same conditions.

The etiology of spastic dysphonia, like that of stuttering, has not definitely been established. Some writers (e.g., Aronson, Brown, Litin, & Pearson, 1968; Aronson & Hartman, 1981; Biller, Som, & Lawson, 1979; Dedo, 1976; McCall, Skolnick, & Brewer, 1971; Robe, Brumlik, & Moore, 1960; Schaefer, Gerling, Finitzo-Hieber, & Freeman, in press) regard it as being primarily neurological, possibly resulting from some degenerative process in the central nervous system. They feel the fact that its onset is during middle age, and that some persons with the disorder exhibit neurological abnormalities, supports their position. Others (e.g., Arnold, 1959; Bloch, 1965; Brodnitz, 1976; Heaver, 1959; Luchinger & Arnold, 1965) regard it as psychological. They feel the fact that its onset appears to be related to some psychological trauma and that persons with it can speak normally at times supports their position. More writers appear to regard its etiology as psychological rather than neurological (Bloodstein, 1984).

While the symptomatology, phenomenology, and possibly etiology, of stuttering and spastic dysphonia seem to be similar, their age of onset and their relative frequencies of occurrence among males and females are not. While, as we have previously noted, most cases of stuttering have their onset in early childhood, most cases of spastic dysphonia begin during middle age. And while stuttering tends to occur far more often in males than in females, spastic dysphonia does not. In fact, several authors (see Arnold, 1959) have reported that it occurs more often in females than in males.

Treatment Strategies

A number of approaches for treating persons who have this disorder have been tried, including psychotherapy (Brodnitz, 1976; D'Asaro, 1978; Fox, 1969), biofeedback (Henschen & Burton, 1978), medication such as a Botulinum injection (Brodnitz, 1976), and surgery (Aminoff, Dedo, & Izedebski, 1978; Dedo, 1976). Results overall do not appear to have been very good. Surgery is the one reported to be the most successful (Salamy & Sessions, 1980).

I am aware of only one report in the literature (Meyers & Anderson, 1985) in which a program for enhancing the fluency of persons who stutter was used with a client who had spastic dysphonia. The approach used was the one developed by Shames & Florance (1980). The authors reported intervention was successful—that is, it resulted in a reduction of vocal fold hyperadduction. Regardless of whether spastic dysphonia is a stuttering-type disorder or simply responds to certain approaches that have been helpful with stutterers, the fact that it may be possible to alleviate the condition without surgery is encouraging!

For further information about spastic dysphonia see Aronson (1973), Aronson et al. (1968), Luchinger & Arnold (1965), and Salamy & Sessions (1980).

ACQUIRED STUTTERING FOLLOWING LARYNGECTOMY

There have been several reports (Freeman & Rosenfield, 1982; Irving & Webb, 1961; Tuck, 1979; Wingate, 1981b) about the postoperative speech fluency of stutterers who have had a laryngectomy. These reports suggest that some persons continue to stutter after relearning to speak using esophageal speech or an electrolarynx.

There is also evidence that suggests stuttering may be acquired following a laryngectomy. Rosenfield and Freeman (1983) have described two cases in which this presumably occurred. The first was of a 71-year-old-man who claimed to have stuttered for one year following a laryngectomy performed at age 59. The second was of a man who was still stuttering when contacted by the authors:

> *C. M. had also been a fluent speaker prior to his laryngectomy. He is 67 years old, right-handed, and has stuttered since his surgery at age 63. There is no family history of stuttering. He has used a Western Electric electrolarynx for more than 3 years. He exhibited dysfluencies including multiple, whole- and part-word repetitions, interjections, and occasional prolongations. He demonstrates struggle behaviors and experiences extreme frustration associated with the disfluency problem. He was independently judged by two experienced speech pathologists to be a stutterer. (Rosenfield & Freeman, 1983, p. 266)*

Since these, to my knowledge, are the only reports of this type of fluency disorder, it is probably a relatively rare phenomenon. However, it apparently is not unusual for laryngectomized patients to be highly disfluent at the early stages of relearning speech (Freeman & Rosenfield, 1982).

STUTTER-LIKE DISFLUENCIES IN MANUAL COMMUNICATION

Many persons who are severely speech impaired because they are deaf, mentally retarded, or autistic use manual communication (signing) alone or in combination with speech. The simultaneous use of both is referred to as "total" communication. There have been a few reports of persons with these disorders who exhibit stutter-like disfluencies while signing (Liles, Lerman, Christensen, & St. Ledger, 1992; Montgomery & Fitch, 1988; Silverman & Silverman, 1971). The types of stutter-like disfluencies observed in manual communication include part-word repetitions, word repetitions, and prolongations. For the persons reported on who used total communication, the signing disfluencies were sometimes accompanied by speech disfluencies and at other times not.

While it appears quite likely that there is a fluency disorder that can affect manual communication, its prevalence, symptomatology, etiology, and management are uncertain. Fortunately, it appears to be quite rare: Montgomery and Fitch (1988) identified only 12 cases in the 9,930 hearing-impaired students they surveyed.

It is not particularly surprising that users of manual communication can develop a fluency disorder. Certainly, conditions that result in neurogenic-acquired stuttering and psychogenic acquired stuttering could as easily affect the musculature of the upper extremities as that of the mouth. Many of the conditions that have been hypothesized to cause stuttering could also do so. These include hypotheses that view stuttering as an anticipatory-struggle behavior or as resulting from demands exceeding capacities (see Chapter 5).

WIND INSTRUMENT STUTTERING

There have been two case reports of stuttering-like behavior occurring during the playing of a wind instrument. One involved the flute (Silverman & Bohlman, 1988) and the other the French horn (Meltzer, 1992). Both persons were stutterers. Meltzer (1992) described the stuttering-like behavior on the French horn as follows:

> *a blocking of the flow of sound as a result of closure and tightening in the throat and a breakdown in coordination of tonguing movements. The frequency of occurrence varied, increasing under conditions of fatigue, stress, anticipation, speed, and the need to maintain a high standard of performance. (p. 260)*

Since playing a wind instrument uses the same muscle groups as does speech—respiratory, laryngeal, and oropharyngeal—it is not particularly surprising that whatever causes stuttering could also interfere with the playing of one.

How might a musician who has such a disorder be helped? The case report by Meltzer (1992) suggests that he or she may benefit from stuttering therapy.

Both the prevalence of such disorders and whether a person who does not stutter can develop one are uncertain. There is a little anecdotal evidence which suggests that such persons can develop them (Meltzer, 1992).

MALINGERED STUTTERING

Speech pathologists have been asked by courts to provide expert testimony about whether a person really has a fluency disorder or is malingering (Shirkey, 1987; Bloodstein, 1988). Shirkey (1987), for example, was asked to provide such testimony about a 33-year-old man accused of a series of sexual assaults on children, whose defense in a previous arrest had been that as a stutterer he could not have committed the crimes because none of the victims stated that their attacker stuttered. And Bloodstein (1988) was asked to provide testimony about a man in his early thirties accused of armed robbery, whose defense was that, being a stutterer, he could not have said fluently: "This is a stickup. Get down on the floor and don't make a move or I'll blow your head off." In both cases it was concluded that the suspect probably was a stutterer because his "moments of stuttering" varied in a manner that was consistent with what had been reported in the literature.

Whenever a person being evaluated has something to gain by being labeled a stutterer, the possibility should be considered that he or she is malingering. While there are no malingering tests for stuttering, both Shirkey (1987) and Bloodstein (1988) offer suggestions about observations a clinician can make to detect it.

DIFFERENTIAL DIAGNOSIS BETWEEN STUTTERING AND OTHER FLUENCY DISORDERS

A clinician will almost always attempt to answer the following question after establishing that a client has a fluency disorder: Which disorder (or disorders) does the client have? The question is phrased in this way because, as a number of writers (including Freund, 1966; Luchinger & Arnold, 1965) have pointed out, a client can have more than one—for example, a combination of stuttering and cluttering.

Information about the symptomatology and phenomenology of stuttering is presented in Chapters 1 and 2 and that of other fluency disorders in this chapter. This information can serve as a guide to help select tasks and formulating questions to ask informants in order to determine the type of disorder.

Distinguishing Stuttering from Cluttering

The disorder in older children and adults is more likely to be cluttering than stuttering if:

1. The client's speaking rate is quite rapid.
2. Because the client is unaware that his or her speaking rate is excessive and that he or she is being abnormally disfluent, he or she is not concerned about it. Consequently, the client neither avoids talking nor does "things" to avoid being disfluent—there are no secondary behaviors.
3. The client does not become more disfluent when he or she feels it is important to speak well. In fact, the opposite may be true. The client may be *more fluent* at these times than he or she is at other times because the act of carefully formulating speech results in a slower speaking rate.

Distinguishing between stuttering and cluttering in young children can be quite difficult because the second and third are also true for children who are beginning to stutter. Furthermore, determining whether a young child's speaking rate is excessive may be difficult.

Daly (1993a) has developed a 33-item checklist "which presents features that numerous clinical researchers believe are indicative of cluttering" (see Appendix C). Each item is rated 0 to 3—the total number of points possible being 99. Daly suggests that a score of 60 or above is usually sufficient to support a diagnosis of cluttering and one between 30 and 60 a diagnosis of cluttering-stuttering. The items on the checklist that Daly indicates are the most indicative of cluttering, if present, are the following: 2, 3, 7, 9, 10, 12, 14, 20, 25, and 33.

Distinguishing Stuttering from Neurogenic-Acquired Stuttering

The disorder in older children and adults is more likely to be neurogenic acquired stuttering than stuttering if:

1. The onset was after the age of ten.
2. An event occurred immediately before the onset of the disorder that resulted in damage to the central nervous system.
3. The amount of abnormal disfluency *does not vary* from day to day and from situation to situation in the same manner as it does in stuttering. There probably is no situation in which the client is completely fluent. Abnormal disfluency is not reduced significantly or eliminated by reading in chorus. Consequently, if a client exhibits little, or no, abnormal disfluency while reading in chorus, the disorder is more likely to be stuttering than neurogenic acquired stuttering.

Distinguishing between stuttering and neurogenic-acquired stuttering in children younger than ten is likely to be quite difficult unless it can be established that damage to the central nervous system resulted in excessive disfluency and that this damage occurred before the onset of the fluency disorder.

Distinguishing Stuttering from Psychogenic-Acquired Stuttering

The disorder in older children and adults is more likely to be psychogenic acquired stuttering than stuttering or neurogenic-acquired stuttering if:

1. The onset was after the age of ten.
2. No event occurred immediately prior to the onset of the disorder that could have resulted in damage to the central nervous system.
3. An event occurred immediately before the onset of the disorder that could have resulted in severe psychological trauma.

4. The amount of abnormal disfluency *does not vary* from day to day and from situation to situation in the same manner as it does in stuttering. There may be no situation in which the client is completely fluent. Abnormal disfluency is not reduced significantly or eliminated by reading in chorus. Consequently, if a client exhibits little, or no, abnormal disfluency while reading in chorus, the disorder is more likely to be stuttering than psychogenic-acquired stuttering.

5. The client is aware of, but *not particularly concerned* about his or her abnormal disfluency. A person who has neurogenic-acquired stuttering is likely to be both aware of it and concerned.

Distinguishing between stuttering and psychogenic-acquired stuttering in children younger than ten is likely to be quite difficult unless the child has been diagnosed as having a psychiatric disorder that could produce abnormal disfluency. Such cases probably are extremely rare judging by the lack of reports of them in the literature.

Identifying Malingering

Establishing "beyond a reasonable doubt" that a person is malingering a fluency disorder is likely to be quite difficult, particularly if the person has read the stuttering literature and is knowledgeable about conditions under which stuttering varies. Malingering should *always* be considered a possibility if a client is likely to benefit in some way from this diagnosis. The benefit might be financial compensation by the person who it is claimed caused the disorder, or eligibility for financial aid (e. g., for vocational rehabilitation), or special consideration in hiring because of it. Malingering a fluency disorder could also be a way to discredit witness identifications if witnesses to a crime reported that the person who committed it was a fluent speaker.

Unfortunately, there are no established guidelines for determining whether a person is malingering a fluency disorder. Consequently, the approach suggested here may not be the best—most effective—one. First determine whether the age of onset, symptomatology, and phenomenology of the fluency disorder claimed is consistent with what is known about the disorder. If they are not consistent with what is known about the disorder, it is likely that the client does not have it. On the other hand, if they are consistent with what is known about the disorder, there are two possibilities. One, the client has the disorder, or two, the client has read enough about the disorder to simulate it. You can ask the client what he or she has read about the disorder. If the client claims to have read nothing about the disorder, you might want to express concern about some aspect of the symptomatology he or she evinced or reported that is not consistent with what is known about it. The client may be thrown off guard and insist that it is consistent with the symptomatology of the disorder, thereby demonstrating knowledge of the literature.

ASSIGNMENTS

Cluttering Simulation

One of the main symptoms of cluttering is tachyphemia—a very rapid speaking rate. Speak to a friend or read a passage at a very rapid rate and record yourself doing so. Listen to the recording. What effect did speaking very rapidly have on your speech fluency? Did you repeat syllables and words more frequently than usual? If your rate of repetition increased, how aware were you of it happening while you were speaking?

APPENDIX A

Wordings and Structures for Paragraphs and Sections in Fluency Disorder Evaluation Reports

Note. A number of paragraphs and sections from evaluation reports of children and adults who have fluency disorders are reproduced in this appendix. These were abstracted from ones submitted to me by the following speech-language pathologists who have national and international reputations as authorities on the treatment of stuttering: Dr. Martin R. Adams, University of Houston; Dr. Oliver Bloodstein, Brooklyn College; Dr. Edward Conture, Syracuse University; Dr. Steven B. Hood, University of South Alabama; Dr. William H. Perkins, University of Southern California; Dr. Richard Shine, East Carolina University; and Dr. Ehud Yahri, University of Illinois at Urbana-Champaign. They are intended to suggest wordings and structures for communicating some types of information in such reports about the fluency disorder. All of the reports, incidentally, contained other types of information—for example, birth and developmental histories and statements of the results of hearing and language tests. Family names were replaced with *Smith* to maintain confidentiality.

IDENTIFYING INFORMATION

NAME: DATE SEEN:
FILE NUMBER: EXAMINER:
BIRTHDATE: PARENTS:
AGE: INFORMANT:
ADDRESS: REFERRAL:
TELEPHONE: REPORT SENT TO:

❖❖❖❖❖❖❖❖❖❖❖❖❖❖❖❖❖❖❖❖❖❖❖❖❖❖❖❖❖❖❖

NAME: DATE OF EVALUATION:
BIRTHDATE: INFORMANT FOR HISTORY:
AGE: CLINIC FILE NUMBER:
SEX: DIAGNOSTIC CODE NUMBER:
ADDRESS: STATEMENT OF DIAGNOSIS:
TELEPHONE:

STATEMENT OF THE PROBLEM

This young boy, accompanied by his father and mother, appeared at the Speech, Hearing, and Language Clinic for a differential diagnosis of a suspected incipient stuttering problem.

❖❖❖❖❖❖❖❖❖❖❖❖❖❖❖❖❖❖❖❖❖❖❖❖❖❖❖❖❖❖❖

Stanley Smith, age eight years-eight months, was seen at this center for a speech and language evaluation. History information was provided by Stanley and his mother. Mrs. Smith indicated that she felt Stanley was becoming concerned about his speech and stated that Stanley has requested finding someone who could "help him with his speech." Of paramount concern to both Stanley and his mother was the increasingly frequent repetitions exhibited in Stanley's speech and his mounting concern over them.

❖❖❖❖❖❖❖❖❖❖❖❖❖❖❖❖❖❖❖❖❖❖❖❖❖❖❖❖❖❖❖

John, a four-year nine-month old male was referred to the Speech and Hearing Clinic for a stuttering evaluation by his parents. His mother expressed concern about his stuttering and indicated that it has worsened during the past year.

❖❖❖❖❖❖❖❖❖❖❖❖❖❖❖❖❖❖❖❖❖❖❖❖❖❖❖❖❖❖❖

Mr. Smith is a personable young man who appeared immediately open, confident, and relaxed in the relationship he established with me. He did almost no stuttering during the interview and could offer no explanation for his fluency in speaking with me. He reports that at times he stutters severely, however. When he tried to imitate his stuttering it seemed to consist of hard contacts of the articulators. He says he feels marked muscular tension when he stutters, especially in the throat area. He is concerned about the fact that his stuttering has been getting worse lately; he feels it is unrealistic to hope for a complete cure, but wants to "contain" the problem and if possible to ameliorate it. Another reason he has for desiring therapy at this time is that he is hoping for advancement in his job. He works for the phone company as a repairman and aspires to a management position in the company. He does not believe that his stuttering would be a bar to such advancement, but feels it would be more appropriate if he stuttered less.

DEVELOPMENTAL HISTORY

In regard to speech development, John's parents reported that the boy produced his first words before the age of 12 months and was speaking in sentences prior to the age of two years. At approximately two years, five months, Mr. and Mrs. Smith began to develop some concern about their son's speech development. Mrs. Smith stated that John was repeating words and syllables at the beginning of a sentence. Recently, he had also begun to experience difficulty with other words within his utterance. This behavior was particularly evident when John was excited or under stress. His parents further reported that John's fluency appeared to break down when he was engaged in competitive conversations with his brother and when John took his turn speaking to his father on the telephone while Mr. Smith was out of town on business.

❖❖❖❖❖❖❖❖❖❖❖❖❖❖❖❖❖❖❖❖❖❖❖❖❖❖❖❖❖❖❖

Joe could not report exactly when he began stuttering, but stated that he was aware of it by age ten. He did not believe that there was any medical or traumatic experience at that time which precipitated his stuttering.

During his high school years, when stress was intensified as a result of increased academic responsibility, Joe's stuttering became more severe. In college, familiar speaking situations and speaking with friends were thought by him to be relatively easy whereas speaking to professors and in front of classes posed more difficulties.

❖❖❖❖❖❖❖❖❖❖❖❖❖❖❖❖❖❖❖❖❖❖❖❖❖❖❖❖❖❖❖

The mother could not recall when Mike spoke his first word or when he started producing sentences. However, she did report that his stuttering behavior was first noticed at approximately two and a half years of age. The mother reported that "at one time his stuttering became better but then he went back to the speech problem." During the last six to eight months, it was reported from his nursery school that the children were having trouble understanding Mike during circle time and that this has caused him to become upset.

The patient is aware of his stuttering and dislikes slowing down or starting over when instructed by a parent. He reportedly is frustrated by his stuttering and dislikes his peers "making fun" of his speech.

The parents view Mike's stuttering as significant and stated that his stuttering has worsened during the past year. His mother is concerned about his self-esteem and aggressive behavior due to constant ridiculing from his peers at school. Initially, their attempts to "help" him overcome stuttering by having him "slow down" or stop and start over again were helpful, but during the past year his attempts to change his speaking behavior have been unsuccessful. At times he gets upset when he is asked to slow down or change his speaking pattern. According to his mother, his stuttering becomes worse when another person is present, especially his older sister. She feels he competes for attention and conversation with his older sister and that this results in his increased stuttering.

❖❖❖❖❖❖❖❖❖❖❖❖❖❖❖❖❖❖❖❖❖❖❖❖❖❖❖❖❖❖❖❖

During a 30-minute interview, Sam provided information about the onset and development of his fluency disorder. Sam reported that he began stuttering around the age of eight, and in second grade he was enrolled in speech therapy for remediation of his disfluencies. He explained that when his family moved to Greenfield, speech therapy was no longer available. He further explained that the period of time during which he did NOT receive any speech therapy at school was from the beginning of third grade until last spring (1988). Susan Jones, speech/language clinician at Greenfield High School, has reportedly provided fluency therapy services to Sam since the spring of 1988.

Sam recalled that his speech disfluencies during elementary school were mostly sound/syllable repetitions. Sam stated that "at first I wouldn't do it that much," and that since elementary school his speech disfluencies have "gotten worse." Sam reported that there were instances when he was unable to "get the word out."

Sam reported becoming the most "conscious" of his speech in junior high. He stated that currently his disfluencies "come and go" and that he is the most disfluent during "one on one" situations. Sam explained that the aspect of his speech fluency that concerns him the most is its effect on his education. He gave the following example: "If I've got to do a speech, I won't do it: then I get a bad grade." Sam reported that he is sometimes "embarrassed" by his speech disfluencies and expressed the hope that the problem will change so that he "will be able to talk clearer."

EVALUATION RESULTS—SPEECH SAMPLE ANALYSES

An analysis of a 566-word sample of Tim's conversational speech revealed a total of 133 disfluencies, or 23.5 stuttered words per 100 words spoken. The breakdown of this figure according to specific disfluency types was as follows:

Part-word repetitions	7.95
Whole-word repetitions	4.77
Phrase repetitions	1.06
Interjections	9.01
Incomplete phrases	0.71
TOTAL	23.50

As can be seen, the predominant types of disfluencies in Tim's speech were interjections and part-word repetitions. The clinician estimated the average repetition to be three or four. Although Tim indicated no specific phonemes on which he had more disfluencies, it was noted that the disfluencies occurred most consistently on words or syllables beginning with the vowel /i/. Tim exhibited quite fluent reading ability when he was asked to read both "The Rainbow Passage" and "My Grandfather." Analysis of these two reading samples revealed only one repetition and one prolongation throughout the 463 words read. Tim's conversational speech was timed. His average rate of speaking 169.5 words per minute, was within the normal range.

Physical behaviors that typically accompany stuttering were observable as Tim spoke. Eye blinking, poor eye contact, and neck and facial muscle tension occurred quite consistently during moments of disfluency. Tim was often observed wringing his hands while he held the rest of his body rather still. Avoidance behaviors observed consisted primarily of interjections used as "starters."

On a seven-point scale for rating severity of stuttering, with one being very mild stuttering and seven being very severe stuttering, Tim's speech was rated by the clinician at five although moments of more severe stuttering did occur.

❖❖❖❖❖❖❖❖❖❖❖❖❖❖❖❖❖❖❖❖❖❖❖❖❖❖❖❖❖❖❖

Joseph engaged in a number of different speaking tasks. He was totally fluent during rote, automatic tasks such as counting, saying the days of the week and the months of the year, and reciting the Pledge of Allegiance. He was normally fluent repeating sentences and reading a passage written for readers at the third-grade level.

Analysis of a 145-word spontaneous speech sample during dialogue yielded 54 disfluent moments (37 percent). Within these 54 disfluencies there were five instances of vocalized pauses and interjections that were "normal" disfluencies. Of particular concern, however, was the fact that syllable repetitions were noted to occur 34 times. For the most part repetitions were disrhythmic and accompanied by mild signs of tension. Most of the syllable repetitions were accompanied by increases in either pitch and/or loudness, and the schwa vowel was often substituted for the correct vowel. For most of the syllable repetitions the number of units ranged from three to five (i.e., *bo-bo-bo-boating, ba-ba-ba-ba-ba-badly*). During 21 of the 34 part-word repetitions, there was some degree of vowel prolongation during the final unit of repetition (row-row-r*ooooo*wing). There were 12 instances of vocalized sound prolongations (*wwwww*indow), 9 of which were also accompanied by increases in either pitch and/or loudness. The remaining two disfluencies were single-unit whole word repetitions. Moments of stuttering were usually between one and two seconds in duration. Avoidance behaviors were not observed.

Joseph's rate of speech was inconsistent. Because of the frequency and duration of disfluencies, his rate of speech in terms of meaningful words spoken was only 84 words per minute. However, this is misleading. Analysis of his articulation rate during fluent utterances yielded a typical range of between seven and nine syllables per second. Therefore, while his speech rate was slow, his fluent articulation rate was very fast.

❖❖❖❖❖❖❖❖❖❖❖❖❖❖❖❖❖❖❖❖❖❖❖❖❖❖❖❖❖❖❖❖

Martin was seen on July 8, 1990, for a speech evaluation. The assessment included obtaining a sample of his speech on videotape during a face-to-face conversation with a stranger and while reading.

The clinician observed that Martin's speech was marked by a high degree of disfluency. During the face-to-face conversation he stuttered on 18 percent of the syllables he uttered and spoke at an average rate of 153 syllables per minute. While reading, Martin averaged a speech rate of 162 syllables per minute with disfluency on 11 percent of his uttered syllables (above 7 percent disfluency is typically considered abnormal; 150 syllables spoken per minute is considered the low end of the normal speech rate range with the average speaker speaking about 225 syllables per minute). Martin's speech rate fell at the lower end of the normal range, in part because of numerous stops resulting from blocks while stuttering.

Martin's speech was characterized by prolongation of sounds and repetition of sounds, whole words, and phrases: It was also observed that he would sometimes be running out of air at the ends of phrases. Accompanying his stuttering struggle were head jerks, general upper body movement, eye blinks, and facial tension. Though Martin related that he typically does not maintain eye contact during a moment of stuttering, during the evaluation his eye contact was excellent.

❖❖❖❖❖❖❖❖❖❖❖❖❖❖❖❖❖❖❖❖❖❖❖❖❖❖❖❖❖❖❖❖

The *Stuttering Severity Instrument* (Riley, 1972) was administered to assess the severity of stuttering based on percentage of stuttered words, duration of the longest instance of stuttering, and physical concomitants.

During a 200-word spontaneous speech sample, Adam stuttered on 14 percent of the words spoken. The longest instance of stuttering was three seconds. Physical concomitants included lip pressing, tense jaw muscles, poor eye contact, and constant looking around. He obtained an overall score of twenty-three, which placed him at the seventy-seventh percentile and resulted in the highest moderate rating of stuttering severity. A score of twenty-four would have placed him in the lowest level of the severe range. Based on reports by the parents that his stuttering is often more severe than it was during the evaluation, it would appear that Adam's stuttering severity sometimes falls at the low end of the severe range.

❖❖❖❖❖❖❖❖❖❖❖❖❖❖❖❖❖❖❖❖❖❖❖❖❖❖❖❖❖❖❖❖

Administration of the *Stocker Probe Technique,* which associates the level of communicative responsibility with the frequency of speech disfluencies, resulted in Dan producing a *total* of nineteen speech disfluencies in response to fifty questions asked in reference to common objects. Dan's typical level of breakdown (the level at which speech disfluencies were *most* frequent) was level IV (eight speech disfluencies per ten questions asked at this level). His typical level of recovery (the level at which speech disfluencies were *least* frequent) was level I (0 speech disfluencies per ten questions asked at this level).

EVALUATION RESULTS—AVOIDANCES, ATTITUDES, AND BELIEFS

Harold was asked to list the people, situations, words, and sounds that he associates with the presence of at least mild stuttering. In response, the patient cited: (1) talking to his mother, grandmother, and grandfather; (2) talking with friends; (3) talking with professors; (4) talking on the phone; (5) answering questions or having to give a report in class; (6) introducing himself; and (7) saying words that begin with /w/ or /a/. Harold was quite candid in admitting that he routinely practices situational and word avoidance. That is, he will consciously seek to evade speaking in certain situations and using certain words. If he has no alternative but to speak, the patient indicated that he would say as little as possible.

Continuing on with the interview, the patient was asked to identify the behaviors that he uses to avoid an expected stuttering or to escape from a stuttering that is in progress. As regards avoidances, Harold replied with: (1) slowing down and breaking words into syllables; (2) taking a deep breath; (3) making word substitutions; (4) interjections; and (5) throat clearings. To escape from a stutter that is in progress, the client said that he might: (1) change to another word; (2) skip over the stuttered word; (3) interrupt the stutter and (a) take a deep breath before re-trying the word; (b) repeat the phrase leading up to the stuttered word; or (c) interject a sound before again attempting the stuttered word. All of these behaviors were observed by the clinician during the evaluation.

❖❖❖❖❖❖❖❖❖❖❖❖❖❖❖❖❖❖❖❖❖❖❖❖❖❖❖❖❖❖

Jerry felt that some situations increase the severity of his stuttering. He has a harder time speaking to a group than to individuals. It is more difficult for him to speak to strangers than to people with whom he is familiar. Jerry did state, however, that he feels that most people generally ignore his stuttering, although some of his students have at times expressed difficulty in listening to and understanding him. Some of the anxiety-producing situations Jerry mentioned were: speaking with people having authority, particularly professors; addressing his class; having to talk after arriving late to a meeting; and some phone conversations.

❖❖❖❖❖❖❖❖❖❖❖❖❖❖❖❖❖❖❖❖❖❖❖❖❖❖❖❖❖❖

Michael reported that he has distinct anticipations of stuttering and often "looks ahead" as he speaks and chooses circumlocutions to avoid stuttering. Yet he deliberately avoids using word substitutions and believes that he always has, by choice. He rarely avoids speaking situations. His most frequent emotional reaction when he stutters is frustration. Fear is a reaction he has only occasionally. He does not seem to be strongly driven to hiding his stuttering. Most of his close associates know that he stutters and he is not excessively troubled by their reactions, although he finds it irritating when listeners supply words for him.

❖❖❖❖❖❖❖❖❖❖❖❖❖❖❖❖❖❖❖❖❖❖❖❖❖❖❖❖❖❖

Results from responses to the *Situational Reaction Questionnaire, Fluency Attitude Scale,* and general background questions revealed that Kevin feels as though his stuttering holds him back in daily life communication interactions as well as to some degree in communicative situations at work. Kevin reported that he is seeking help now because he wants to express himself "more freely."

Kevin seems to be very strongly motivated to improve his communication ability in order to experience greater personal satisfaction—to say what he wants to say and participate in speaking situations in which he would like to be involved with greater confidence and ease of speaking.

SUMMARY AND RECOMMENDATIONS

The general picture is that of a typical case of adult stuttering that has fallen somewhat short of its potential development as a serious personal problem. There is an absence of continual fear and shame and systematic avoidance. Andrew's greatest fear is that the problem will continue to become more severe.

I outlined for Andrew the two major philosophies of stuttering therapy, the "talk differently" and the "stutter differently" approaches, emphasizing the advantages and disadvantages of each as objectively as possible, on the assumption that the choice should always lie with the stutterer. Without hesitation, he expressed his preference for the stutter-differently method. He expressed a strong aversion to any approach that attempted to train him to speak in an unnatural manner. He was also emphatic in stating that his goal was not normal speech but a reduction in the severity of his stuttering. He expressed considerable enthusiasm about the idea of learning to stutter with less effort and tension. Accordingly, I suggested that we try the Van Riper techniques of cancellation and pullouts.

❖❖❖❖❖❖❖❖❖❖❖❖❖❖❖❖❖❖❖❖❖❖❖❖❖❖❖❖❖❖❖

Throughout the diagnostic session Jerry exhibited moderate to severe stuttering. Although the speech therapy he received 2½ years ago had been successful, it is apparent that he needs additional therapy. Jerry's stuttering clearly interferes with his personal and academic life and his professional aspirations. Because he is a teaching assistant at present, it seems apparent that there is a need for him to obtain help for his stuttering. Jerry has expressed a desire to begin speech therapy and stated that his main goal is to be able to go before a class "without stuttering much" and to be able "to handle it better." It is recommended, therefore, that he be enrolled in speech therapy.

❖❖❖❖❖❖❖❖❖❖❖❖❖❖❖❖❖❖❖❖❖❖❖❖❖❖❖❖❖❖❖

This young man is presently exhibiting a stuttering problem of no worse than moderate severity. The problem seems to be weakly associated with anxiety, but closely connected to problems with the prompt, easy initiation and maintenance of voicing. Roy's clinical picture is further complicated by his extensive use of word and situational avoidance and by his employment of other "tricks" that are designed to minimize or altogether mask the stuttering.

It was recommended to the client that he place himself on our clinic's waiting list for therapy this coming fall. Roy was agreeable to this suggestion.

When therapy is undertaken, it should involve two procedures that are utilized simultaneously. These procedures are training in breathstream management and conscious suppression of all escape/avoidance behaviors. Treatment should be instituted on as intensive a basis as possible, certainly no less frequently than two, 1-hour clinic visits per week.

APPENDIX B

Organizations for Persons Interested in Stuttering

Note: All of these organizations desire participation by speech-language pathologists as well as stutterers. There are comparable ones in other countries, including both Eastern and Western Europe, Canada, Australia, and Japan.

COMPULSIVE STUTTERERS ANONYMOUS, P. O. Box 1406, Park Ridge, Illinois 60068
This is a relatively new organization that has adapted the Alcoholics Anonymous 12-step program to stuttering.

THE NATIONAL COUNCIL ON STUTTERING, P. O. Box 344, Rochelle, Illinois 61068.
The National Council on Stuttering (NCOS), which was founded in 1974, is a voluntary, nonprofit, self-help organization devoted to promoting a better understanding of the problems of stuttering. The objectives of NCOS include, but are not limited to, gathering information about stuttering, increasing public awareness, generating support for clinical research, assisting in the formation of new chapters, and establishing programs to help people understand and cope with the problem of stuttering [abstracted from the organization's statement of purpose]. The NCOS holds annual meetings and publishes a quarterly journal.

THE NATIONAL STUTTERING PROJECT, 4601 Irving Street, San Francisco, California 94122-1020.
The National Stuttering Project, which began in 1977, is the largest of the self-help groups. It has more than 65 active support group chapters for teenagers and adults in the United States. Most of them meet twice a month. Twenty percent of its members are speech-language pathologists. It sponsors an annual convention and a monthly newsletter. For further information about he organization, see the January 1990 issue of *Asha*.

SPEAK EASY INTERNATIONAL FOUNDATION, 233 Concord Drive, Paramus, New Jersey 07652.
This organization, like the National Council on Stuttering and the National Stuttering Project, is a self-help group for persons who stutter. It sponsors an annual convention and a newsletter.

SPEECH FOUNDATION OF AMERICA, P. O. Box 11749, Memphis, Tennessee 38111
This organization publishes low-cost books on stuttering for stutterers, their parents, and speech-language pathologists. Write for a catalog.

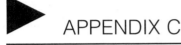

APPENDIX C

Evaluation Forms and Tasks

1. The Rainbow Passage
2. "Arthur the Young Rat"
3. Sentence Repetition Task
4. The S-Scale
5. Stutterers Self-Ratings of Reactions to Speech Situations
6. Stuttering Problem Profile
7. Inventory of Communication Attitudes
8. Problem Profile for Elementary-School-Age Children Who Stutter about Talking
9. Physician's Screening Procedure for Children Who May Stutter
10. Stuttering Severity Instrument
11. Iowa Scale of Severity of Stuttering
12. Checklist of Stuttering Behavior
13. Perceptions of Self Semantic Differential Task
14. Southern Illinois University Speech Situation Checklist
15. Disfluency Descriptor Digest
16. Children's Attitudes about Talking—Revised (CAT-R)
17. The Cooper Chronicity Prediction Checklist
18. Daly's Checklist for Possible Cluttering—Experimental Edition

THE RAINBOW PASSAGE

When the sunlight strikes raindrops in the air, they act like a prism and form a rainbow. A rainbow is a division of white light into many beautiful colors. These take the shape of a long round arch, with its path high above, and its two ends apparently beyond the horizon. There is, according to legend, a boiling pot of gold at one end. People look, but no one ever finds it. When a man looks for something beyond his reach, his friends say he is looking for the pot of gold at the end of the rainbow.

Throughout the centuries men have explained the rainbow in various ways. Some have accepted it as a miracle without physical explanation. To the Hebrews it was a token that there would be no more universal floods. The Greeks used to imagine that it was a sign from the gods to foretell war or heavy rain. The Norsemen considered the rainbow as a bridge over which the gods passed from earth to their home in the sky. Other men have tried to explain the phenomenon physically. Aristotle thought that the rainbow was caused by reflection of the sun's rays by the rain. Since then physicists have found that it is not reflection, but refraction of the raindrops which causes the rainbow. Many complicated ideas about the rainbow have been formed. The difference in the rainbow depends considerably upon the size of the water drops, and the width of the color band increases as the size of the drops increases. The actual primary rainbow observed is said to be the effect of superposition of a number of bows. If the red of the second bow falls upon the green of the first, the result is to give a bow with an abnormally wide yellow band, since red and green light when mixed form yellow. This is a very common type of bow, one showing mainly red and yellow, with little or no green or blue.

[Reproduced from Fairbanks, 1960, p. 127.]

ARTHUR THE YOUNG RAT

Once, a long time ago, there was a young rat named Arthur who could never make up his flighty mind. Whenever his swell friends used to ask him to go out and play with them, he would only answer airily, "I don't know." He wouldn't try to say yes or no either. He would always shrink from making a specific choice.

His proud Aunt Helen scolded him: "Now look here," she stated, "no one is going to aid or care for you if you carry on like this. You have no more mind than a stray blade of grass."

That very night there was a big thundering crash and in the foggy morning some zealous men—with twenty boys and girls—rode up and looked at the fallen barn. One of them slipped back a broken board and saw a squashed young rat, quite dead, half in and half out of his hole. Thus, in the end the poor shirker got his just dues. Oddly enough his Aunt Helen was glad. "I hate such oozy, oily sneaks," said she.

[Reproduced from Darley & Spriestersbach, 1978, p. 276.]

SENTENCE REPETITION TASK

The child is instructed to repeat each of the following sentences after the examiner.

1. Mother is cooking dinner.
2. Grandmother likes to receive letters.
3. Father's swimming suit has black and white stripes.
4. My sister really likes painting pictures.
5. Please give me the yellow balloon.
6. It was chilly at the football game.
7. Peter picked some green peppers.
8. Bring the broom and sweep the floor.
9. The wind blew briskly.
10. Frank likes to read sports magazines.
11. The baby carriage has been painted white.
12. David rode his bicycle to school.
13. On Sundays Christians go to church.
14. The bell on the fire engine rings loudly.
15. We had fresh bread for lunch on Tuesday and Wednesday.
16. The sun shone brightly today.

THE S-SCALE

The response for each statement that indicates an "undesirable" attitude is printed in brackets following it.

1. I usually feel that I am making a favorable impression when I talk. [F]
2. It is easy for me to talk to important people. [F]
3. More than anything else I would like to be able to talk better. [T]
4. You can't gain much by arguing. [T]
5. I find it easy to talk with almost anyone. [F]
6. I find it very easy to look at my audience while speaking to a group. [F]
7. I have felt self-conscious when reciting in class. [T]
8. A person who is my teacher or my boss is hard to talk to. [T]
9. I am often in places where I need to introduce one person to another. [F]
10. I would like to introduce the speaker at a meeting. [F]
11. I never did volunteer much to recite in class. [T]
12. Even the idea of giving a talk in public makes me afraid. [T]
13. Some words are harder than others for me to say. [T]
14. I would rather not introduce myself to a stranger. [T]
15. I forget all about myself shortly after I begin to give a speech. [F]
16. I am a good mixer. [F]

17. People sometimes feel uncomfortable when I am talking to them. [T]
18. I dislike introducing one person to another. [T]
19. I often ask questions in group discussions. [F]
20. I find it easy to keep control of my voice when speaking. [F]
21. I become suddenly afraid when called upon to speak. [T]
22. I do not mind speaking before a group. [F]
23. I find it easier to talk with persons younger than me. [T]
24. I do not talk well enough to do the kind of work I'd really like to do. [T]
25. My speaking voice is rather pleasant and easy to listen to. [F]
26. I am sometimes embarrassed by the way I talk. [T]
27. I face most speaking situations with complete confidence. [F]
28. There are few people I can talk with easily. [T]
29. I talk better than I write. [F]
30. My speech is the same as always. [F]
31. I wish it did not bother me to talk to people. [T]
32. It is easier to answer questions in class than to ask them. [T]
33. I often feel nervous while talking. [T]
34. In school I found it very hard to talk before the class. [T]
35. I find it hard to make talk when I meet new people. [T]
36. I often have to search for the words I want. [T]
37. I feel pretty confident about my speaking ability. [F]
38. I wish I could say things as clearly as others do. [T]
39. Even though I knew the right answer I often failed to give it because I was afraid to speak out. [T]

[Reproduced from Erickson, 1969, pp. 717–718.]

STUTTERER'S SELF-RATINGS OF REACTIONS TO SPEECH SITUATIONS

The four, five-point scales used for rating speaking situations are defined as follows (Darley & Spriestersbach, 1978, pp. 317–318):

A. Avoidance:

1. I never try to avoid this situation and have no desire to avoid it.
2. I don't try to avoid this situation, but sometimes I would like to.
3. More often than not I do not try to avoid this situation, but sometimes I do try to avoid it.
4. More often than not I do try to avoid this situation.
5. I avoid this situation every time I possibly can.

B. Reaction [enjoyment of speaking in the situation]

　　1. I definitely enjoy speaking in this situation.
　　2. I would rather speak in this situation than not.
　　3. It's hard to say whether I'd rather speak in this situation than not.
　　4. I'd rather not speak in this situation.
　　5. I very much dislike speaking in this situation.

C. Stuttering [or substitute another type of abnormal disfluency behavior]:

　　1. I don't stutter at all (or only rarely) in this situation.
　　2. I stutter mildly (for me) in this situation.
　　3. I stutter with average severity (for me) in this situation.
　　4. I stutter more than average (for me) in this situation.
　　5. I stutter severely (for me) in this situation.

D. Frequency:

　　1. This is a situation I meet very often, two or three times a day, or even more, on the average.
　　2. I meet this situation at least once a day with rare exceptions (except Sunday perhaps).
　　3. I meet this situation from three to five times a week on the average.
　　4. I meet this situation once a week, with few exceptions, and occasionally I meet it twice a week.
　　5. I rarely meet this situation, certainly not as often as once a week.

The speaking situations rated include the following (Darley & Spriestersbach, 1978, pp. 318–319):

1. Ordering in a restaurant
2. Introducing myself (face to face)
3. Telephoning to ask the price, train fare, etc.
4. Buying a plane, train, or bus ticket
5. Short class recitation (ten words or less)
6. Telephoning for a taxi
7. Introducing one person to another
8. Buying something from a store clerk
9. Conversation with a good friend
10. Talking with an instructor after class or in his office
11. Long distance telephone call to someone I know
12. Conversation with my father
13. Asking a person for a date (or talking to a person who asks me for a date)

14. Making a short speech
15. Giving my name over the telephone
16. Conversation with my mother
17. Asking a secretary if I can see her employer
18. Going to a house and asking for someone
19. Making a speech to an unfamiliar audience
20. Participating in a committee meeting
21. Asking an instructor a question in class
22. Saying hello to a friend going by
23. Asking for a job
24. Telling a person a message from someone else
25. Telling a funny story with one stranger in the crowd
26. Playing games requiring speech
27. Reading aloud to friends
28. Participating in a bull session
29. Dinner conversation with strangers
30. Talking with my barber (or beauty operator)
31. Telephoning to make an appointment, or arrange a meeting place with someone
32. Answering roll call in class
33. Asking at a desk for a book, or card to be filled out, etc.
34. Talking with someone I don't know well while waiting for a bus or class, etc.
35. Talking with other players during a playground game
36. Taking leave of a hostess
37. Conversation with a friend while walking along the street
38. Buying stamps at a post office
39. Giving directions or information to strangers
40. Taking leave of a girl (boy) after a date

Means for adult male stutterers in terms of the twenty-fifth, fiftieth, and seventy-fifth percentile values for each of the four modes of response.

Mode of Response	Twenty-fifth Percentile	Fiftieth Percentile	Seventy-fifth Percentile
Avoidance	1.82	2.20	2.80
Reaction	2.10	2.56	2.97
Stuttering	2.08	2.53	2.98
Frequency	3.48	3.88	4.11

Source: Adapted from Shumak, 1955, p. 356

STUTTERING PROBLEM PROFILE

NAME: AGE: DATE:

ADDRESS:

Instructions

On the following pages are a list of statements made by stutterers about their stuttering problem following a period of therapy. In order to help you and your clinician to define goals for therapy, please circle the numbers of those statements that you would like to be able to make at the termination of therapy *that you don't feel you could make now.* If there are statements you would like to be able to make that aren't included in the list, write them on the last page.

1. I am usually willing to stutter openly.
2. I have learned to speak on exhalation rather than on inhalation.
3. I don't usually have trouble with the first sounds of words.
4. I no longer have a great deal of difficulty speaking in school.
5. I am able to give myself assignments and carry them out to my own satisfaction.
6. I am usually willing to use the telephone.
7. I am as cheerful as most people.
8. I don't usually experience a great mounting of tension and feeling of panic before speaking engagements.
9. I repeat sounds, syllables, and words infrequently.
10. I have a strong desire to do something about my stuttering problem.
11. I used to be quiet and shy. Now I tend to be outgoing.
12. My attitude toward my stuttering is no longer one of embarrassment.
13. I am not in a rush to respond when talking with people.
14. I don't usually experience emotional depression after stuttering in front of other people.
15. I can usually control the level of tensing when involved in speaking situations.
16. I can read relatively fluently.
17. I have learned to live with my problem.
18. I have learned not to be afraid of people.
19. I no longer have the feeling that stuttering is a miserable abnormality.
20. I am putting more emphasis on communicating well than on not stuttering.
21. I have learned how to stutter in a way that is more acceptable to the listener.
22. I have gained a better overall understanding of the problem.
23. I am confident that if I work at it, I can do something about my stuttering.
24. I understand how fluent speakers react to stutterers and why.
25. I usually don't hold myself back from talking when with a group of people.
26. I am not as ashamed as I used to be because of my stuttering.

27. I usually don't stutter much when giving a formal report to a group of people.
28. I have gained increased courage to participate in conversations, answer phone calls, and talk to strangers.
29. I am reasonably tolerant of nonfluency in general.
30. I usually don't avoid feared words and situations.
31. I no longer have a feeling of hopelessness about my stuttering.
32. My mental attitude toward my stuttering has changed. The gist of my present attitude is "true acceptance of the fact that I *am* a stutterer."
33. I talk as much as most people.
34. When around other people, I usually don't hold back my feelings because of fear of stuttering.
35. I usually am not preoccupied with myself.
36. I am usually willing to discuss my problem with other people.
37. I no longer object to my therapy program.
38. I have expanded my activities, both social and business.
39. I usually don't have strong feelings of shame and embarrassment when I block.
40. I now feel I could change what I do when I stutter if I would wake up and do it.
41. I no longer anticipate stuttering on certain sounds.
42. I am convinced that I can talk without having to struggle.
43. I don't usually become very anxious when I have to initiate a phone call.
44. My breathing while speaking usually isn't irregular.
45. When I stutter, related movements such as hand jerks and eye blinkings rarely occur.
46. I no longer speak at an excessive rate.
47. I usually am not afraid of public speaking.
48. I find it relatively easy to ask a clerk for something in a store.
49. I can purposely speak the way I want in the majority of situations.
50. I would be willing to become an officer in a club where I would have to give speeches.
51. I have learned that speaking can be an enjoyable experience.
52. I don't usually worry about entering speaking situations.
53. I don't usually become extremely depressed when in a period of "regression" in my speech.
54. I no longer consider myself an oddity because I stutter.
55. I usually am willing to say what I feel like saying.
56. I usually am not afraid to stutter in front of people.
57. My self-confidence has increased considerably.
58. It doesn't bother me to hear other stutterers speak.
59. I try to avoid changing words I think I will stutter on.
60. Words that I used to use as "starters" have all but completely disappeared.
61. I am getting involved in many speaking situations.
62. I believe I can overcome my problem to the extent I can live comfortably with it.

63. I look upon my stuttering as something that can be changed or modified.
64. I have as many friends as most people.
65. I have learned to modify some of the overt behavior, e.g., facial grimaces.
66. I am relatively relaxed in speaking situations.
67. I am sure I can completely conquer the problem.
68. I recognize the worth of experimenting and playing around with my stuttering.
69. I don't usually experience feelings of failure when in a period of "regression" in my speech.
70. I no longer try to avoid looking at the person with whom I am talking when I am stuttering.
71. I now rarely anticipate stuttering.
72. I feel that I have learned to accept the fact that I stutter.
73. I have quit being a lone wolf.
74. I do not react violently to my nonfluencies.
75. I feel fairly confident I can do something about my stuttering.
76. I have finally accepted the fact I am a stutterer. Before I never felt like I was one and always tried to "hide" it.
77. I push myself to enter situations in which I know I will stutter instead of avoiding them.
78. I probably talk to as many people as most persons.
79. I am usually willing to modify my stuttering blocks outside the therapy situation in the manner recommended by my therapist.
80. I usually don't worry very much about the reactions of others when I have a speech block.
81. I am paying more attention to my strengths than my weaknesses.
82. I tend to be relatively relaxed when giving a formal report to a group of people.
83. I usually am not afraid to approach people and talk to them.
84. I realize that improving my speech must be a day-to-day affair with specific goals and assignments set up.
85. I have accepted a certain amount of nonfluency as normal speech behavior.
86. I recite in the classroom as much as most students.

Additional Statements

[Reproduced from Silverman, 1980b.]

INVENTORY OF COMMUNICATION ATTITUDES

Response Scales of the Inventory of Communication Attitudes

Affective Scale 1

1 ___ I definitely enjoy speaking in this situation.
2 ___
3 ___
4 ___
5 ___
6 ___
7 ___ I hate speaking in this situation.

Behavioral Scale 2

1 ___ My speech skills are excellent in this situation.
2 ___
3 ___
4 ___
5 ___
6 ___
7 ___ My speech skills are poor in this situation.

Cognitive-A Scale 3

1 ___ Most speakers definitely enjoy speaking in this situation.
2 ___
3 ___
4 ___
5 ___
6 ___
7 ___ Most speakers hate speaking in this situation.

Cognitive-B Scale 4

1 ___ Most speakers' speech skills are excellent in this situation.
2 ___
3 ___
4 ___
5 ___
6 ___
7 ___ Most speakers' speech skills are poor in this situation.

Frequency Scale 5

1 ___ I meet this situation 2 or 3 times a day, or more, on the average.
2 ___
3 ___
4 ___
5 ___
6 ___
7 ___ I never meet this situation.

Thirteen Situational Subscales and Associated Items of the Inventory of Communication Attitudes

Subscale 1: Telephone Conversations
    Item 01 Telephoning to ask a price, train fare, etc.
    Item 02 Telephoning to make an appointment with a stranger.
    Item 03 Talking with a salesperson on the telephone.
Subscale 2: Argument/Conflict with a Friend
    Item 04 Refusing a friend a favor
    Item 05 Confronting a friend who has failed to fulfill an agreement.
    Item 06 Criticizing a friend for a mistake he or she has made.
Subscale 3: Argument/Conflict with a Stranger
    Item 07 Arguing with a salesperson about an overcharge.
    Item 08 Arguing with a service person to provide additional service or to lower the cost of service.
    Item 09 Complaining to a waiter/waitress about poor service.
Subscale 4: One-to-One Conversation with a Family Member
    Item 10 Talking with my father.
    Item 11 Talking with my mother.
    Item 12 Talking with a family member while riding in a car.
Subscale 5: One-to-One Conversation with an Authority Figure
    Item 13 Telling my doctor what is ailing me.
    Item 14 Talking with a lawyer.
    Item 15 Talking with a store manager.
Subscale 6: Group Conversation with Known Group (Informal)
    Item 16 Telling a funny story to a group of 2 to 8 friends.
    Item 17 Talking with a group of 2 to 8 friends at a party.
    Item 18 Carrying on a conversation with 2 to 8 friends during a card, golf, or other game.
Subscale 7: Group Conversations with Unknown Group (Informal)
    Item 19 Talking with 2 to 8 strangers during dinner.
    Item 20 Taking part in a discussion group of 2 to 8 strangers.
    Item 21 Starting off a discussion in a group of 2 to 8 strangers.

Subscale   8: Formal Presentations
    Item 22 Making a short speech (1 or 2 minutes) at work or in a class.
    Item 23 Making a 5- to 10-minute speech at work or in a class.
    Item 24 Acting as a spokesperson or representative of a group in a meeting at work or in a class.
Subscale   9: Questioning a Friend or Family Member to Obtain Information or to Elicit Action
    Item 25 Asking a friend for a ride.
    Item 26 Asking a family member for money (a small loan).
    Item 27 Asking a family member for advice.
Subscale   10: Questioning a Stranger to Obtain Information or to Elicit Action
    Item 28 Asking a stranger for the time of a movie or other event.
    Item 29 Asking for stamps at the post office.
    Item 30 Asking a waiter/waitress for help.
Subscale   11: Questioning an Authority Figure to Obtain Information or to Elicit Action
    Item 31 Asking a policeman for directions or information.
    Item 32 Asking a question of a boss at work or an instructor in class.
    Item 33 Asking a question of an authority at a forum or a meeting.
Subscale   12: Situations Involving Time Constraints
    Item 34 Asking a secretary to see his or her employer when I am late for an appointment.
    Item 35 Asking for flight or bus information when I am late for that plane or bus.
    Item 36 Talking to a store clerk when a number of other customers are waiting for help.
Subscale   13: Situations Involving Memorized Content or Unchangeable Content
    Item 37 Telling someone my address.
    Item 38 Telling someone my telephone number.
    Item 39 Telling someone my name.

[Reproduced from Watson, 1987, pp. 404–405.]

PROBLEM PROFILE FOR ELEMENTARY-SCHOOL-AGE CHILDREN WHO STUTTER ABOUT TALKING

Below are the aspects of talking sampled and some examples of questions that would be asked about each:

"Whom Do You Like to Talk to?" Questions Whom do you like to talk to at home; at school? Who don't you like to talk to at home; at school? Who do you think likes to talk with you at home; at school? Who do you think doesn't like to talk with you at home; at school? Questions of this kind can also be asked in terms of a 3-point scale, such as, who likes to talk to you best at home, the next best, the least best? After each answer you can obtain additional information by asking questions such as "Why do you think this is so?"

"Who Talks the Most?" Questions Who talks the most (the least) at home? Whom do you talk to the most (the least) at home; at school? Whom does your father, mother, brother,... talk to the most (the least) at home? Again, these questions can be put on a scale whereby the child ranks the relative amount each member of the family talks. The same scale can be used to find the relative amount the child talks in comparison with other children at home or at school. Where appropriate, follow his answer with "Why?"

"Who Interrupts?" Questions Who interrupts the most at home, school, play? Who interrupts the least? This question can be pursued by asking who interrupts father, mother, brother, the most? Who interrupts you the most (the least)? Whom do you interrupt the most (the least) at home; at school? An answer obtained to any question can [and probably should] be pursued by asking "why" questions.

"Who Are Good Talkers?" Questions Who's the best talker at home? Who's the next best talker? Who's the poorest talker at home? Why do you consider him or her to be a good talker? Why do you consider (the ones named toward the bottom of the list) not to be very good talkers? If the child does not include himself, you can ask directly about where he puts himself on the scale of "good talker" or "poor talker." The same question can be asked about his school environment.

"When Do You Want to Talk Well?" Questions Are there times when you want to talk extra well? Where? Why? Are there times when you don't care particularly how you talk? Where? Why? Do you think this is true about other people who talk?

"Where Do You Want to Talk More than You Do?" Questions In school, on the playground, at parties, when company comes, do you talk more than, less than, or about the same amount as other children in your class? Are there times when you wish you could talk more but aren't permitted to? Why do you think this is so? Does this happen with other children? Why?

"Who Listens?" Questions Who pays the most (the least) attention to you when you talk at home; at school? What do you like listeners to do when you talk to them? How do you want them to listen? For example, do you want them to look down; to look at you; to smile; to frown; to interrupt you; to talk for you? Who does the most and the least of those things that you (like) (don't like) at home; at school? Why do you think they do it?

[Reproduced from Williams, 1978, pp. 68–70.]

PHYSICIAN'S SCREENING PROCEDURE FOR CHILDREN WHO MAY STUTTER

Child's Name _____ File _____

Date of Birth _____ Exam Date _____ Age ____

	Normal	Borderline	Abnormal	Very Abnormal
AREA A Types of Disfluencies	1. Repeats phrases or whole words. 2. Interjects "uh" while thinking.	3. Repeats the first sound of a word 2 or 3 times without tension.	4. Repeats sound 4 or more times before getting the word out.	5. Child has tense voice during the repetitions. 6. Child has "hard" blocks. Gets stuck on words.
AREA B Other behaviors during abnormal disfluencies				1. Tries to change words for fear of stuttering. 2. Child struggles to get word out as seen in facial grimaces and/or hand, arm or foot movements.
AREA C Frequency of abnormal disfluencies		1. Infrequent (less than 2%).	2. Frequent (one in every 2-3 sentences).	3. Very frequent (one or more per sentence).
AREA D Child's reactions to the abnormal disfluencies	1. None. Seems unaware of them.		2. Child just keeps on trying.	3. Child gives up trying to say the sentence or asks, "Why can't I talk right?"

	Normal	Borderline	Abnormal	Very Abnormal
AREA E Other people's reactions to the abnormal disfluencies.	1. No one is bothered by the disfluencies		2. Parents are afraid he/she will not outgrow the stuttering.	3. Child is very upset by teasing or other listener reactions.
AREA F How long since the abnormal disfluencies were first noticed?		1. They began less than four months ago.	2. They began 4 to 12 months ago.	3. They began more than 12 months ago.

Examiner's Comments: _____

_____

_____

Note the number of "Abnormal" and "Very abnormal" symptoms on the right-hand half of the page.

1 or 2 symptoms? __ (Monitor)   3 or more symptoms? __ (Refer)

Examiner: _____

[Reproduced from Riley & Riley, 1989, p. 64.]

STUTTERING SEVERITY INSTRUMENT

Frequency (Use A or B, not both)

A. For readers. Use 1 and 2				B. For nonreaders	
1. Job Task		2. Reading Task		Picture Task	
Percent-age	Task Score	Percent-age	Task Score	Percent-age	Task Score
1	2	1	2	1	4
2–3	3	2–3	2	2–3	6
4	4	4–5	5	4	8
5–6	5	6–9	6	5–6	10
7–9	6	10–16	7	7–9	12
10–14	7	17–26	8	10–14	14
15–28	8	27 and up	9	15–28	16
29 and up	9			29 and up	18

Total
Frequency
A 1 & 2
or
B

Duration

Estimated Length of Three Longest Blocks	Task Score
Flecting	1
One half second	2
One full second	3
2 to 9 seconds	4
10 to 30 seconds (by second hand)	5
30 to 60 seconds	6
More than 60 seconds	7

Total
Duration
Score

Physical Concomitants

Evaluating Scale: 0 = none; 1 = not noticeable unless looking for it;
2 = barely noticeable to casual observer; 3 = distracting; 4 = very
distracting; 5 = severe and painful looking.

1. Distracting Sounds. Noisy breathing, whistling,
   sniffing, blowing, clicking sounds.................................. 0 1 2 3 4 5

2. Facial grimaces. Jaw jerking, tongue protruding, lip
   pressing, jaw muscles tense.. 0 1 2 3 4 5

3. Head movement. Back, forward, turning away, poor eye
   contact, constant looking around.................................... 0 1 2 3 4 5

4. Extremities movement. Arm and hand movement, hands
   about face, torso movement, leg movements, foot tap-
   ping or swinging... 0 1 2 3 4 5

Total
Physical
Concomitant
Score

[Reproduced from Riley, 1972, p. 321.]

IOWA SCALE OF SEVERITY OF STUTTERING

Speaker_____ Age ____ Sex _____ Date _____

Rater_____ Identification_____

Instructions:
Indicate your identification by some such term as "speaker's clinician," "clinical observer," "clinical student," or "friend," "mother," "classmate," et cetera. Rate the severity of the speaker's stuttering on a scale from 0 to 7, as follows:

0 No stuttering
1 *Very mild*—stuttering on less than 1 percent of words; very little relevant tension; disfluencies generally less than one second in duration; patterns of disfluency simple; no apparent associated movements of body, arms, legs, or head.
2 *Mild*—stuttering on 1 to 2 percent of words; tension scarcely perceptible; very few, if any, disfluencies last as long as a full second; patterns of disfluency simple; no conspicuous associated movements of body, arms, legs, or head.
3 *Mild to moderate*—stuttering on about 2 to 5 percent of words; tension noticeable but not very distracting; most disfluencies do not last longer than a full second; patterns of disfluency mostly simple; no distracting associated movements.
4 *Moderate*—stuttering on about 5 to 8 percent of words; tension occasionally distracting; disfluencies average about one second in duration; disfluency patterns characterized by an occasional complicating sound or facial grimace; an occasional distracting associated movement.
5 *Moderate to severe*—stuttering on about 8 to 12 percent of words; consistently noticeable tension; disfluencies average about 2 seconds in duration; a few distracting sounds and facial grimaces; a few distracting associated movements.
6 *Severe*—stuttering on about 12 to 25 percent of words; conspicuous tension; disfluencies average 3 to 4 seconds in duration; conspicuous distracting sounds and facial grimaces; conspicuous distracting associated movements.
7 *Very severe*—stuttering on more than 25 percent of words; very conspicuous tension; disfluencies average more than 4 seconds in duration; very conspicuous distracting sounds and facial grimaces; very conspicuous distracting associated movements.

[Reproduced from Sherman, 1952.]

CHECKLIST OF STUTTERING BEHAVIOR

Name _____ Age_____ Sex _____

Observer _____ Date _____

Instruction to Observer

Observe the stutterer as he or she speaks or reads aloud. Focus your attention on such disfluencies and related reactions as you would classify as stuttering. Observe these reactions as they are associated with the speaking of specific words. Write each such word at the top of a column and make a check mark in the appropriate space to indicate each type of disfluency or other reaction observed. Note by the use of 1, 2, 3, et cetera, the sequencing of behaviors. Under "Supplementary Observations" add descriptive details concerning any of the numbered items checked, and comment on apparent emotionality of the speaker, general degree of tension, relevant remarks made by the speaker, et cetera.

Types of Reaction	*Word 1*	*Word 2*	*Word 3*	*Word 4*	*Word 5*	*Word 6*
1. Repeating part of word	____	____	____	____	____	____
2. Repeating whole monosyllabic word	____	____	____	____	____	____
3. Repeating this and other word(s)	____	____	____	____	____	____
4. Saying "uh—uh" or the like	____	____	____	____	____	____
5. Prolonging sound(s)	____	____	____	____	____	____
6. Pausing in the middle of word	____	____	____	____	____	____
7. Failing to complete the word	____	____	____	____	____	____
8. Holding breath	____	____	____	____	____	____
9. Gasping	____	____	____	____	____	____
10. Inhaling irregularly	____	____	____	____	____	____
11. Exhaling irregularly	____	____	____	____	____	____
12. Speaking on exhausted breath	____	____	____	____	____	____
13. Delay in starting word	____	____	____	____	____	____
14. Pressing lips together	____	____	____	____	____	____
15. Pressing tongue against teeth or palate	____	____	____	____	____	____
16. Closing eyes	____	____	____	____	____	____
17. Protruding tongue	____	____	____	____	____	____
18. Enlarging eyes	____	____	____	____	____	____

Types of Reaction	Word 1	Word 2	Word 3	Word 4	Word 5	Word 6
19. Opening mouth irrelevantly	___	___	___	___	___	___
20. Dilating nostrils	___	___	___	___	___	___
21. Turning head sideways	___	___	___	___	___	___
22. Bending head downward	___	___	___	___	___	___
23. Moving head up or back	___	___	___	___	___	___
24. Moving hands or fingers	___	___	___	___	___	___
25. Moving legs or feet	___	___	___	___	___	___
26. Moving body	___	___	___	___	___	___
27. Other (specify)	___	___	___	___	___	___
28. _____	___	___	___	___	___	___
29. _____	___	___	___	___	___	___
30. _____	___	___	___	___	___	___

Supplementary Observations:

[Reproduced from Darley & Spriestersbach, 1978, pp. 307–308.]

PERCEPTIONS OF SELF
SEMANTIC DIFFERENTIAL TASK

Below are some rating scales each with nine points. I would like you to evaluate
YOURSELF, as you typically are, on each of these scales. Please circle the number
on the scale that best describes yourself, on each scale.

	1	2	3	4	5	6	7	8	9
1. Open									Guarded
2. Nervous	1	2	3	4	5	6	7	8	9 Calm
3. Cooperative	1	2	3	4	5	6	7	8	9 Uncooperative
4. Shy	1	2	3	4	5	6	7	8	9 Bold
5. Friendly	1	2	3	4	5	6	7	8	9 Unfriendly
6. Self-conscious	1	2	3	4	5	6	7	8	9 Self-assured
7. Tense	1	2	3	4	5	6	7	8	9 Relaxed
8. Sensitive	1	2	3	4	5	6	7	8	9 Insensitive
9. Anxious	1	2	3	4	5	6	7	8	9 Composed
10. Pleasant	1	2	3	4	5	6	7	8	9 Unpleasant
11. Withdrawn	1	2	3	4	5	6	7	8	9 Outgoing
12. Quiet	1	2	3	4	5	6	7	8	9 Loud
13. Intelligent	1	2	3	4	5	6	7	8	9 Dull
14. Talkative	1	2	3	4	5	6	7	8	9 Reticent

	1	2	3	4	5	6	7	8		9
15.	Avoiding									Approaching

	1	2	3	4	5	6	7	8	9
16.	Fearful								Fearless

	1	2	3	4	5	6	7	8	9
17.	Aggressive								Passive

	1	2	3	4	5	6	7	8	9
18.	Afraid								Content

	1	2	3	4	5	6	7	8	9
19.	Introverted								Extroverted

	1	2	3	4	5	6	7	8	9
20.	Daring								Hesitant

	1	2	3	4	5	6	7	8	9
21.	Secure								Insecure

	1	2	3	4	5	6	7	8	9
22.	Emotional								Bland

	1	2	3	4	5	6	7	8	9
23.	Perfectionistic								Careless

	1	2	3	4	5	6	7	8	9
24.	Bragging								Self-derogatory

	1	2	3	4	5	6	7	8	9
25.	Inflexible								Flexible

[Reproduced from Kalinowski et al., 1987, pp. 329–331.]

SOUTHERN ILLINOIS UNIVERSITY
SPEECH SITUATION CHECKLIST

Instructions: The items in this checklist refer to speech situations, situations where you are involved in talking. Talking in these situations may or may not currently cause you some negative emotion, e.g., fear, tension, anxiety, or other unpleasant feelings. In the column as indicated put the number that best describes how much each of these speech situations disturbs you nowadays.

> 0 = not relevant
> 1 = not at all
> 2 = a little
> 3 = a fair amount
> 4 = much
> 5 = very much

Rating	Speech Situation
1.	Talking on the telephone
2.	Talking to a stranger
3.	Giving your name
4.	Talking with a young child
5.	Saying a sound or word that has in the past been troublesome
6.	Placing an order in a restaurant
7.	Talking to an animal
8.	Placing a person-to-person telephone call
9.	Talking with a close friend
10.	Arguing with parents
11.	Talking with a sales clerk
12.	Talking in a rap or bull session
13.	Being criticized
14.	Meeting someone for the first time
15.	Talking after being teased about your speech
16.	Saying hello
17.	Reading an unchangeable passage aloud
18.	Being misunderstood
19.	Answering a specific question
20.	Asking for information
21.	Being interviewed for a job

Rating	Speech Situation
22.	Trying to get across your own point of view
23.	Introducing yourself
24.	Giving directions
25.	Talking when "high"
26.	Talking to hairdresser
27.	Talking when trying to make a good impression
28.	Talking when generally happy
29.	Talking with teachers
30.	Making an appointment with a secretary
31.	Asking the teacher a question
32.	Answering questions about your speech
33.	Being asked to repeat your answer
34.	Being asked to give your name
35.	Making introductions
36.	Being asked to give personal information
37.	Asking if someone is at home
38.	Buying a plane, bus, or train ticket to a specific place
39.	Telling a taxicab driver where to take you
40.	Asking a gas station attendant for a specific amount of gas
41.	Speaking before a group
42.	Making an appointment
43.	Giving a prepared speech
44.	Being rushed when speaking
45.	Apologizing
46.	Being with a member of the opposite sex
47.	Refuting a criticism
48.	Giving a telephone number
49.	Giving an ad lib report
50.	Returning a call
51.	Selling a product

[Reproduced from Hanson, Gronhovd, & Rice, 1981, pp. 354–355.]

DISFLUENCY DESCRIPTOR DIGEST

THE UNIVERSITY OF ALABAMA
DEPARTMENT OF COMMUNICATIVE DISORDERS,

**PERSONALIZED FLUENCY CONTROL THERAPY
DISFLUENCY DESCRIPTOR DIGEST,
For the Identification of
Appropriate Fluency Initiating Gestures**

CLIENT _____ FILE NO. _____

CLINICIAN _____ DATE _____

Directions: Below are statements describing behavior frequently observed in the disfluent speech of stutterers. Place a check (✓) in the box preceding the statement if the behavior is present in the client's stuttering pattern even if the behavior occurs only occasionally.

☐ 1. Disfluencies are characterized by obvious "struggle behavior" in the laryngeal area prior to speech onset.

☐ 2. Frequently the disfluency is characterized by obvious articulatory posturings of the jaw, lips, or tongue prior to the initiation of sound.

☐ 3. Speech appears monotone with abnormally little variation in intensity and pitch.

☐ 4. The onset and the termination of speech sounds in continued speech appears abnormally abrupt.

☐ 5. The breathing pattern for speech appears to be more "clavicular" or "thoracic" than abdominal.

☐ 6. Articulatory movements appear abnormally rapid.

☐ 7. The habitual pitch level appears too high or low for the individual's age, sex, and size.

☐ 8. The voice quality appears "harsh," "husky," or "hoarse."

☐ 9. In general, the rate of speech appears rapid.

☐ 10. Disfluencies frequently are characterized by rapid and repetitious articulatory movements of the jaw, lips, or tongue.

☐ 11. During periods of disfluency, the breathing pattern appears asynchronous and disruptive to fluent speech.

☐ 12. Disfluencies frequently are characterized by fixed articulatory placements of the jaw, lips, or tongue resulting in a complete closure of the vocal tract.

☐ 13. Disfluencies frequently appear to originate at the level of the larynx with an inability to initiate phonation.

☐ 14. Inhalation prior to the speech attempt appears abnormally rapid.

☐ 15. Inhalation prior to the speech attempt appears insufficient.

☐ 16. Inhalation prior to the speech attempt appears abnormally prolonged.

☐ 17. Speech appears abnormally soft with respect to loudness.

☐ 18. Disfluencies appear to occur at the end of an exhalation—client appears "out-of-breath."

☐ 19. Pauses are observed between the cessation of inhalation and the initiation of phonation.

☐ 20. Speech appears abnormally loud.

Directions: Now place a check before those numbers in the box below that correspond to the statement numbers that you checked above. When finished you might be able to identify more clearly which FIG or FIGs will be most helpful for your client.

FIG Fluency Initiating Gesture	Numbers of statements above describing behavior modified by the FIG
Slow Speech	☐6 ☐9 ☐10
Smooth Speech	☐4 ☐8 ☐12
Easy Onset	☐1 ☐2 ☐7 ☐12 ☐13 ☐19
Deep Breath	☐5 ☐7 ☐11 ☐14 ☐15 ☐16 ☐18
Syllable Stress	☐3 ☐11 ☐12
Loudness Control	☐3 ☐8 ☐17 ☐20

[Reproduced from Cooper, 1982, p. 357.]

CHILDREN'S ATTITUDES ABOUT TALKING—REVISED (CAT-R)

Read each sentence carefully so you can say if it is true or false for you. The sentences are about your talking. If you feel that the sentence is right, circle "True." If you think the sentence about your talking is not right, circle "False." Remember, circle "False" if you think the sentence is wrong and "True" if you think it is right.

1.	I don't talk right.	**True**	False
2.	I don't mind asking the teacher a question in class	True	**False**
3.	Sometimes words will stick in my mouth when I talk.	**True**	False
4.	People worry about the way I talk.	**True**	False
5.	It is harder for me to give a report in class than it is for most of the other kids.	**True**	False
6.	My classmates don't think I talk funny.	True	**False**
7.	I like the way I talk.	True	**False**
8.	People sometimes finish my words for me.	**True**	False
9.	My parents like the way I talk.	True	**False**
10.	I find it easy to talk to most everyone.	True	**False**
11.	I talk well most of the time.	True	**False**
12.	It is hard for me to talk to people.	**True**	False
13.	I don't talk like other kids.	**True**	False
14.	I don't worry about the way I talk.	True	**False**
15.	I don't find it easy to talk.	**True**	False
16.	My words come out easily.	True	**False**
17.	It is hard for me to talk to strangers.	**True**	False
18.	The other kids wish they could talk like me.	True	**False**
19.	Some kids make fun of the way I talk.	**True**	False
20.	Talking is easy for me.	True	**False**
21.	Telling someone my name is hard for me.	**True**	False
22.	Words are hard for me to say.	**True**	False
23.	I talk well with most everyone.	True	**False**
24.	Sometimes I have trouble talking.	**True**	False
25.	I would rather talk than write.	True	**False**
26.	I like to talk.	True	**False**
27.	I wish I could talk like other kids.	**True**	False
28.	I am afraid the words won't come out when I talk.	**True**	False
29.	I don't worry about talking on the phone.	True	**False**
30.	People don't seem to like the way I talk.	**True**	False
31.	I let others talk for me.	**True**	False
32.	Reading out loud in class is easy for me.	True	**False**

(The answers in "bold" indicate a negative attitude toward talking.)

[Reproduced from De Nil & Brutten, 1991a, pp. 65–66.]

THE COOPER CHRONICITY
PREDICTION CHECKLIST

Instructions: To be completed for children ages three to eight. Answers to questions require the assistance of the child's parents. Each item should be explained and discussed with the parents. Place a check (✓) on the appropriate blank.

	Yes	No	Unknown

I.   Historical Indicators of Chronicity

    1. Is there a history of chronic stuttering in the family? ____ ____ ____

    2. Is the severity (frequency, duration, consistency) of the disfluencies increasing? ____ ____ ____

    3. Did the disfluencies begin with blockings rather than with easy repetitions? ____ ____ ____

    4. Have the child's disfluencies persisted since being observed (as opposed to being episodic with long periods of normal fluency)? ____ ____ ____

    5. Has the child been disfluent for two or more years? ____ ____ ____

II. Attitudinal Indicators of Chronicity

    1. Does the child perceive himself or herself to be disfluent? ____ ____ ____

    2. Does the child experience communicative fear because of the disfluencies? ____ ____ ____

    3. Does the child believe the disfluency problem to be getting worse? ____ ____ ____

    4. Does the child avoid speaking situations? ____ ____ ____

    5. Does the child express anger or frustration because of the disfluencies? ____ ____ ____

III. Behavioral Indicators of Chronicity

    1. Do sound prolongations or hesitations occur among the disfluencies? ____ ____ ____

    2. Are the repetitions more frequently whole word or phrase repetitions rather than part-word repetitions? ____ ____ ____

    3. Are the part-word repetitions accompanied by visible tension or stress? ____ ____ ____

    4. Do the part-word repetitions occur more than three times on the same word? ____ ____ ____

    5. Is the rapidity of the syllable repetitions faster than normal? ____ ____ ____

    6. Is the schwa vowel inappropriately inserted in the syllable repetition? ____ ____ ____

    7. Is the air flow during the repetitions often interrupted? ____ ____ ____

    8. Do prolongations last longer than one second? ____ ____ ____

    9. Do prolongations occur on more than one word in a hundred during periods of disfluency? ____ ____ ____

    10. Are the prolongations uneven or interrupted as opposed to being smooth? ____ ____ ____

    11. Is there observable tension during the prolongation? ____ ____ ____

12. Are the terminations of the prolongations sudden as
opposed to being gradual?   ___ ___ ___
13. During prolongations of voiced sounds is the
airflow interrupted?   ___ ___ ___
14. Are the silent pauses prior to the speech
attempt unusually long?   ___ ___ ___
15. Are the inflection patterns restricted and monotone? ___ ___ ___
16. Is there loss of eye contact during the moment of
disfluency?   ___ ___ ___
17. Are there observable and/or distracting extraneous
facial or body movements during the moment of
disfluency?   ___ ___ ___

Total 'Yes' Responses   ___

Instructions: Place a check on the appropriate blank.

Predictive of Recovery: 0–6   ___

Requiring Vigilance: 7–15   ___

Predictive of Chronicity: 16–27   ___

Caution: The categorization of scores used on this checklist is based on an interpretation of data reported by McClelland and Cooper (*Journal of Fluency Disorders,* 1978) and on clinical observation. It is not based on longitudinal studies. Judgments as to probable stuttering chronicity should not be based solely on the scoring of this checklist.

From: Cooper, E. B., & Cooper, C. S. (1985). *Cooper personalized fluency therapy handbook* (rev.). Allen, TX: DLM Teaching Resources. Used with permission from DLM Teaching Resources.

[Reproduced from Gordon & Luper, 1992.]

DALY'S CHECKLIST FOR POSSIBLE CLUTTERING—EXPERIMENTAL EDITION

Client's Name_____ Date _____

Instructions: Please respond to each descriptive statement below. Your answers should reflect how well you believe the statement describes the child/adult:

STATEMENT TRUE FOR CLIENT	*Not at all* 0	*Just a little* 1	*Pretty much* 2	*Very much* 3
1. Repeats syllables, words, phrases	0	1	2	3
2. Started talking late; onset of words and sentences delayed	0	1	2	3
3. Fluency disruptions started early; no remissions; never very fluent	0	1	2	3
4. Speech very disorganized; confused wording	0	1	2	3
5. Silent gaps or hesitations common; interjections; many "filler" words	0	1	2	3
6. Stops before saying initial vowel; no tension; drawn-out vowels	0	1	2	3
7. Rapid rate (speaks too fast); tachylalia; speaks in spurts	0	1	2	3
8. Extrovert; high verbal output; compulsive talker	0	1	2	3
9. Jerky breathing pattern, respiratory dysrhythmia	0	1	2	3
10. Slurred articulation (omits sounds or unstressed syllables)	0	1	2	3
11. Mispronunciation of /r/, /l/, and sibilants	0	1	2	3
12. Speech better under pressure; e.g., during short periods of heightened attention	0	1	2	3
13. Difficulty following directions; impatient/uninterested listener	0	1	2	3
14. Distractible; attention span problems; poor concentration	0	1	2	3
15. Story-telling difficulty; (trouble sequencing events)	0	1	2	3
16. Demonstrates word-finding difficulties resembling anomia	0	1	2	3
17. Inappropriate reference by pronouns is common	0	1	2	3
18. Improper language structure; poor grammar and syntax	0	1	2	3
19. Clumsy and uncoordinated; motor activities accelerated (or hasty)	0	1	2	3

STATEMENT TRUE FOR CLIENT	*Not at all* 0	*Just a little* 1	*Pretty much* 2	*Very much* 3
20. Reading disorder is a prominent disability	0	1	2	3
21. Disintegrated and fractionated writing; poor motor control	0	1	2	3
22. Writing shows transposition of letters and words (omits letters and syllables)	0	1	2	3
23. Left-right confusion; delayed hand preference	0	1	2	3
24. Initial loud voice; trails off to a murmer; mumbles	0	1	2	3
25. Seems to think faster than he can talk or write	0	1	2	3
26. Above average in mathematical and abstract reasoning abilities	0	1	2	3
27. Poor rhythm, timing, or musical ability (may dislike singing)	0	1	2	3
28. Improper stress patterns of speech; poor melodic accenting of syllables	0	1	2	3
29. Appears younger than age; small and/or immature	0	1	2	3
30. Other family member with same/similar problem; heredity	0	1	2	3
31. Untidy; careless, hasty; impulsive or forgetful	0	1	2	3
32. Impatient, superficial, and/or short-tempered	0	1	2	3
33. Lack of self-awareness; unconcerned attitude over inappropriateness of many behaviors and responses	0	1	2	3

TOTAL SCORE _____

DIAGNOSIS _____

Other Relevant Information Determined by Interviewer:

(Circle correct answer)

Identified in school as learning disabled.   Yes No   Recommended for testing   Don't know

Current receiving speech/language therapy Yes No   Recommended   Don't know

Comments: _____
_____
_____

Clinician _____

Experimental Edition by
David A. Daly, 1991

[Reproduced from Daly, 1993a]

References

Abe, K., Yokoyama, R., & Yorifuji, S. (1992). On stuttering-like hesitation resulting from infarct in the midbrain and the mesial thalami [Japanese]. *Rinsho Shinkeigaku,* 32(8), 822–825.

Abe, K., Yokoyama, R., & Yorifuji, S. (1993). Repetitive speech disorder resulting from infarcts in the paramedian thalami and midbrain. *Journal of Neurology, Neurosurgery, & Psychiatry,* 56, 1024–1026.

Accordi, M., Bianchi, R., Consolaro, C., Tronchin, F., DeFilippi, R., Pasqualon, L., Ugo, E., & Croatto, L. (1983). L'Eziopatogenesi della balbuzie: Studio statistico su 2802 casi. *Acta Phoniatrica Latina,* 5, 171–180.

Adamczyk, B. (1994). Stuttering therapy with the "Echo Method." *Journal of Fluency Disorders,* 19, 147.

Adams, M. R. (1981). The speech production abilities of stutterers: Recent, ongoing and future research. *Journal of Fluency Disorders,* 6, 311–326

Adams, M. R. (1982). A case report on the use of flooding in stuttering therapy. *Journal of Fluency Disorders,* 7, 343–353.

Adams, M. R. (1983). Learning from negative outcomes in stuttering therapy: I. Getting off on the wrong foot. *Journal of Fluency Disorders,* 8, 147–153.

Adams, M. R. (1984). Stuttering theory, research, and therapy: A five-year retrospective and look ahead. *Journal of Fluency Disorders,* 9, 103–113.

Adams, M. R. (1990). The demands and capacities model I: Theoretical elaborations. *Journal of Fluency Disorders,* 15, 135–141.

Adams, M. R. (1992). Childhood stuttering under "positive" conditions. *American Journal of Speech-Language Pathology,* 1(3), 5–6.

Adams, M. R., & Hayden, P. (1976). The ability of stutterers and nonstutterers to initiate and terminate phonation during production of an isolated vowel. *Journal of Speech and Hearing Research,* 19, 290–296.

Adams, M. R., & Ramig, P. (1980). Vocal characteristics of normal speakers and stutterers during oral reading. *Journal of Speech and Hearing Research,* 23, 457–469.

Adams, M. R., & Runyan, C. M. (1981). Stuttering and fluency: Exclusive events or points on a continuum? *Journal of Fluency Disorders,* 6, 197–218.

Adams, M. R., Sears, R. L., & Ramig, P. R. (1982). Vocal changes in stutterers and nonstutterers during monotoned speech. *Journal of Fluency Disorders,* 7, 21–35.

Aguirrebengoa, L. (1994). Prevention of stuttering: Parents of stuttering children. *Journal of Fluency Disorders,* 19, 148–149.

Ainsworth, S., & Fraser-Gruss, J. (1981). *If Your Child Stutters: A Guide for Parents.* Memphis, TN: Speech Foundation of America.

Ajuriaguerra, J. R. De, Diakine, H. De Gobineau, Narlian, S., & Stambak, M. (1958). Le Bégaiement. *Presse Medicale,* 66, 953–956.

Alfonso, P. J. (1990). Subject definition and selection criteria for stuttering research in adult subjects. *Asha Reports* (Number 18), 15–24.

Alm, P. (1994). Study groups for stutterers: A valuable part of stuttering therapy? *Journal of Fluency Disorders,* 19, 149.

Ambrose, N. G., & Yairi, E. (1994). The development of awareness of stuttering in preschool children. *Journal of Fluency Disorders.* 19, 229–245.

Ambrose, N. G., Yairi, E., & Cox, N. (1993). Genetic aspects of early childhood stuttering. *Journal of Speech and Hearing Research,* 36, 701–706.

American Speech-Language-Hearing Association (March 1995). Guidelines for practice in stuttering treatment. *Asha,* 37 (Supplement 4), 26–35.

Aminoff, M. J., Dedo, H. H., & Izedebski, K. (1978). Clinical aspects of spastic dysphonia. *Journal of Neurology, Neurosurgery, and Psychiatry,* 41, 361–365.

Amman, J. O. C. (1700). *A Dissertation on Speech.* (Reprinted 1965) New York: Stechert-Hafner.

Ammons, R., & Johnson, W. (1944). The construction and application of a test of attitude toward stuttering. *Journal of Speech and Hearing Disorders,* 9, 39–49.

Amster, B. (1994). Perfectionism and stuttering. *Journal of Fluency Disorders,* 9, 150.

Amster, B., & Wark, J. (1994). The effect of verapamil on school-age stuttering children. *Journal of Fluency Disorders,* 9, 150.

Anderson, D. (1994). He stammers! That's a pity!: Historical perceptions of stuttering as reflected in the arts. *Journal of Fluency Disorders,* 19, 150.

Anderson, J. M., Hood, S. B., & Sellers, D. E. (1988). Central auditory processing abilities of adolescent and preadolescent stuttering and nonstuttering children. *Journal of Fluency Disorders,* 13, 199–214.

Andrews, G. (1984). The epidemiology of stuttering. In R. F. Curlee & W. H. Perkins (Eds.), *The Nature and Treatment of Stuttering: New Directions.* San Diego, CA: College-Hill.

Andrews, G., & Craig, A. (1982). Stuttering: Overt and covert measurement of the speech of treated stutterers. *Journal of Speech and Hearing Disorders,* 47, 96–99.

Andrews, G., & Craig, A. (1988). Prediction of outcome after treatment for stuttering. *British Journal of Psychiatry,* 153, 236–240.

Andrews, G., Craig, A., Feyer, A.-M., Hoddinott, S., Howie, P., & Neilson, M. (1983). Stuttering: A review of research findings and theories circa 1982. *Journal of Speech and Hearing Disorders,* 48, 226–246.

Andrews, G., & Cutler, J. (1974). Stuttering therapy: The relation between changes in symptom level and attitude. *Journal of Speech and Hearing Disorders,* 39, 312–319.

Andrews, G., & Dozsa, M. (1977). Haloperidol and the treatment of stuttering. *Journal of Fluency Disorders,* 2, 217–224.

Andrews, G., & Harris, M. (1964). *The Syndrome of Stuttering.* London: William Heinemann Medical Books.

Andrews, G., Howie, P. M., Dozsa, M., & Guitar, B. E. (1982). Stuttering: Speech pattern characteristics under fluency-inducing conditions. *Journal of Speech and Hearing Research,* 25, 208–216.

Andrews, G., & Ingham, R. J. (1972). Stuttering: An evaluation of follow-up procedures for syllable-timed speech/token system therapy. *Journal of Communication Disorders,* 5, 307–319.

Andrews, G., & Tanner, S. (1982a). Stuttering treatment: An attempt to replicate the regulated-breathing method. *Journal of Speech and Hearing Disorders,* 47, 138–140.

Andrews, G., & Tanner, S. (1982b). Stuttering: The results of 5 days treatment with an airflow technique. *Journal of Speech and Hearing Disorders,* 47, 427–429.

Andy, O. J., & Bhatnagar, S. C. (1991). Thalamic-induced stuttering (surgical observations). *Journal of Speech and Hearing Research,* 34, 796–800.

Andy, O. J., & Bhatnagar, S. C. (1992). Stuttering acquired from subcortical pathologies and its alleviation from thalamic perturbation. *Brain and Language,* 42(4), 385–401.

Appelt, A. (1911). *Stammering and its Permanent Cure.* London: Methuen.

Aram, D. M., Meyers, S. C., & Ekelman, B. L. (1990). Fluency of conversational speech in children with unilateral brain lesions. *Brain and Language,* 38, 105–121.

Ardila, A., & Lopez, M. V. (1986). Severe stuttering associated with right hemisphere disease. *Brain and Language,* 27, 239–246.

Arnold, G. E. (1959). Spastic dysphonia: I. Changing interpretations of a persistent affliction. *Logos,* 2, 3–14

Arnold, G. E. (1965). Cluttering: Tachyphemia. In R. Luchinger & G. E. Arnold (Eds.), *Voice-Speech-Language.* Belmont, CA: Wadsworth.

Arnott, N. (1828). *Elements of Physics.* Edinburgh: Adams.

Aronson, A. E. (1973). *Psychogenic Voice Disorders; An Interdisciplinary Approach to Detection, Diagnosis, and Therapy.* Philadelphia: W. B. Saunders.

Aronson, A. E. (1990). *Clinical Voice Disorders, An Interdisciplinary Approach.* New York: Thieme.

Aronson, A. E., Brown, J. R., Litin, E. M., & Pearson, J. S. (1968). Spastic dysphonia: I. Voice, neurological, and psychiatric aspects. *Journal of Speech and Hearing Disorders, 33,* 203–218.

Aronson, A. E., & Hartman, D. (1981). Adductor spastic dysphonia as a sign of essential (voice) tremor. *Journal of Speech and Hearing Disorders, 46,* 52–58.

Atkins, C. P. (1988). Perceptions of speakers with minimal eye contact: Implications for stutterers. *Journal of Fluency Disorders, 13,* 429–436.

Attanasio, J. S. (1987a). A case of late-onset or acquired stuttering in adult life. *Journal of Fluency Disorders, 12,* 287–290.

Attanasio, J. S. (1987b). The dodo was Lewis Carroll, you see: Reflections and speculations. *Journal of Fluency Disorders, 12,* 107–118.

Azrin, N. H., & Nunn, R. G. (1974). A rapid method of eliminating stuttering by a regulated breathing approach. *Behavior Research and Therapy, 12,* 279–286.

Azrin, N. H., Nunn, R. G., & Frantz, S. E. (1979). Comparison of regulated breathing vs. abbreviated desensitization on reported stuttering episodes. *Journal of Speech and Hearing Disorders, 44,* 331–339.

Baken, R. J., McManus, D. A., & Cavallo, S. A. (1983). Prephonatory chest wall posturing in stutterers. *Journal of Speech and Hearing Research, 26,* 444–450.

Bakker, K., & Brutten, G. J. (1990). Speech-related reaction times of stutterers and nonstutterers: Diagnostic implications. *Journal of Speech and Hearing Disorders, 55,* 295–299.

Balasubramanian, V., & Hayden, P. (1994). Acquired stuttering following bilateral parietal lobe lesion: A case report. *Journal of Fluency Disorders, 19,* 152.

Barbara, D. A. (1982). *The Psychodynamics of Stuttering.* Springfield, IL: Charles C. Thomas.

Barber, J. (1981). *The Development and Evaluation of an Instrument for Assessing Stutterers' Communication Attitudes.* Unpublished doctoral dissertation, Northwestern University, Chicago.

Barber, V. (1939). Studies in the psychology of stuttering: XV. Chorus reading as a distraction in stuttering. *Journal of Speech Disorders, 4,* 371–383.

Baumgartner, J. M., & Brutten, G. J. (1983). Expectancy and heart rate as predictors of the speech performance of stutterers. *Journal of Speech and Hearing Research, 26,* 383–388.

Bebout, L., & Arthur, B. (1992). Cross-cultural attitudes toward speech disorders. *Journal of Speech and Hearing Research, 35,* 45–52.

Beech, H. R., & Fransella, F. (1968). *Research and Experiment in Stuttering.* New York: Pergamon.

Bell, A. M. (1853). *Observations on Defects of Speech, the Cure of Stammering, and the Principles of Elocution.* London: Hamilton-Adams.

Bellak, L. (1954). *The Thematic Apperception Test and the Children's Apperception Test in Clinical Use.* New York: Grune & Stratton.

Bender, J. F. (1939). *The Personality Structure of Stuttering.* New York: Pitman.

Benecken, J. (1994). On the nature and clinical relevance of a stigma: "The stutterer." *Journal of Fluency Disorders,* 19, 154.

Berlin, A. J. (1954). An exploratory attempt to isolate types of stuttering. Unpublished doctoral dissertation, Northwestern University.

Berlin, C. I. (1960). Parents' diagnoses of stuttering. *Journal of Speech and Hearing Research,* 3, 372–379.

Berlin, S., & Berlin, L. (1964). Acceptability of stuttering and control patterns. *Journal of Speech and Hearing Disorders,* 29, 436–441.

Bernstein-Ratner, N., & Benitez, M. (1985). Linguistic analysis of a bilingual stutterer. *Journal of Fluency Disorders,* 10, 211–219

Bhatnagar, S. C., & Andy, O. J. (1989). Alleviation of acquired stuttering with human centremedian thalamic stimulation. *Journal of Neurology, Neurosurgery, and Psychiatry,* 52, 1182–1184.

Biller, H. F., Som, M. L., & Lawson, W. (1979). Laryngeal nerve crush for spastic dysphonia. Paper presented at the annual meeting of the American Laryngological Association, Los Angeles.

Black, J. A. (1987). A comparative study of the perception of freedom-in-leisure between stuttering and nonstuttering individuals. *Journal of Fluency Disorders,* 12, 239–248.

Blackburn, W. B. (1931). Study of voluntary movements in stutterers and normal speakers. *Psychological Monographs,* 41, 1–13.

Blaesing, L. (1982). A multidisciplinary approach to individualized treatment of stuttering. *Journal of Fluency Disorders,* 7, 203–218.

Blankenship, J., & Kay, C. (1964). Hesitation phenomena in English speech: A study in distribution. *Word,* 20, 360–373.

Blanton, S., & Blanton, M. G. (1936). *For Stutterers.* New York: D. Appleton-Century.

Bloch, E. L. & Goodstein, L. D. (1971). Functional speech disorders and personality: A decade of research. *Journal of Speech and Hearing Disorders,* 36, 295–314.

Bloch, P. (1965). Neuro-psychiatric aspects of spastic dysphonia. *Folia Phoniatrica,* 17, 301–364.

Blood, G. W. (1993). Treatment efficacy in adults who stutter: Review and recommendations. *Journal of Fluency Disorders,* 18, 303–318.

Blood, G. W., & Blood, I. M. (1989a). Laterality preferences in adult female and male stutterers. *Journal of Fluency Disorders,* 14, 1–10.

Blood, G. W., & Blood, I. M. (1989b). Multiple data analysis of dichotic listening advantages of stutterers. *Journal of Fluency Disorders,* 14, 97–107.

Blood, G. W., Blood, I. M., & Hood, S. B. (1987). The development of ear preferences in stuttering and nonstuttering children: A longitudinal study. *Journal of Fluency Disorders,* 12, 119–131.

Blood, G. W., & Seider, R. (1981). The concomitant problems of young stutterers. *Journal of Speech and Hearing Disorders,* 24, 31–33.

Bloodstein, O. (1950). A rating scale study of conditions under which stuttering is reduced or absent. *Journal of Speech and Hearing Disorders,* 15, 29–36.

Bloodstein, O. (1958). Stuttering as an anticipatory struggle reaction. In J. Eisenson (Ed.), *Stuttering: A Symposium.* New York: Harper & Brothers, 1–69.

Bloodstein, O. (1960). The development of stuttering: II. Developmental phases. *Journal of Speech and Hearing Disorders,* 25, 366–376.

Bloodstein, O. (1961). The development of stuttering: III. Theoretical and clinical implications. *Journal of Speech and Hearing Disorders,* 26, 67–82.

Bloodstein, O. (1975). Stuttering as tension and fragmentation. In J. Eisenson (Ed.), *Stuttering: A Second Symposium.* New York: Harper & Row, pp. 1–95.

Bloodstein, O. (1984). *Speech Pathology: An Introduction* (2nd Ed.). Boston: Houghton Mifflin.

Bloodstein, O. (1987). *A Handbook on Stuttering* (4th ed.). Chicago: National Easter Seal Society.

Bloodstein, O. (1988). Verification of stuttering in a suspected malingerer. *Journal of Fluency Disorders,* 13, 83–88.

Bloodstein, O. (1990). On pluttering, skivering, and floggering: A commentary. *Journal of Speech and Hearing Disorders,* 55, 392–393.

Bloodstein, O., & Grossman, M. (1981). Early stutterings: Some aspects of their form and distribution. *Journal of Speech and Hearing Research,* 24, 298–302.

Bloodstein, O., & Schreiber, L. R. (1957). Obsessive-compulsive reactions in stutterers. *Journal of Speech and Hearing Disorders,* 22, 33–39.

Bloom, C. M., & Silverman, F. H. (1973). Do all stutterers adapt? *Journal of Speech and Hearing Research,* 16, 518–521.

Bloom, L. (1978). Notes for a history of speech pathology. *Psychoanalytic Review,* 65, 433–463.

Bluemel, C. S. (1932). Primary and secondary stammering. *Quarterly Journal of Speech,* 18, 187–200.

Bluemel, C. S. (1935). *Stammering and Allied Disorders.* New York: Macmillan.

Bluemel, C. S. (1957). *The Riddle of Stuttering.* Danville, IL: Interstate Publishing Company.

Boberg, E. (1976). Intensive group therapy program for stutterers. *Human Communication,* 1, 29–42.

Boberg, E. (1981). *The Maintenance of Fluency.* New York: Elsevier.

Boberg, E., Ewart, B., Mason, G., Lindsay, K., & Wynn, S. (1978). Stuttering in the retarded: II. Prevalence of stuttering in EMR and TMR children. *Mental Retardation Bulletin,* 6, 67–76.

Boberg, E., Howie, P., & Woods, L. (1979). Maintenance of fluency: A review. *Journal of Fluency Disorders,* 4, 93–116.

Boberg, E., & Sawyer, L. (1977). The maintenance of fluency following intensive therapy. *Human Communication,* 2, 21–28.

Boberg, E., Yeudall, L. T., Schopflocher, D., & Bo-Lassen, P. (1983). The effect of an intensive behavioral program on the distribution of EEG alpha power in stutterers during the processing of verbal and visuospatial information. *Journal of Fluency Disorders,* 8, 245–263.

Boberg, J. M., & Boberg, E. (1990). The other side of the block: The stutterer's spouse. *Journal of Fluency Disorders,* 15, 61–75.

Boehmler, R. M. (1958). Listener responses to non-fluencies. *Journal of Speech and Hearing Research,* 1, 132–141.

Boehmler, R. M., & Boehmler, S. I. (1989). The cause of stuttering: What is the question? *Journal of Fluency Disorders,* 14, 447–450.

Bogue, B. N. (1926). *Stammering: Its Cause and Cure.* Indianapolis, IN: Published by the author.

Bonin, B., Ramig, P., & Prescott, T. (1985). Performance differences between stuttering and nonstuttering subjects on a sound fusion task. *Journal of Fluency Disorders,* 10, 291–300.

Boome, E. J., & Richardson, M. A. (1931). *The Nature and Treatment of Stammering.* London: Methuen & Co.

Boone, D. R. (1987). *Human Communication and Its Disorders.* Englewood Cliffs, NJ: Prentice-Hall.

Borden, G. L., Baer, T., & Kenney, M. K. (1985). Onset of voicing in stuttered and fluent utterances. *Journal of Speech and Hearing Research,* 28, 363–372.

Bradford, D. (1963). Studies in tachyphemia: VII. A framework of therapeusis for articulation therapy with tachyphemia and/or general language disability. *Logos,* 6, 59–65.

Brady, J. P. (1968). A behavioral approach to the treatment of stuttering. *American Journal of Psychiatry,* 125, 843–848.

Brady, J. P. (1969). Studies on the metronome effect on stuttering. *Behavior Research and Therapy,* 7, 197–204.

Brady, J. P. (1971). Metronome-conditioned speech retraining for stuttering. *Behavior Therapy,* 2, 129–150.

Brady, J. P. (1991). The pharmacology of stuttering: A critical review. *American Journal of Psychiatry,* 148, 1309–1316.

Brady, J. P. (1994). The role of pharmacology in the treatment of stuttering. *Journal of Fluency Disorders,* 19, 158.

Brady, W. A., & Hall, D. E. (1976). The prevalence of stuttering among school-age children. *Language, Speech, and Hearing Services in Schools,* 7, 75–81.

Brauneis, E. (1994). The use of acupuncture in a holistic approach to the treatment of stuttering. *Journal of Fluency Disorders,* 19, 158.

Breuer, J., & Freud, S. (1936). *Studies in Hysteria* (Nervous and Mental Disease Monograph Series No. 61). New York: Nervous and Mental Disease Publishing Company.

Brill, A. A. (1923). Speech disturbances in nervous and mental diseases. *Quarterly Journal of Speech,* 9, 129–135.

Brodnitz, F. S. (1976). Spastic dysphonia. *Annals of Otology, Rhinology, and Laryngology,* 85, 212–213.

Broida, H. (1963). An empirical study of sex-role identification and sex-role preference in stuttering. *Speech Monographs,* 30, 242–243.

Brown, C. J., Zimmerman, G. N., Linville, R. N., & Hegmann, J. P. (1990). Variations in self-paced behaviors in stutterers and nonstutterers. *Journal of Speech and Hearing Research,* 33, 317–323.

Brown, G., & Cullinan, W. L. (1981). Word-retrieval difficulty and disfluent speech in adult anomic speakers. *Journal of Speech and Hearing Research,* 24, 358–365.

Brown, S. F. (1938). Stuttering with relation to word accent and word position. *Journal of Abnormal and Social Psychology,* 33, 112–120.

Brown, S. F. (1945). The loci of stutterings in the speech sequence. *Journal of Speech Disorders,* 10, 181–192.

Brown, S. F., & Hull, H. C. (1942). A study of some social attitudes of a group of 59 stutterers. *Journal of Speech Disorders,* 7, 323–324.

Brown, S. F., & Shulman, E. E. (1940). Intramuscular pressure in stutterers and non-stutterers. *Speech Monographs,* 7, 63–74.

Brunner, W., & Frank, F. (1976). Das pulstelemetrische Verhalten von Stotterern, geheilten Stotterern und Sprachgesunden. *Folia Phoniatrica,* 28, 174–181.

Brutten, G. J. (1951). *Anxiety as a Personality Factor among Stutterers.* Unpublished master's thesis, Brooklyn College.

Brutten, G. J. (1975). Stuttering: Topography, assessment, and behavior-change strategies. In J. Eisenson (Ed.), *Stuttering: A Second Symposium.* New York: Harper & Row, pp. 199–262.

Brutten, G. J. (1985). *Communication Attitude Scale.* Carbondale, IL: Speech Clinic, Southern Illinois University.

Brutten, G. J., & Dunham, S. L. (1989). The Communication Attitude Test: A normative study of grade school children. *Journal of Fluency Disorders,* 14, 371–377.

Brutten, G. J., & Shoemaker, D. J. (1967). *The Modification of Stuttering.* Englewood Cliffs, NJ: Prentice-Hall.

Brutten, G. J., & Shoemaker, D. J. (1974). *Speech Situation Checklist.* Carbondale, IL: Speech Clinic, Southern Illinois University.

Brutten, G. J., & Trotter, A. C. (1985). Hemispheric interference: A dual-task investigation of youngsters who stutter. *Journal of Fluency Disorders,* 10, 77–85.

Bryngelson, B. (1952). Suggestions in the theory and treatment of dysphemia and its symptom, stuttering. *The Speech Teacher,* 1, 131–136.

Bryngelson, B., Chapman, M. E., & Hansen, O. K. (1955). *Know Yourself: Guide for Those Who Stutter* (4th ed.). Minneapolis, MN: Burgess Publishing Company.

Bullen, A. K. (1945). A cross-cultural approach to the problem of stuttering. *Child Development,* 16, 1–88.

Burley, P. M., & Morley, R. (1987). Self-monitoring processes in stutterers. *Journal of Fluency Disorders,* 12, 71–78.

Burley, P. M., & Rinaldi, W. (1986). Effects of sex of listener and of stutterer on ratings of stuttering speakers. *Journal of Fluency Disorders,* 11, 329–333.

Byrd, K., & Cooper, E. B. (1989). Expressive and receptive language skills in stuttering children. *Journal of Fluency Disorders,* 14, 121–126.

Byrne, A., Byrne, M. K., & Zibin, T. O. (1993). Transient neurogenic stuttering. *International Journal of Eating Disorders,* 14, 511–514.

Cannito, M. P., Vogel, D., Deal, J. L. & Watson, B. C. (1995). Disfluency and disordered speech motor control. *Journal of Fluency Disorders,* 20, 80–85.

Canter, G. (1971). Observations on neurogenic stuttering: A contribution to differential diagnosis. *British Journal of Disorders of Communication,* 6, 139–143.

Carlisle, J. A. (1985). *Tangled Tongue: Living with a Stutter.* Toronto: University of Toronto Press.

Carlisle, J. A. (1987). Self-help groups and client perception. *Human Communication Canada,* 3, 23–27.

Carp, F. M. (1962). Psychosexual development of stutterers. *Journal of Projective Techniques,* 26, 388–391.

Caruso, A. J., Conture, E. G., & Colton, R. H. (1988). Selected temporal parameters of coordination associated with stuttering in children. *Journal of Fluency Disorders,* 13, 57–82.

Cash, T. F., & Pruzinsky, T. (Eds.) (1990). *Body Images.* New York: Guilford Press.

Cerf, A., & Prins, D. (1974). Stutterers ear preference for dichotic syllables. Paper presented at the annual meeting of the American Speech and Hearing Association, Las Vegas, NV.

Chaney, C. F. (1969). Loci of disfluencies in the speech of nonstutterers. *Journal of Speech and Hearing Research,* 12, 667–668.

Chapman, A. H., & Cooper, E. B. (1973). Nature of stuttering in a mentally retarded population. *American Journal of Mental Deficiency,* 78, 153–157.

Chen, W. H., & Peng, M. C. (1993). Acquired stuttering in a patient with encephalitis. *Kaohsiung Journal of Medical Sciences,* 9(3), 183–185.

Cherry, C., & Sayers, B. (1956). Experiments upon the total inhibition of stammering by external control and some clinical results. *Journal of Psychosomatic Research,* 1, 233–246.

Christensen, J. E., & Lingwall, J. B. (1983). The relationship between treatment exposure times and changes in stuttering frequency during contingent stimulation. *Journal of Fluency Disorders,* 8, 275–281.

Christensen, J. M. (1992). Did primitive man really talk like an ape? *Journal of Speech and Hearing Research,* 35, 805.

Cicero (1942). *Cicero de Oratore* [E. W. Sutton, Trans.]. London: Heinemann.

Clark, R. M. (1964). Our enterprising predecessors and Charles Sydney Bluemel. *Asha,* 6, 108–114.

Code of Ethics of the American Speech-Language-Hearing Association (1991). *Asha,* 33 (3), 103–104.

Cohen, L. R., Thompson, P. F., Ruppel, R. W., & Flaherty, R. P. (1975). Assertive training: An adjunct to fluency shaping. *Journal of Fluency Disorders, 1,* 10–25.

Colcord, R. D., & Gregory, H. H. (1987). Perceptual analyses of stuttering and non-stuttering children's fluent speech productions. *Journal of Fluency Disorders, 12,* 185–195.

Collins, C. R., & Blood, G. W. (1990). Acknowledgment and severity of stuttering as factors influencing nonstutterers' perceptions by stutterers. *Journal of Speech and Hearing Disorders, 55,* 75–81.

Columbus, P. J. (1992). Don't call me Billy Budd! *Journal of Fluency Disorders, 17,* 205–209.

Commodore, R. W., & Cooper, E. B. (1978). Communicative stress and stuttering frequency during normal, whispered, and articulation-without-phonation speech modes. *Journal of Fluency Disorders, 3,* 1–12.

Conture, E. G. (1990a). Childhood stuttering: What it is and who does it. *Asha Reports* (Number 18), 2–14.

Conture, E. G. (1990b). *Stuttering* (2nd ed.). Englewood Cliffs, NJ: Prentice-Hall.

Conture, E. G., Colton, R. H., & Gleason, J. R. (1988). Selected temporal aspects of coordination during fluent speech of young stutterers. *Journal of Speech and Hearing Research, 31,* 640–653.

Conture, E. G., & Edwards, M. (1994). Childhood stuttering and disordered phonology. *Journal of Speech and Hearing Research, 19,* 164.

Conture, E. G., & Fraser, J. (1989). *Stuttering and Your Child: Questions and Answers.* Memphis, TN: Speech Foundation of America.

Conture, E. G., & Guitar, B. E. (1993). Evaluating efficacy of treatment of stuttering: School-age children. *Journal of Fluency Disorders, 18,* 253–287.

Conture, E. G., & Kelly, E. M. (1991). Young stutterers' nonspeech behavior during stuttering. *Journal of Speech and Hearing Research, 34,* 1041–1056.

Conture, E. G., Louko, L. J., & Edwards, M. L. (1993). Simultaneously treating stuttering and disordered phonology in children: Experimental treatment, preliminary findings. *American Journal of Speech-Language Pathology, 2(3),* 72–81.

Conture, E. G., McCall, G. N., & Brewer, D. W. (1977). Laryngeal behavior during stuttering. *Journal of Speech and Hearing Research, 20,* 661–668.

Conture, E. G., Schwartz, H. D., & Brewer, D. W. (1985). Laryngeal behavior during stuttering: A further study. *Journal of Speech and Hearing Research, 28,* 233–240.

Cooper, E. B. (1968). A therapy process for the adult stutterer. *Journal of Speech and Hearing Disorders, 33,* 246–260.

Cooper, E. B. (1972). Recovery from stuttering in a junior and senior high school population. *Journal of Speech and Hearing Research, 15,* 632–638.

Cooper, E. B. (1973). The development of a stuttering chronicity prediction checklist: A preliminary report. *Journal of Speech and Hearing Disorders, 38,* 215–223.

Cooper, E. B. (1978). Facilitating parental participation in preparing the therapy component of the stutterer's Individualized Education Program. *Journal of Fluency Disorders,* 3, 221–228.

Cooper, E. B. (1979). Intervention procedures for the young stutterer. In H. H. Gregory (Ed.), *Controversies About Stuttering Therapy.* Baltimore: University Park Press, pp. 63–96.

Cooper, E. B. (1982). A disfluency descriptor digest for clinical use. *Journal of Fluency Disorders,* 7, 355–358.

Cooper, E. B. (1986). Treatment of stuttering: Future trends. *Journal of Fluency Disorders,* 11, 317–327.

Cooper, E. B. (1987). The chronic perseverative stuttering syndrome: Incurable stuttering. *Journal of Fluency Disorders,* 12, 381–388.

Cooper, E. B. (1993a). Chronic perseverative stuttering syndrome: A harmful or helpful construct? *American Journal of Speech-Language Pathology,* 2(3), 11–15, 21–22.

Cooper, E. B. (1993b). Red herrings, dead horses, straw men, and blind alleys: Escaping the stuttering conundrum. *Journal of Fluency Disorders,* 18, 375–387.

Cooper, E. B., Cady, B. B., & Robbins, C. J. (1970). The effect of the verbal stimulus words *wrong, right,* and *tree* on the disfluency rates of stutterers and nonstutterers. *Journal of Speech and Hearing Research,* 13, 239–244.

Cooper, E. B., & Cooper, C. S. (1985a). Clinician attitudes toward stuttering: A decade of change (1973–1983). *Journal of Fluency Disorders,* 10, 19–33.

Cooper, E. B., & Cooper, C. S. (1985b). *Cooper Personalized Fluency Control Therapy Handbook.* Allen, TX: DLM Teaching Resources.

Cooper, E. B., & Rustin, L. (1985). Clinician attitudes toward stuttering in the United States and Great Britain: A cross-cultural study. *Journal of Fluency Disorders,* 10, 1–17.

Cordes, A. K., & Ingham, R. J. (1994). The reliability of observational data: II. Issues in the identification and measurement of stuttering events. *Journal of Speech and Hearing Research,* 37, 279–294.

Cordes, A. K., & Ingham, R. J. (1995a). Judgments of stuttered and nonstuttered intervals by recognized authorities in stuttering research. *Journal of Speech and Hearing Research,* 38, 33–41.

Cordes, A. K., & Ingham, R. J. (1995b). Stuttering includes both within-word and between-word disfluencies. *Journal of Speech and Hearing Research,* 38, 382–386.

Coriat, I. H. (1931). The nature and analytical treatment of stuttering. *Proceedings of the American Speech Correction Association,* 1, 151–156.

Coriat, I. H. (1933). Psychoanalytic concept of stammering. *Nervous Child,* 2, 167–171.

Costello, J. M. (1975). The establishment of fluency with time-out procedures: The case studies. *Journal of Speech and Hearing Disorders,* 15, 216–231.

Costello, J. M., & Hurst, M. R. (1981). An analysis of the relationship among stuttering behaviors. *Journal of Speech and Hearing Research,* 24, 247–256.

Cox, M. D. (1982). The stutterer and stuttering: Neuropsychological correlates. *Journal of Fluency Disorders,* 7, 129–140.

Cox, M. D. (1986). The psychologically maladjusted stutterer. In K. O. St. Louis (Ed.), *The Atypical Stutterer.* Orlando, FL: Academic Press.

Cox, N. J., Seider, R. A., & Kidd, K. K. (1984). Some environmental factors and hypotheses for stuttering in families with several stutterers. *Journal of Speech and Hearing Research,* 27, 543–548.

Craig, A. R. (1990). An investigation into the relationship between anxiety and stuttering. *Journal of Speech and Hearing Disorders,* 55, 290–294.

Craig, A. R., & Calver, P. (1991). Following up on treated stutterers: Studies of perceptions of fluency and job status. *Journal of Speech and Hearing Research,* 34, 279–284.

Craig, A. R., & Cleary, P. J. (1982). Reduction of stuttering of young male stutterers by electromyographic feedback. *Biofeedback and Self Regulation,* 7, 241–255.

Craven, D. C., & Ryan, B. P. (1984). The use of a portable delayed auditory feedback unit in stuttering therapy. *Journal of Fluency Disorders,* 9, 237–243.

Cross, D., & Luper, H. L. (1979). Voice reaction time of stuttering and nonstuttering children and adults. *Journal of Fluency Disorders,* 4, 59–77.

Cross, D., & Luper, H. L. (1983). Relation between finger reaction time and voice reaction time in stuttering and nonstuttering children and adults. *Journal of Speech and Hearing Research,* 26, 356–361.

Crowe, T. A., & Robinson, T. L. Jr. (1993). Prevention in stuttering: Do we have an ounce to give? *Asha,* 35(11), 53–54.

Culatta, R., & Leeper, L. (1988). Dysfluency isn't always stuttering. *Journal of Speech and Hearing Disorders,* 53, 486–488.

Cullinan, W. L. (1988). Consistency measures revisited. *Journal of Fluency Disorders,* 13, 1–9.

Culp, D. (1984). The preschool fluency development program: Assessment and treatment. In M. Peins (Ed.), *Contemporary Approaches in Stuttering Therapy.* Boston: Little, Brown.

Culton, G. L. (1986). Speech disorders among college freshmen: A 13-year survey. *Journal of Speech and Hearing Disorders,* 51, 3–7.

Curlee, R. F. (1993a). The early history of the behavior modification of stuttering: From laboratory to clinic. *Journal of Fluency Disorders,* 18, 13–25.

Curlee, R. F. (1993b). *Stuttering and Related Fluency Disorders.* New York: Thieme Medical Publishers.

Curry, F., & Gregory, H. (1969). The performance of stutterers on dichotic listening tasks thought to reflect cerebral dominance. *Journal of Speech and Hearing Research,* 12, 73–81.

Dalton, P., & Hardcastle, W. J. (1977). *Disorders of Fluency and Their Effects on Communication.* London: Elsevier North-Holland.

Daly, D. A. (1981). Differentiating stuttering subgroups with Van Riper's developmental tracks: A preliminary study. *Journal of the National Student Speech and Hearing Association,* 9, 89–101.

Daly, D. A. (1986). The clutterer. In K. O. St. Louis (Ed.), *The Atypical Stutterer.* Orlando, FL: Academic Press.

Daly, D. A. (1987). Use of the home VCR to facilitate transfer of fluency. *Journal of Fluency Disorders,* 12, 103–106.

Daly, D. A. (1988). *The Freedom of Fluency: A Therapy Program for the Chronic Stutterer.* Moline, IL: LinguiSystems.

Daly, D. A. (1992). Helping the clutterer: Therapy considerations. In F. Myers & K. O. St. Louis (Eds.), *Cluttering: A Clinical Perspective.* Leicester, England: Far Communications, 107–121.

Daly, D. A. (1993a). Cluttering: Another fluency syndrome. In R. Curlee (Ed.), *Stuttering and Related Disorders of Fluency.* New York: Thieme Medical Publishers, 179–204.

Daly, D. A. (1993b). Cluttering: The orphan of speech-language pathology. *American Journal of Speech-Language Pathology,* 2(2), 6–8.

Daly, D. A., Thompson, J. D., & Simon, C. A. (1985). Treatment of cluttering with stutter-free speech and mental imagery. Paper presented at the annual meeting of the American Speech-Language-Hearing Association in Cincinnati, OH.

Darley, F. L. (1955). The relationship of parental attitudes and adjustments to the development of stuttering. In W. Johnson & R. Leutenegger (Eds.), *Stuttering in Children & Adults.* Minneapolis: University of Minnesota Press.

Darley, F. L., & Spriestersbach, D. C. (1978). *Diagnostic Methods in Speech Pathology* (2nd ed.). New York: Harper & Row.

Darwin, E. (1800). *Zoonomia.* London.

D'Asaro, M. J. (1978). Spastic dysphonia: A non-surgical intervention. Paper presented at the annual meeting of the American Speech-Language-Hearing Association, San Francisco.

Davis, D. (1939). The relation of repetitions in the speech of young children to certain measures of language maturity and situational factors: Part I. *Journal of Speech Disorders,* 4, 303–318.

Davis, G. A. (1993). *A Survey of Adult Aphasia* (Second Edition). Englewood Cliffs, NJ: Prentice-Hall.

Deal, J. L. (1982). Sudden onset of stuttering: A case report. *Journal of Speech and Hearing Disorders,* 47, 301–304.

Deal, J. L., & Doro, J. M. (1987). Episodic hysterical stuttering. *Journal of Speech and Hearing Disorders,* 52, 299–300.

Decker, T. N., Healey, E. C., & Howe, S. W. (1982). Brainstem auditory electrical response characteristics of stutterers and nonstutterers: A preliminary report. *Journal of Fluency Disorders,* 7, 385–401.

Dedo, H. (1976). Recurrent laryngeal section for spastic dysphonia. *Annals of Otology, Rhinology, and Laryngology,* 85, 451–459.

De Keyser, J. (1973). The stuttering of Lewis Carroll. In Y. Lebrun & R. Hoops (Eds.), *Neurolinguistic Approaches to Stuttering.* The Hague: Mouton, 32–36.

Dembowski, J., & Watson, B. C. (1991). Preparation time and response complexity effects of stutterers' and nonstutterers' LRT. *Journal of Speech and Hearing Research,* 34, 49–59.

Dempsey, G. L., & Granich, M. (1978). Hypno-behavioral therapy in the case of a traumatic stutterer: A case report. *International Journal of Clinical and Experimental Hypnosis.* 26, 125–133.

Denhardt, R. (1890). *Das Stottern. Eine Psychose.* Leipzig: Ernst Keil's Nachfolger.

De Nil, L. F., & Brutten, G. J. (1990). Speech-associated attitudes: Stuttering, voice disordered, articulation disordered, and normal speaking children. *Journal of Fluency Disorders,* 15, 127–134.

De Nil, L. F., & Brutten, G. J. (1991a). Speech-associated attitudes of stuttering and nonstuttering children. *Journal of Speech and Hearing Research,* 34, 60–66.

De Nil, L. F., & Brutten, G. J. (1991b). Voice onset times of stuttering and nonstuttering children: The influence of externally and linguistically imposed time pressure. *Journal of Fluency Disorders,* 16, 143–158.

Denny, M., & Smith, A. (1992). Gradations in a pattern of neuromuscular activity associated with stuttering. *Journal of Speech and Hearing Research,* 35, 1216–1229.

Devore, J. E., Nandur, M. S., & Manning, W. H. (1984). Projective drawings and children who stutter. *Journal of Fluency Disorders,* 9, 217–226.

Dewar, A., Dewar, A. D., & Anthony, J. F. K. (1976). The effects of auditory feedback masking on concomitant moments of stuttering. *British Journal of Disorders of Communication,* 11, 95–102.

Dewar, A., Dewar, A. D., & Barnes, H. E. (1976). Automatic triggering of auditory feedback masking in stammering and cluttering. *British Journal of Disorders of Communication,* 11, 19–26.

DiCarlo, L., Katz, J., & Batkin, S. (1959). An exploratory investigation of the effect of meprobamate on stuttering behavior. *Journal of Nervous and Mental Diseases,* 128, 558–561.

Dickson, S. (1971). Incipient stuttering and spontaneous remission of stuttered speech. *Journal of Communication Disorders,* 4, 99–110.

Diedrich, W. M. (1984). Cluttering: Its diagnosis. In W. Winitz (Ed.), *Treating Articulation Disorders: For Clinicians by Clinicians.* Baltimore: University Park Press.

Dietrich, S., Barry, S. J., & Parker, D. E. (1995). Middle latency auditory responses in makes who stutter. *Journal of Speech and Hearing Research,* 38, 5–17.

Diggs, C. C. (1990). Self-help for communication disorders. *Asha,* 32 (1), 32–34.

Doody, I., Kalinowski, J., Armson, J., & Stuart, A. (1993). Stereotypes of stutterers and nonstutterers in three rural communities in Newfoundland. *Journal of Fluency Disorders,* 18, 363–373.

Dopheide, B. (1987). Competencies expected of beginning clinicians working with children who stutter. *Journal of Fluency Disorders,* 12, 157–166.

Duncan, M. H. (1949). Home adjustment of stutterers and non-stutterers. *Journal of Speech Disorders,* 14, 195–198.

Dunlap, K. (1917). The stuttering boy. *Journal of Abnormal Psychology,* 12, 44–48.

Dunlap, K. (1932). *Habits: Their Making and Unmaking.* New York: Liveright.

Eldridge, M. (1968). *The History of the Treatment of Speech Disorders.* Baltimore: Williams & Wilkins.

Emerick, L. L. (1960). Extensional definition and attitude toward stuttering. *Journal of Speech and Hearing Research,* 3, 181–186.

Erickson, R. L. (1969). Assessing communication attitudes among stutterers. *Journal of Speech and Hearing Research,* 12, 711–724.

Fagan, L. B. (1931). The relation of dextral training to the onset of stuttering. *Quarterly Journal of Speech,* 17, 73–76.

Fairbanks, G. (1960). *Voice and Articulation Drillbook* (2nd ed.). New York: Harper & Brothers.

Fenichel, O. (1945). *The Psychoanalytic Theory of Neurosis.* New York: W. W. Norton.

Ferrand, C. T., Gilbert, H. R., & Blood, G. W. (1991). Selected aspects of central processing and vocal motor function in stutterers and nonstutterers: P300, laryngeal shift, and vibratory onset. *Journal of Fluency Disorders,* 16, 101–115.

Finkelstein, P., & Weisberger, S. E. (1954). The motor proficiency of stutterers. *Journal of Speech and Hearing Disorders,* 19, 52–58.

Finn, P., & Ingham, R. J. (1994). Stutterers' self-ratings of how natural speech sounds and feels. *Journal of Speech and Hearing Research,* 37, 326–340.

Fitzgerald, H. E., Cooke, P. A., Greiner, J. R. (1984). Speech and bimanual hand organization in adult stutterers and nonstutterers. *Journal of Fluency Disorders,* 9, 51–65.

Fitzgerald, H. E., Djurdjic, S. D., & Maguin, E. (1992). Assessment and sensitivity to interpersonal stress in stutterers. *Journal of Communication Disorders,* 25, 31–42.

FitzSimons, R. (1962). *The New Boy on Hillside Street.* New York: Springer Publishing Company.

Flanagan, B., Goldiamond, I., & Azrin, N. (1958). Operant stuttering: The control of stuttering behavior through response-contingent consequences. *Journal of Experimental Analysis of Behavior,* 1, 173–177.

Fleet, W. S., & Heilman, K. M. (1985). Acquired stuttering from a right hemisphere lesion in a right-hander. *Neurology,* 35, 1343–1346.

Fletcher, J. M. (1914). An experimental study of stuttering. *Journal of Applied Psychology,* 25, 201–249.

Fossler, H. R. (1932). Disturbances in breathing during stuttering. *Psychological Monographs,* 43, 218–275.

Fox, D. R. (1969). Spastic dysphonia: A case presentation. *Journal of Speech and Hearing Disorders,* 34, 275–279.

Francis, J. G. (1984). Stopping stuttering starting with hypnosis. *Australian Journal of Clinical and Experimental Hypnosis,* 12, 9–21.

Franken, M. C., Boves, L., Peters, H. F. M., & Webster, R. L. (1992). Perceptual evaluation of the speech before and after fluency shaping stuttering therapy. *Journal of Fluency Disorders,* 17, 223–241.

Franken, M. C., Boves, L., Peters, H. F. M., & Webster, R. L. (1995). Perceptual rating instrument for speech evaluation of stuttering treatment. *Journal of Speech and Hearing Research,* 38, 280–288.

Frankl, V. E. (1939). Zur medikamentosen Unterstutzung der Psychotherapie bei Neurosen. *Schweizer Archiv fur Neurologie und Psychiatrie,* 43, 26–31.

Frankl, V. E. (1985). *Man's Search for Meaning.* New York: Washington Square Press. [Note: While most of the book is relevant for speech-language pathologists, pages 145–152 are particularly relevant for the management of stuttering.]

Fransella, F. (1972). *Personal Change and Reconstruction: Research on a Treatment of Stuttering.* New York: Academic Press.

Fraser, J., & Perkins, W. H. (Eds.) (1987). *Do You Stutter: A Guide for Teens.* Memphis, TN: Speech Foundation of America.

Fraser, M. (Ed.) (no date). *If Your Child Stutters: A Guide for Parents.* Memphis, TN: Speech Foundation of America.

Fraser, M. (Ed.) (no date). *Self-therapy for the Stutterer.* Memphis, TN: Speech Foundation of America.

Fraser, M. (Ed.) (no date). *Self-therapy for the Stutterer: One Approach.* Memphis, Tennessee: Speech Foundation of America.

Fraser, M. (Ed.) (1972). *To the Stutterer.* Memphis, TN: Speech Foundation of America.

Fraser, M. (Ed.) (1987). *Self-therapy for the Stutterer* (5th ed.). North Hollywood, CA: Wilshire Book Company.

Freeman, F. J. (1979). Phonation in stuttering: A review of current research. *Journal of Fluency Disorders,* 4, 79–89.

Freeman, F. J. (1982). Stuttering. In N. J. Lass, L. V. McReynolds, J. L. Northern, & D. E. Yoder (Eds.), *Speech, Language, and Hearing* (Vol. 2). Philadelphia: W. B. Saunders.

Freeman, F. J., & Rosenfield, D. B. (1982). A research note on "source" in dysfluency. *Journal of Fluency Disorders,* 7, 295–296.

Freeman, F. J., & Ushijima, T. (1978). Laryngeal muscle activity during stuttering. *Journal of Speech and Hearing Research,* 21, 538–562.

Freund, H. (1966). *Psychopathology and the Problems of Stuttering.* Springfield, IL: Charles C. Thomas.

Froeschels, E. (1943). Pathology and therapy of stuttering. *Nervous Child,* 2, 148–161.

Froeschels, E. (1950). A technique for stutterers—ventriloquism. *Journal of Speech and Hearing Disorders,* 15, 336–337.

Fruewald, E. (1936). Intelligence ratings of severe college stutterers compared with that of others entering universities. *Journal of Speech Disorders,* 1, 47–51.

Fucci, D., Petrosino, L., Gorman, P., & Harris, D. (1985). Vibrotactile magnitude production scaling: A method for studying sensory-perceptual responses of stutterers and fluent speakers. *Journal of Fluency Disorders,* 10, 69–75.

Fukawa, T., Yoshioka, H., Ozawa, E., & Yoshida, S. (1988). Differences of susceptibility to delayed auditory feedback between stutterers and nonstutterers. *Journal of Speech and Hearing Research,* 31, 475–479.

Gaines, N. D., Runyan, C. M., & Meyers, S. C. (1991). A comparison of young stutterers' fluent versus stuttered utterances on measures of length and complexity. *Journal of Speech and Hearing Research,* 34, 37–42.

Garber, S. F., & Martin, R. R. (1977). Effect of noise and increased vocal intensity on stuttering. *Journal of Speech and Hearing Research,* 20, 233–240.

Gens, G. W. (1950). Correlation of neurological findings, psychological analyses, and speech disorders among institutionalized epileptics. *Training School Bulletin,* 47, 3–18.

Georgieva, D. (1994). Speech situations increasing stuttering in 13- to 16-year-old persons. *Journal of Fluency Disorders,* 19, 175.

Gerstman, H. L. (1983). The concatenation of stuttering to negative behavioral events: A clinical insight. *Journal of Fluency Disorders,* 8, 169–173.

Geschwind, N., & Galaburda, A. M. (1985). Cerebral lateralization: Biological mechanisms, associations, and pathology: I. A hypothesis and a program for research. *Archives of Neurology,* 42, 429–459.

Glauber, I P. (1958). The psychoanalysis of stuttering. In J. Eisenson (Ed.), *Stuttering: A Symposium.* New York: Harper & Brothers, pp. 71–119.

Glauber, I. P. (1982). *Stuttering: A Psychoanalytic Understanding.* New York: Human Sciences Press.

Goda, S. (1961). Stuttering manifestations following spinal meningitis. *Journal of Speech and Hearing Disorders,* 26, 392–393.

Goldberg, B. (1989). Historic treatment of stuttering: From pebbles to psychoanalysis. *Asha,* 31 (6/7), 71.

Goldiamond, I. (1965). Stuttering and fluency as manipulable operant response classes. In L. Krasner & L. P. Ullman (Eds.), *Research in Behavior Modification.* New York: Holt, Rinehart, & Winston.

Goldman-Eisler, F. (1968). *Psycholinguistics: Experiments in Spontaneous Speech.* New York: Academic Press.

Goldsand, J. G. (1944). Sensory perseveration in stutterers and non-stutterers. *Journal of Speech Disorders,* 9, 180.

Goodstein, L. D. (1958). Functional speech disorders and personality: A survey of the research. *Journal of Speech and Hearing Research,* 1, 359–376.

Gordon, P. A., & Luper, H. L. (1992a). The early identification of beginning stuttering I: Protocols. *American Journal of Speech-Language Pathology,* 1(3), 43–53.

Gordon, P. A., & Luper, H. L. (1992b). The early identification of beginning stuttering II: Problems. *American Journal of Speech-Language Pathology,* 1(4), 48–55.

Gottlober, A. B. (1953). *Understanding Stuttering.* New York: Grune & Stratton.

Gregory, H. H. (1968). Applications of learning theory concepts in the management of stuttering. In Hugo H. Gregory (Ed.), *Learning Theory and Stuttering Therapy.* Evanston, IL: Northwestern University Press, pp. 107–128.

Gregory, H. H. (1969). *An Assessment of the Results of Stuttering Therapy.* Evanston, IL: Department of Communicative Disorders, Northwestern University.

Gregory, H. H. & Hill, D. (1984). Stuttering therapy for children. In W. Perkins (Ed.), *Stuttering Disorders.* New York: Thieme-Stratton.

Greiner, J. R., Fitzgerald, H. E., Cooke, P. A., & Djurdjic, S. D. (1985). Assessment of sensitivity to interpersonal stress in stutterers and nonstutterers. *Journal of Communication Disorders,* 18, 215–225.

Grewel, F. (1970). Cluttering and its problems. *Folia Phoniatrics,* 22, 301–310.

Guitar, B. (1975). Reduction of stuttering frequency using analog electromyographic feedback. *Journal of Speech and Hearing Research,* 18, 672–685.

Guitar, B. (1976). Pre-treatment factors associated with outcome of stuttering therapy. *Journal of Speech and Hearing Research,* 19, 590–600.

Guitar, B., & Bass, C. (1978). Stuttering therapy: The relationship between attitude change and long-term outcome. *Journal of Speech and Hearing Disorders,* 43, 392–400.

Guitar, B., Schaefer, H. K., Donahue-Kilburg, G., & Bond, L. (1992). Parent verbal interactions and speech rate: A case study in stuttering. *Journal of Speech and Hearing Research,* 35, 742–754.

Gutzmann, H. (1939). Erbbiologische, soziologische und organische Faktoren die Sprachstörungen begunstigen. *Archive für Stimmheilkunde,* 3, 133–136.

Haefner, R. (1929). *The Educational Significance of Left-Handedness.* New York: Teachers College, Columbia University Press.

Hafford, J. (1941). A comparative study of the salivary pH of the normal speaker and stutterer. *Journal of Speech Disorders,* 6, 173–184.

Hageman, C. F., & Greene, P. N. (1989). Auditory comprehension of stutterers on a competing message task. *Journal of Fluency Disorders,* 14, 109–120.

Hahn, E. F. (1956). *Stuttering: Significant Theories and Therapies* (2nd Ed.). Stanford, CA: Stanford University Press.

Hall, J. W., & Jerger, J. (1978). Central auditory function in stutterers. *Journal of Speech and Hearing Research,* 21, 324–337.

Hall, K. D., & Yairi, E. (1992). Fundamental frequency, jitter, and shimmer in preschoolers who stutter. *Journal of Speech and Hearing Research,* 35, 1002–1008.

Halvorson, J. A. (1971). The effects on stuttering frequency of pairing punishment (response cost) with reinforcement. *Journal of Speech and Hearing Research,* 14, 356–364.

Ham, R. E. (1986). *Techniques of Stuttering Therapy.* Englewood Cliffs, NJ: Prentice-Hall.

Ham, R. E. (1988). Unison speech and rate control therapy. *Journal of Fluency Disorders,* 13, 115–126.

Ham, R. E. (1989). What are we measuring? *Journal of Fluency Disorders,* 14, 231–243.

Ham, R. E. (1990a). Clinician preparation: Experiences with pseudostuttering. *Journal of Fluency Disorders,* 15, 305–315.

Ham, R. E. (1990b). *Therapy of Stuttering: Preschool Through Adolescence.* Englewood Cliffs, NJ: Prentice-Hall.

Hamilton, P. G. (1940). *The Visual Characteristics of Stutterers During Silent Reading.* Unpublished doctoral dissertation, Columbia University Teachers College.

Hammer, C. S. (1994). Working with families of Chamorro and Carolinian cultures. *American Journal of Speech-Language Pathology, 3*(3), 5–12.

Hamre, C. (1992a). Stuttering prevention: I. Primacy of identification. *Journal of Fluency Disorders,* 3–23.

Hamre, C. (1992b). Stuttering prevention: II. Progression. *Journal of Fluency Disorders, 17,* 63–79.

Hand, C. R., & Haynes, W. O. (1983). Linguistic processing and reaction time differences in stutterers and nonstutterers. *Journal of Speech and Hearing Research, 26,* 181–185.

Hanna, R., & Owen, N. (1977). Facilitating transfer and maintenance of fluency in stuttering therapy. *Journal of Speech and Hearing Disorders, 42,* 65–76.

Hannley, M., & Dorman, M. F. (1982). Some observations on auditory function and stuttering. *Journal of Fluency Disorders, 7,* 93–108.

Hanson, B. R., Gronhovd, L. D., & Rice, P. L. (1981). A shortened form of the Southern Illinois University Speech Situation Checklist for the identification of speech-related anxiety. *Journal of Fluency Disorders, 6,* 351–360.

Hardin, C. B., Pindzola, R. H., & Haynes, W. O. (1992). A tachistoscopic study of hemispheric processing in stuttering and nonstuttering children. *Journal of Fluency Disorders, 17,* 265–281.

Harle, M. (1946). Dynamic interpretation and treatment of acute stuttering in a young child. *American Journal of Orthopsychiatry, 15,* 156–162.

Harrison, H. S. (1947). A study of the speech of sixty institutionalized epileptics. *Speech Monographs, 14,* 210.

Harvey, J. E., Culatta, R., Halikas, J. A., Sorenson, J., Luxenberg, M., & Pearson, V. (1992). The effects of carbamazepine on stuttering. *Journal of Nervous and Mental Disease, 180*(7), 451–457.

Hasbrouck, J. M., & Lowry, F. (1989). Elimination of stuttering and maintenance of fluency by means of airflow, tension reduction, and discriminative stimulus control procedures. *Journal of Fluency Disorders, 14,* 165–183.

Hayden, P. A., Adams, M. R., & Jordahl, N (1982). The effects of pacing and masking on stutterers' and nonstutterers' speech initiation times. *Journal of Fluency Disorders, 7,* 9–19.

Hayden, P. A., Jordahl, N., & Adams, M. R. (1982). Stutterers' voice initiation times during conditions of novel stimulation. *Journal of Fluency Disorders, 7,* 1–7.

Healey, E., & Gutkin, B. (1984). Analysis of stutterers' voice onset times and fundamental frequency contours during fluency. *Journal of Speech and Hearing Research, 27,* 219–225.

Healey, E., Mallard, A., & Adams, M. (1976). Factors contributing to the reduction of stuttering while singing. *Journal of Speech and Hearing Research, 19,* 475–480.

Healey, E. C., & Ramig, P. R. (1986). Acoustic measures of stutterers' and nonstutterers' fluency in two speech contexts. *Journal of Speech and Hearing Research,* 29, 325–331.

Heaver, L. (1959). Spastic dysphonia: II. Psychiatric considerations. *Logos,* 2, 15–24.

Hedges, D. W., Umar, F., Mellon, C. D., Herrick, L. C., Hanson, M. L., & Wahl, M. J. (1995). Direct comparison of the family history method and the family study method using a large stuttering pedigree. *Journal of Fluency Disorders,* 20, 25–33.

Hegde, M. N. (1972). Stuttering, neuroticism and extraversion. *Behavior Research and Therapy,* 10, 385–397.

Hegde, M. N. (1978). Fluency and fluency disorders: Their definition, measurement, and modification. *Journal of Fluency Disorders,* 3, 51–71.

Helm, N. A., Butler, R. B., & Benson, D. (1978). Acquired stuttering. *Neurology,* 28, 1159–1165.

Helm, N. A., Butler, R. B., & Canter, G. J. (1980). Neurogenic acquired stuttering. *Journal of Fluency Disorders,* 5, 269–279.

Helm, N. A., Yeo, R., Geschwind, M., Freedman, M., & Wenstein, C. (1986). Stuttering: Disappearance and reappearance with acquired brain lesions. *Neurology,* 36, 1109–1112.

Helm-Estabrooks, N. (1986). Diagnosis and management of neurogenic stuttering in adults. In K. O. St. Louis (Ed.), *The Atypical Stutterer.* Orlando, FL: Academic Press.

Helm-Estabrooks, N. (1993). Stuttering associated with acquired neurological disorders. In R. E. Curlee (Ed.), *Stuttering and Related Disorders of Fluency.* New York: Thieme Medical Publishers, 205–219.

Heltman, H. J., & Peacher, G. M. (1943). Misarticulation and diadokokinesis in the spastic paralytic. *Journal of Speech Disorders,* 8, 137–145.

Henschen, T. L., & Burton, N. G. (1978). Treatment of spastic dysphonia by EMG biofeedback. *Biofeedback and Self Regulation,* 3, 91–96.

Herodotus (1821). *Herodotus II.* London: S. & R. Bentley.

Hertrich, I., & Ackermann, H. (1994). Acquired stuttering in Parkinson syndrome. *Journal of Fluency Disorders,* 19, 179.

Hill, H. (1944a). Stuttering: I. A critical review and evaluation of biochemical investigations. *Journal of Speech Disorders,* 9, 245–261.

Hill, H. (1944b). Stuttering: II. A review and integration of physiological data. *Journal of Speech Disorders,* 9, 289–324.

Hillis, J. W. (1993). Ongoing assessment in the management of stuttering: A clinical perspective. *American Journal of Speech-Language Pathology,* 2(1), 24–37.

Hippocrates (1923a). *Aphorisms* [W. H. S. Jones, Trans.]. London: Heinemann.

Hippocrates (1923b). *Precepts* [W. H. S. Jones, Trans.]. London: Heinemann.

Hippocrates (1923c). *The Sacred Disease* [W. H. S. Jones, Trans.]. London: Heinemann.

Hoepfner, T. (1911). Stottern-als assoziative Aphasie. *Zeitschrift für Pathopsychologie,* 1, 448–452.

Hoops, R., & Wilkinson, P. (1973). Group ratings of stuttering severity. In Y. Lebrun & R. Hoops (Eds.), *Neurolinguistic Approaches to Stuttering*. The Hague: Mouton.

Horii, Y., & Ramig, P. R. (1987). Pause and utterance durations and fundamental frequency characteristics of repeated oral readings by stutterers and nonstutterers. *Journal of Fluency Disorders, 12*, 257–270.

Horlick, R. S., & Miller, M. H. (1960). A comparative personality study of a group of stutterers and hard of hearing patients. *Journal of General Psychology, 63*, 259–266.

Horner, J., & Massey, E. W. (1983). Progressive disfluency associated with right hemisphere disease. *Brain and Language, 18*, 71–85.

Horovitz, L. J., Johnson, S. B., Pearlman, R. C., Schaffer, E. J., & Hedin, A. K. (1978). Stapedial reflex and anxiety in fluent and disfluent speakers. *Journal of Speech and Hearing Research, 21*, 762–767.

Howie, P. M. (1981). Concordance for stuttering in monozygotic and dizygotic twin pairs. *Journal of Speech and Hearing Research, 24*, 317–321.

Howie, P. M., Tanner, S., & Andrews, G. (1981). Short- and long-term outcome in an intensive treatment program for adult stutterers. *Journal of Speech and Hearing Disorders, 46*, 104–109.

Howie, P. M., Woods, C. L., & Andrews, G. (1982). Relationship between covert and overt speech measures immediately before and immediately after stuttering treatment. *Journal of Speech and Hearing Disorders, 47*, 419–422.

Hubbard, C. P., & Prins, D. (1994). Word familiarity, syllabic stress pattern, and stuttering. *Journal of Speech and Hearing Research, 37*, 564–571.

Hubbard, C. P., & Yairi, E. (1988). Clustering of disfluencies in the speech of stuttering and nonstuttering preschool children. *Journal of Speech and Hearing Research, 31*, 228–233.

Hulit, L. M. (1989). A stutterer like me. *Journal of Fluency Disorders, 14*, 209–214.

Hulit, L. M., & Haasler, S. K. (1989). Influence of suggestion on the nonfluencies of normal speakers. *Journal of Fluency Disorders, 14*, 359–369.

Hulit, L. M., & Wirtz, L. (1994). The association of attitudes toward stuttering with selected variables. *Journal of Fluency Disorders, 19*, 247–267.

Hunt, H. (1861). *Stammering and Stuttering, Their Nature and Treatment*. [A facsimile was published in 1967 by Hafner Publishing Company, New York.]

Hurst, M., & Cooper, E. B. (1983a). Employer attitudes toward stuttering. *Journal of Fluency Disorders, 8*, 1–12.

Hurst, M., & Cooper, E. B. (1983b). Vocational rehabilitation counselors' attitudes toward stuttering. *Journal of Fluency Disorders, 8*, 13–27.

Hutchinson, J. M. (1975). Aerodynamic patterns of stuttered speech. In L. M. Webster & L. C. Furst (Ed.), *Vocal Tract Dynamics and Disfluency*. New York: Speech and Hearing Institute.

Hutchinson, J. M., & Watkin, K. L. (1976). Jaw mechanics during release of the stuttering moment: Some initial observations and interpretations. *Journal of Communication Disorders, 9*, 269–279.

Ingham, J. C. (1993). Current status of stuttering and behavior modification—I: Recent trends in the application of behavior modification in children and adults. *Journal of Fluency Disorders,* 18, 27–55.

Ingham, R. J. (1975). Operant methodology in stuttering therapy. In J. Eisenson (Ed.), *Stuttering: A Second Symposium.* New York: Harper & Row, 333–399.

Ingham R. J. (1982). The effects of self-evaluation training on maintenance and generalization during stuttering treatment. *Journal of Speech and Hearing Disorders,* 47, 271–280.

Ingham, R. J. (1984). *Stuttering and Behavior Therapy: Current Status and Experimental Foundations.* San Diego: College-Hill.

Ingham, R. J. (1990a). Commentary on Perkins (1990) and Moore and Perkins (1990): On the valid role of reliability in identifying "What Is Stuttering?" *Journal of Speech and Hearing Disorders,* 55, 394–397.

Ingham, R. J. (1990b). Research on stuttering treatment for adults and adolescents: A perspective on how to overcome a malaise. *ASHA Reports,* 18, 91–95.

Ingham, R. J. (1993a). Current status of stuttering and behavior modification—II. Principal issues and practices in stuttering therapy. *Journal of Fluency Disorders,* 18, 57–79.

Ingham, R. J. (1993b). Transfer and maintenance of treatment gains of chronic stutterers. In R. F. Curlee (Ed.), *Stuttering and Related Disorders of Fluency.* New York: Thieme Medical Publishers, 166–178.

Ingham, R. J., & Andrews, G. (1973). An analysis of a token economy in stuttering therapy. *Journal of Applied Behavior Analysis,* 6, 219–229.

Ingham, R. J., & Cordes, A. K. (1992). Interclinic differences in stuttering-event counts. *Journal of Fluency Disorders,* 17, 171–176.

Ingham, R. J., Cordes, A. K., Ingham, J. C., & Gow, M. L. (1995). Identifying the onset and offset of stuttering events. *Journal of Speech and Hearing Research,* 38, 315–326.

Ingham, R. J., Gow, M., & Costello, J. M. (1985). Stuttering and speech naturalness: Some additional data. *Journal of Speech and Hearing Disorders,* 50, 217–219.

Ingham, R. J., Martin, R. R., Haroldson, S. K., Onslow, M., & Leney, M. (1985). Modification of listener-judged naturalness in the speech of stutterers. *Journal of Speech and Hearing Research,* 28, 495–504.

Ingham, R. J., & Packman, A. (1979). A further evaluation of the speech of stutterers during chorus- and nonchorus-reading conditions. *Journal of Speech and Hearing Research,* 22, 784–793.

Ingham, R. J., Southwood, H., & Horsburgh, G. (1981). Some effects of the Edinburgh masker on stuttering during oral reading and spontaneous speech. *Journal of Fluency Disorders,* 6, 135–154.

Irving, R. W., & Webb, N. W. (1961). Teaching esophageal speech to pre-operative severe stutterer. *Annals of Otology, Rhinology, and Laryngology,* 70, 1069–1079.

Irwin, J., & Duffy, J. K. (1955). *Speech and Hearing Hurdles.* Columbus, OH: School and College Service.

Jacobson, E. (1938). *Progressive Relaxation.* Chicago: University of Chicago Press.

James, J. E. (1981). Punishment of stuttering: Contingency and stimulus parameters. *Journal of Communication Disorders, 14,* 375–386.

Jäncke, L. (1994). Variability and duration of voice onset time and phonation in stuttering and nonstuttering adults. *Journal of Fluency Disorders, 19,* 21–37.

Jayaram, M. (1984). Distribution of stuttering in sentences: Relationship to sentence length and clause position. *Journal of Speech and Hearing Research, 27,* 338–341.

Jensen, P. H., Sheehan, J. G., Williams, W. N., & Lapointe, L. L. (1975). Oral sensory-perceptual integrity of stutterers. *Folia Phoniatrica, 17,* 38–45.

Johannsen, H. S., & Victor, C. (1986). Visual information processing in the left and right hemispheres during unilateral tachistoscopic stimulation of stutterers. *Journal of Fluency Disorders, 11,* 285–291.

Johnson, G. F. (1987a). A clinical study of Porky Pig cartoons. *Journal of Fluency Disorders, 12,* 235–238.

Johnson, G. F. (1987b). Ten commandments for long-term maintenance of acceptable self-help skills for persons who are hard-core stutterers. *Journal of Fluency Disorders, 12,* 9–18.

Johnson, W. (1930). *Because I Stutter.* New York: Appleton-Century-Crofts.

Johnson, W. (1932). The influence of stuttering on the personality. *University of Iowa Studies in Child Welfare, 5* (5).

Johnson, W. (1946). *People in Quandaries.* New York: Harper & Brothers.

Johnson, W. (1958). Introduction: The six men and the stuttering. In J. Eisenson (Ed.), *Stuttering: A Symposium.* New York: Harper & Brothers, xi–xxiv.

Johnson, W. (1961). Measurement of oral reading and speaking rate and disfluency of adult male and female stutterers and nonstutterers. *Journal of Speech and Hearing Disorders Monograph 7,* 1–20.

Johnson, W., & Associates (1959). *The Onset of Stuttering: Research Findings and Implications.* Minneapolis, MN: University of Minnesota Press.

Johnson, W., Darley, F. L., & Spriestersbach, D. C. (1963). *Diagnostic Methods in Speech Pathology.* New York: Harper & Row.

Johnson, W., & Knott, J. R. (1937a). Certain objective clues related to the precipitation of the moments of stuttering. *Journal of Speech Disorders, 2,* 17–19.

Johnson, W., & Knott, J. R. (1937b). Studies in the psychology of stuttering: I. The distribution of moments of stuttering in successive readings of the same material. *Journal of Speech Disorders, 2,* 17–19.

Johnson, W., & Rosen, B. (1937). Studies in the psychology of stuttering: VII. The effect of certain changes in speech pattern upon frequency of stuttering. *Journal of Speech Disorders, 2,* 105–109.

Johnson, W., & Sinn, A. (1937). Studies in the psychology of stuttering: V. Frequency of stuttering with expectation of stuttering controlled. *Journal of Speech Disorders*, 2, 98–100.

Johnson, W., & Solomon, A. (1937). Studies in the psychology of stuttering: IV. A quantitative study of expectation of stuttering as a process involving a low degree of consciousness. *Journal of Speech Disorders*, 2, 95–97.

Johnson, W., Young, M. A., Sachs, J. L., & Bedell, G. N. (1959). Effects of hyperventilation and tetany on the speech fluency of stutterers and nonstutterers. *Journal of Speech and Hearing Research*, 2, 203–215.

Johnston, S. J., Watkin, K. L., & Macklem, P. T. (1993). Lung volume changes during relatively fluent speech in stutterers. *Journal of Applied Physiology*, 75(2), 696–703.

Jones, R. (1966). Observations on stammering after localized cerebral injury. *Journal of Neurology, Neurosurgery, and Psychiatry*, 29, 192–195.

Kalinowski, J., Armson, J., Roland-Mieszkowski, M., Stuart, A., & Gracco, V. L. (1993). Effects of alterations in auditory feedback and speech rate on stuttering frequency. *Language and Speech*, 36(1), 1–16.

Kalinowski, J., Noble, S., Armson, J., & Stuart, A. (1994). Pretreatment and posttreatment speech naturalness ratings of adults with mild and severe stuttering. *American Journal of Speech-Language Pathology*, 3(2), 61–66.

Kalinowski, L. S., Lerman, J. W., & Watt, J. (1987). A preliminary examination of the perception of self and others in stutterers and nonstutterers. *Journal of Fluency Disorders*, 12, 317–331.

Kamhi, A. G. (1982). The problem of relapse in stuttering: Some thoughts on what might cause it and how to deal with it. *Journal of Fluency Disorders*, 7, 459–467.

Kamhi, A. G., & McOsker, T. G. (1982). Attention and stuttering: Do stutterers think too much about speech? *Journal of Fluency Disorders*, 7, 309–321.

Kampman, K., & Brady, J. P. (1993). Bethanechol in the treatment of stuttering. *Journal of Clinical Psychopharmacology*, 13(4), 284–285.

Karlin, I. W., & Sobel, A. E. (1940). A comparative study of the blood chemistry of stutterers and non-stutterers. *Speech Monographs*, 7, 75–84.

Katsovskaia, I. I. K. (1962). The problem of children's stuttering. *Deafness, Speech, and Hearing Abstracts*, 2, 296.

Katz, L. (1966). *Dependency and Immaturity in Stuttering Children*. Unpublished master's thesis, Brooklyn College.

Katz, M. (1977). Survey of patented anti-stuttering devices. In R. W. Rieber (Ed.), *The Problem of Stuttering: Theory and Therapy*. New York: Elsevier, 181–206.

Keane, V. E. (1972). The incidence of speech and language problems in the mentally retarded. *Mental Retardation*, 10, 3–8.

Kelly, E. M., & Conture, E. G. (1988). Acoustic and perceptual correlates of adult stutterers' typical and imitated stutterings. *Journal of Fluency Disorders,* 13, 233–252.

Kelly, E. M., & Conture, E. G. (1992). Speaking rate, response time latencies, and interrupting behaviors of young stutterers, nonstutterers, and their mothers. *Journal of Speech and Hearing Research,* 35, 1256–1267.

Kelly, G. A. (1932). Some common factors in reading and speech disabilities. *Psychological Monographs,* 43, 175–201.

Kelly, G. A. (1955). *The Psychology of Personal Constructs.* New York: Norton.

Kent, L. R., & Williams, D. E. (1959). Use of meprobamate as an adjunct to stuttering therapy. *Journal of Speech and Hearing Disorders,* 24, 64–70.

Kent, R. D. (1983). Facts about stuttering: Neurologic perspectives. *Journal of Speech and Hearing Disorders,* 48, 249–255.

Kidd, K. K. (1977). A genetic perspective on stuttering. *Journal of Fluency Disorders,* 2, 259–269.

Kidd, K. K., Kidd, J. R., & Records, M. A. (1978). The possible causes of the sex ratio in stuttering and its implications. *Journal of Fluency Disorders,* 3, 13–23.

King, P. T. (1961). Perseveration in stutterers and nonstutterers. *Journal of Speech and Hearing Research,* 4, 346–357.

Klencke, H. (1860). *Die Heilung des Stotterns.* Leipzig.

Klingbeil, G. M. (1939). The historical background of the modern speech clinic. *Journal of Speech and Hearing Disorders,* 4, 115–132.

Knott, J., Johnson, W., & Webster, M. (1937). Studies in the psychology of stuttering: II. A quantitative evaluation of expectation of stuttering in relation to the occurrence of stuttering. *Journal of Speech Disorders,* 2, 20–22.

Köpf, A., & Christmann, O. (1994). German Stutterers' Self-Help Association and its contribution to the prevention of stuttering. *Journal of Fluency Disorders,* 19, 186.

Kopp, G. A. (1934). Metabolic studies of stutterers: I. Biochemical study of blood composition. *Speech Monographs,* 1, 117–132.

Kopp, H. (1946). Psychosomatic study of fifty stuttering children: II. Ozeretzky tests. *American Journal of Orthopsychiatry,* 16, 114–119.

Kraaimaat, F., Janssen, P., & Brutten, G. J. (1988). The relationship between stutterers' cognitive and autonomic anxiety and therapy outcome. *Journal of Fluency Disorders,* 13, 107–113.

Krauss-Lehrman, T., & Reeves, L. (1989). Attitudes toward speech-language pathology and support groups: Results of a survey of members of the National Stuttering Project. *Texas Journal of Audiology and Speech Pathology,* 15(1), 22–25.

Kroll, R. M., & De Nil, L. (1994). Locus of control and client performance variables as predictors of stuttering treatment outcome. *Journal of Fluency Disorders,* 19, 186–187.

Kroll, R. M., & Hood, S. B. (1974). Differences in stuttering adaptation between oral reading and spontaneous speech. *Journal of Communication Disorders, 7,* 227–237.

Kuhr, A., & Rustin, L. (1985). The maintenance of fluency after intensive in-patient therapy: Long-term follow-up. *Journal of Fluency Disorders,* 10, 229–236.

Kurshev, V. A. (1968). Issledovanie vnerechenovo dykhaniya u zaikayushchikhsya. *Zh. Nevropatol. Psikhiat.,* 68, 1840–1841.

Kushner, H. S. (1981). *Why Bad Things Happen to Good People.* New York: Avon Books.

Ladouceur, R., Caron, C., & Caron, G. (1989). Stuttering severity and treatment outcome. *Journal of Behavior Therapy and Experimental Psychiatry,* 20, 49–56.

Ladouceur, R., Coté, C., Leblond, G., & Bluchard, L. (1982). Evaluation of regulated-breathing method and awareness training in the treatment of stuttering. *Journal of Speech and Hearing Disorders,* 47, 422–426.

Langlois, A., & Long, S. H. (1988). A model for teaching parents to facilitate fluent speech. *Journal of Fluency Disorders,* 13, 163–172.

Lanyon, R. I. (1967). The measurement of stuttering severity. *Journal of Speech and Hearing Research,* 10, 836–843.

Lanyon, R. I. (1977). Effect of biofeedback-based relaxation on stuttering during oral reading and spontaneous speech. *Journal of Consulting and Clinical Psychology,* 45, 860–866.

Lanyon, R. I., & Barocas, V. S. (1975). Effects of contingent events on stuttering and fluency. *Journal of Clinical and Consulting Psychology,* 43, 786–793.

Lanyon, R. I., Barrington, C. C., & Newman, A. C. (1976). Modification of stuttering through EMG biofeedback: A preliminary study. *Behavior Therapy,* 7, 96–103.

Lanyon, R. I., Goldsworthy, R. J., & Lanyon, B. P. (1978). Dimensions of stuttering and relationship to psychopathology. *Journal of Fluency Disorders,* 3, 103–113.

Lanyon, R. I., Lanyon, B. P., & Goldsworthy, R. J. (1979). Outcome predictors in the behavioral treatment of stuttering. *Journal of Fluency Disorders,* 4, 131–139.

LaSalle, L. R., & Conture, E. G. (1991). Eye contact between young stutterers and their mothers. *Journal of Fluency Disorders,* 16, 173–199.

Lay, T. (1982a). Nonspecific elements in therapy with stutterers. *Journal of Fluency Disorders,* 7, 479–486.

Lay, T. (1982b). Stuttering: Training the therapist. *Journal of Fluency Disorders,* 7, 63–69.

Leach, E. (1969). Stuttering: Clinical application of response-contingent procedures. In B. B. Gray & G. England (Eds.), *Stuttering and the Conditioning Therapies.* Monterey, CA: Monterey Institute of Speech and Hearing.

Leahy, M. M. (1994). Attempting to ameliorate student therapists' negative stereotype of the stutterer. *European Journal of Disorders of Communication,* 29(1), 39–49.

Lebrun, Y., & Bayle, M. (1973). Surgery in the treatment of stuttering. In Y. Lebrun & R. Hoops (Eds.), *Neurolinguistic Approaches to Stuttering.* The Hague: Mouton, pp. 82–89.

Lebrun, Y., & Leleux, C. (1985). Acquired stuttering following right brain damage in dextrals. *Journal of Fluency Disorders,* 10, 137–141.

Lebrun, Y., Leleux, C., & Retif, J. (1987). Neurogenic stuttering. *Acta Neurochirurgica,* 85, 103–109.

Lebrun, Y., Leleux, C., Rousseau, J., & Devreux, F. (1983). Acquired stuttering. *Journal of Fluency Disorders,* 8, 323–330.

Lebrun, Y., & Van Borsel, J. (1990). Final sound repetitions. *Journal of Fluency Disorders,* 15, 107–113.

Lees, R. M. (1988). The effect of foreperiod length on the acoustic voice reaction times of stutterers. *Journal of Fluency Disorders,* 13, 157–162.

Leith, W. R., & Timmons, J. L. (1983). The stutterer's reaction to the telephone as a speaking situation. *Journal of Fluency Disorders,* 8, 233–243.

Lemert, E. M. (1953). Some Indians who stutter. *Journal of Speech and Hearing Disorders,* 18, 168–174.

Lemert, E. M. (1962). Stuttering and social structure in two Pacific societies. *Journal of Speech and Hearing Disorders,* 27, 3–10.

Lerman, J. W., Powers, G. R., & Rigrodsky, S. (1965). Stuttering patterns observed in a sample of mentally retarded individuals. *Training School Bulletin,* 62, 27–32.

Levin, H., & Silverman, I. (1965). Hesitation phenomena in children's speech. *Language and Speech,* 8, 67–85.

Levina, R. Y. (1968). Study and treatment of stammering among children. *Journal of Learning Disabilities,* 2, 24–30.

Liebetrau, R. M., & Daly, D. A. (1981). Auditory processing and perceptual abilities of "organic" and "functional" stutterers. *Journal of Fluency Disorders,* 6, 219–231.

Liles, B. Z., Lerman, J., Christensen, L., & St. Ledger, J. (1992). A case description of verbal and signed disfluencies of a 10-year-old boy who is retarded. *Language, Speech, and Hearing Services in Schools,* 23, 107–112.

Lindsay, J. S. (1989). Relationship of developmental disfluency and episodes of stuttering to the emergence of cognitive stages in children. *Journal of Fluency Disorders,* 14, 271–284.

Linebaugh, C. W. (1984). Mild aphasia. In A. Holland (Ed.), *Language Disorders in Adults.* San Diego, CA: College-Hill, 113–131.

Lockhart, M. S., & Robertson, A. W. (1977). Hypnosis and speech therapy as a combined therapeutic approach to the problem of stammering. *British Journal of Disorders of Communication,* 12, 97–108.

Logan, K. J., & Conture, E. G. (1995). Length, grammatical complexity, and rate differences in stuttered and fluent conversational utterances of children who stutter. *Journal of Fluency Disorders,* 20, 35–61.

Louko, L., Edwards, M. L., & Conture, E. (1990). Phonological characteristics of young stutterers and their normally fluent peers: Preliminary observations. *Journal of Fluency Disorders,* 15, 191–210.

Louttit, C. M., & Halls, E. C. (1936). Survey of speech defects among public school children of Indiana. *Journal of Speech Disorders,* 1, 73–80.

Lowinger, L. (1952). The psychodynamics of stuttering: An evaluation of the factors of aggression and guilt feelings in a group of institutionalized children. *Dissertation Abstracts,* 12, 725.

Luchinger, R, & Arnold, G. E. (1965). *Voice-Speech-Language.* Belmont, CA: Wadsworth.

Ludlow, C. L., & Braun, A. (1993). Research evaluating the use of neuropharmacological agents for treating stuttering: Possibilities and problems. *Journal of Fluency Disorders,* 18, 169–182.

Ludlow, C. L., & Dooman, A. G. (1992). Genetic aspects of idiopathic speech and language disorders. *Otolaryngologic Clinics of North America,* 25(5), 979–994.

Ludlow, C. L., Rosenberg, J., Salazar, A., Grafman, J., & Smutok, M. (1987). Site of penetrating brain lesions causing chronic acquired stuttering. *Annals of Neurology,* 22, 60–66.

Luper, H. L. (1968). An appraisal of learning theory concepts in understanding and treating stuttering in children. In H. H. Gregory (Ed.), *Learning Theory and Stuttering Therapy.* Evanston, IL: Northwestern University Press, 84–106.

Luterman, D. (1984). *Counseling the Communicatively Disordered and Their Families.* Boston: Little, Brown.

Macfarlane, F. K. (1990). The use of hypnosis in speech therapy: A questionnaire study. *British Journal of Disorders of Communication,* 25, 227–246.

MacFarlane, W. B., Hanson, M., Walton, W., & Mellon, C. D. (1991). Stuttering in five generations of a single family: A preliminary report including evidence supporting a sex-modified mode of transmission. *Journal of Fluency Disorders,* 16, 117–123.

Maclay, H., & Osgood, C. E. (1959). Hesitation phenomena in spontaneous English. *Word,* 15, 19–44.

Maestas, A. G., & Erickson, J. G. (1992). Mexican immigrant mothers' beliefs about disabilities. *American Journal of Speech-Language Pathology,* 1(4), 5–10.

Mahr, G., & Leith, W. (1992). Psychogenic stuttering of adult onset. *Journal of Speech and Hearing Research,* 35, 283–286.

Maier, S. F., & Seligman, M. E. P. (1976). Learned helplessness: Theory and evidence. *Journal of Experimental Psychology: General,* 105, 3–46.

Mallard, A. R., Hicks, D. M., & Riggs, D. E. (1982). A comparison of stutterers and nonstutterers in a task of controlled voice onset. *Journal of Speech and Hearing Research,* 25, 287–290.

Mallard, A. R., & Kelley, J. S. (1982). The Precision Fluency Shaping Program: Replication and evaluation. *Journal of Fluency Disorders,* 7, 287–294.

Mallard, A. R., & Meyer, L. A. (1979). Listener preferences for stuttered and syllable-timed speech production. *Journal of Fluency Disorders, 4,* 117–121.

Manders, E., & Bastijns, P. (1988). Sudden recovery from stuttering after an epileptic attack: A case report. *Journal of Fluency Disorders, 13,* 421–425.

Manning, W. H. (1977). In pursuit of fluency. *Journal of Fluency Disorders, 2,* 53–56.

Manning, W. H., & Beachy, T. (1994). Humor and the treatment of fluency disorders. *Journal of Fluency Disorders, 19,* 191–192.

Manning, W. H., Dailey, D., & Wallace, S. (1984). Attitude and personality characteristics of older stutterers. *Journal of Fluency Disorders, 9,* 207–215.

Manning, W. H., & Monte, K. L. (1981). Fluency breaks in older speakers: Implications for a model of stuttering throughout the life cycle. *Journal of Fluency Disorders, 6,* 35–48.

Manning, W. H., & Shirkey, E. (1980). Fluency and the aging process. In D. S. Beasley & A. D. Davis (Eds.), *Aging: Communication Processes and Disorders.* New York: Grune & Stratton.

Manning, W. H., Trutna, P. A., & Shaw, C. K. (1976). Verbal versus tangible reward for children who stutter. *Journal of Speech and Hearing Disorders, 41,* 52–62.

Market, K. W., Montague, J. C., Jr., Buffalo, M. D., & Drummond, S. S. (1990). Acquired stuttering: Descriptive data and treatment outcome. *Journal of Fluency Disorders, 15,* 21–33.

Martin, R. R. (1993). The future of behavior modification of stuttering: What goes around comes around. *Journal of Fluency Disorders, 18,* 81–108.

Martin, R. R., & Haroldson, S. K. (1979). Effects of five experimental treatments on stuttering. *Journal of Speech and Hearing Research, 22,* 132–146.

Martin, R. R., & Haroldson, S. K. (1981). Stuttering identification: Standard definition and moment of stuttering. *Journal of Speech and Hearing Research, 24,* 59–63.

Martin, R. R., & Haroldson, S. K. (1982). Contingent self-stimulation for stuttering. *Journal of Speech and Hearing Disorders, 47,* 407–413.

Martin, R. R., & Haroldson, S. K. (1988). An experimental increase in stuttering frequency. *Journal of Speech and Hearing Research, 31,* 272–274.

Martin, R. R., Haroldson, S. K., & Triden, K. A. (1984). Stuttering and speech naturalness. *Journal of Speech and Hearing Disorders, 49,* 53–58.

Martin, R. R., Haroldson, S. K., & Woessner, G. L. (1988). Perceptual scaling of stuttering severity. *Journal of Fluency Disorders, 13,* 27–47.

Martin, R. R., Johnson, L. J., Siegel, G. M., & Haroldson, S. K. (1985). Auditory stimulation, rhythm, and stuttering. *Journal of Speech and Hearing Research, 28,* 497–498.

Martin, R. R., Juhl, P., & Haroldson, S. K. (1972). An experimental treatment with two preschool stuttering children. *Journal of Speech and Hearing Research, 15,* 743–752.

Martin, R. R., Lawrence, B. A., Haroldson, S. K., & Gunderson, D. (1981). Stuttering and oral stereognosis. *Perceptual and Motor Skills, 53,* 155–162.

Martin, R. R., & Siegel, G. M. (1966a). The effects of response contingent shock on stuttering. *Journal of Speech and Hearing Research, 9,* 340–352.

Martin, R. R., & Siegel, G. M. (1966b). The effects of simultaneously punishing stuttering and rewarding fluency. *Journal of Speech and Hearing Research, 9,* 466–475.

Martin, R. R., Siegel, G. M., Johnson, L. J., & Haroldson, S. K. (1984). Sidetone amplification, noise, and stuttering. *Journal of Speech and Hearing Research, 27,* 518–527.

Matsuda, M. (1989). Working with Asian parents: Some communication strategies. *Topics in Language Disorders, 9*(3), 45–53.

Mavlov, L. (1994). Mechanisms of fluency disorders in neocerebellar dysarthria and premotor articulatory apraxia. *Journal of Fluency Disorders, 19,* 192–193.

Maxwell, D. L. (1982). Cognitive and behavioral self-control strategies. *Journal of Fluency Disorders, 7,* 403–432.

Maxwell, R., & Paterson, J. (1958). Meprobamate in the treatment of stuttering. *British Medical Journal, 179,* 873–874.

Mazzucchi, A., Moretti, G., Carpeggiani, P., Parma, M., & Paini, P. (1981). Clinical observations on acquired stuttering. *British Journal of Disorders of Communication, 16,* 19–30.

McCall, G. N., Skolnick, M. L., & Brewer, D. W. (1971). A preliminary report on some atypical movement patterns in the tongue, palate, hypopharynx and larynx of patients with spasmodic dysphonia. *Journal of Speech and Hearing Disorders, 36,* 466.

McClean, M. D. (1990). Neuromotor aspects of stuttering: Levels of impairment and disability. *ASHA Reports, 18,* 64–71.

McClean, M. D., Goldsmith, H., & Cerf, A. (1984). Lower-lip EMG and displacement during bilabial disfluencies in adult stutterers. *Journal of Speech and Hearing Research, 27,* 342–349.

McClean, M. D., & McLean, A., Jr. (1985). Case report of stuttering acquired in association with phenytoin use for post-head-injury seizures. *Journal of Fluency Disorders, 10,* 241–255.

McCord, H. (1955). Hypnotherapy and stuttering. *Journal of Clinical and Experimental Hypnosis, 3,* 210–214.

McCroskey, R. L. (1957). Effect of speech on metabolism: A comparison between stutterers and non-stutterers. *Journal of Speech and Hearing Disorders, 22,* 46–52.

McDonough, A., & Quesal, R. W. (1988). Locus of control orientation of stutterers and nonstutterers. *Journal of Fluency Disorders, 13,* 97–106.

McDowell, E. D. (1928). *The Educational and Emotional Adjustment of Stuttering Children.* New York: Columbia University Teachers College.

McFarlane, S. C., & Shipley, K. G. (1981). Latency of vocalization onset for stutterers and nonstutterers under conditions of auditory and visual cueing. *Journal of Speech and Hearing Disorders,* 46, 307–312.

McKeehan, A. B. (1994). Student experiences with fluency facilitating speech strategies. *Journal of Fluency Disorders,* 19, 113–123

McLaughlin, S. F., & Cullinan, W. L. (1989). Disfluencies, utterance length, and linguistic complexity in nonstuttering children. *Journal of Fluency Disorders,* 14, 17–36.

McLean-Muse, A., Larson, C. R., & Gregory, H. H. (1988). Stutterers' and nonstutterers' voice fundamental frequency changes in response to auditory stimuli. *Journal of Speech and Hearing Research,* 31, 549–555.

Meltzer, A. (1992). Horn stuttering. *Journal of Fluency Disorders,* 17, 257–264.

Meltzer, H. (1944). Personality differences between stuttering and non-stuttering children as indicated by the Rorschach Test. *Journal of Psychology,* 17, 39–59.

Metraux, R. (1950). Speech profiles of the preschool child 18–54 months. *Journal of Speech & Hearing Disorders,* 15, 37–53.

Meyer, V., & Comley, J. (1969). A preliminary report on the treatment of stammer by the use of rhythmic stimulation. In B. B. Gray & F. England (Eds.), *Stuttering and the Conditioning Therapies.* Monterey, CA: Monterey Institute for Speech and Hearing.

Meyer, V., & Mair, J. M. M. (1963). A new technique to control stammering. *Behavioral Research and Therapy,* 1, 251–254.

Meyers, I., & Anderson, D. (1985). A stuttering therapy program with spastic dysphonia—A single case study. *The South African Journal of Communication Disorders,* 32, 31–36.

Meyers, S. C. (1986). Qualitative and quantitative differences and patterns of variability in disfluencies emitted by preschool stutterers and nonstutterers during dyadic conversations. *Journal of Fluency Disorders,* 11, 293–306.

Meyers, S. C., Hall, N. E., & Aram, D. M. (1990). Fluency and language recovery in a child with a left hemisphere lesion. *Journal of Fluency Disorders,* 15, 159–173.

Miller, D. T., & Turnbill, W. (1986). Expectancies and interpersonal processes. *Annual Review of Psychology,* 37, 233–257.

Miller, S. (1982). Airflow therapy program: Facts and/or fancy. *Journal of Fluency Disorders,* 7, 187–202.

Miller, S., & Watson, B. C. (1992). The relationship between communication attitude, anxiety, and depression in stutterers and nonstutterers. *Journal of Speech and Hearing Research,* 35, 789–798.

Moeller, D. (1975). *Speech Pathology and Audiology: Iowa Origins of a Discipline.* Iowa City: University of Iowa Press.

Montgomery, B. M., & Fitch, J. L. (1988). The prevalence of stuttering in the hearing-impaired school age population. *Journal of Speech and Hearing Disorders,* 53, 131–135.

Moore, J. C., & Rigo, T. G. (1983). An awareness approach to the covert symptoms of stuttering. *Journal of Fluency Disorders,* 8, 133–145.

Moore, M. A. S., & Adams, M. R. (1985). The Edinburgh Masker: A clinical analog study. *Journal of Fluency Disorders,* 10, 281–290.

Moore, S. E., & Perkins, W. H. (1990). Validity and reliability of judgments of authentic and simulated stuttering. *Journal of Speech and Hearing Disorders,* 55, 383–391.

Moore, W. E. (1938). A conditioned reflex study of stuttering. *Journal of Speech Disorders,* 3, 163–183.

Moore, W. E. (1946). Hypnosis in a system of therapy for stuttering. *Journal of Speech and Hearing Disorders,* 11, 117–122.

Moore, W. H., Jr. (1976). Bilateral tachistoscopic word perception of stutterers and normal subjects. *Brain and Language,* 3, 434–442.

Moore, W. H., Jr. (1984). Hemispheric alpha asymmetries during an electromyographic biofeedback procedure for stuttering: A single-subject experimental design. *Journal of Fluency Disorders,* 9, 143–162.

Moore, W. H., Jr. (1986). Hemispheric alpha asymmetries of stutterers and nonstutterers for the recall and recognition of words and connected reading passages: Some relationships to severity of stuttering. *Journal of Fluency Disorders,* 11, 71–89.

Moore, W. H., Jr. (1990). Pathophysiology of stuttering: Cerebral activation differences in stutterers vs. nonstutterers. *ASHA Reports,* 18, 72–80.

Morgenstern, J. J. (1956). Socio-economic factors in stuttering. *Journal of Speech and Hearing Disorders,* 21, 25–33.

Morley, M. E. (1957). *The Development and Disorders of Speech in Childhood.* Edinburgh: Livingstone.

Mowrer, D. (1987). Reported use of a Japanese accent to promote fluency. *Journal of Fluency Disorders,* 12, 19–39.

Mowrer, O. H. (1968a). A resume of basic principles of learning. In H. H. Gregory (Ed.), *Learning Theory and Stuttering Therapy.* Evanston, IL: Northwestern University Press, 3–20.

Mowrer, O. H. (1968b). Stuttering as simultaneous admission and denial; or, What is the stutterer "saying"? In H. H. Gregory (Ed.), *Learning Theory and Stuttering Therapy.* Evanston, IL: Northwestern University Press, 67–71.

Muellerleile, S. (1981). Portable delayed auditory feedback device: A preliminary report. *Journal of Fluency Disorders,* 6, 361–363.

Murdoch, B. E., Killin, H., & McCaul, A. (1989). A kinematic analysis of respiratory function in a group of stutterers pre- and posttreatment. *Journal of Fluency Disorders,* 14, 323–350.

Murphy, A. T., & Fitzsimons, R. M. (1960). *Stuttering and Personality Dynamics: Play Therapy, Projective Therapy, and Counseling.* New York: Ronald Press.

Murray, F. P., & Edwards, S. G. (1980). *A Stutterer's Story.* Danville, IL: Interstate Printers and Publishers.

Myers, F., & St. Louis, K. O. (Eds.) (1992). *Cluttering: A Clinical Perspective.* Leicester, England: Far Communications.

Mygind, H. (1898). Über die Ursachen des Stotterns. *Archive für Laryngologie und Rhinologie,* 8, 294–307.

Nadoleczny, M. (1926). *Kurzes Lehrbuch der Sprach- und Stimmheilkunde mit Besonderer Berucksichtigung des Kindesalters.* Leipzig: Verlag Von F. C. W. Vogel.

Nagafuchi, M. (1994). Acquired stuttering due to damage to the left premotor area. *Journal of Fluency Disorders,* 19, 195.

Nagel, R., & Van Eupen, A-K. (1994). Presentation of a cognitive training program for stuttering children: "Think-Wise!" *Journal of Fluency Disorders,* 19, 196.

Nass, R., Schreter, B., & Heier, L. (1994). Acquired stuttering after a second stroke in a two-year-old. *Developmental Medicine and Child Neurology,* 36(1), 73–78.

Neilson, P. D., Quinn, P. T., & Neilson, M. D. (1976). Auditory tracking measures of hemispheric asymmetry in normals and stutterers. *Australian Journal of Human Communication Disorders,* 4, 121–126.

Newman, L. L. (1987). The effects of punishment of repetitions and the acquisition of "stutter-like" behaviors in normal speakers. *Journal of Fluency Disorders,* 12, 51–62.

Newman, P. W., Harris, R. W., & Hilton, L. M. (1989). Vocal jitter and shimmer in stuttering. *Journal of Fluency Disorders,* 14, 87–95.

Nippold, M. A. (1990). Concomitant speech and language disorders in stuttering children: A critique of the literature. *Journal of Speech and Hearing Disorders,* 55, 51–60.

Nippold, M. A., & Schwartz, I. E. (1990). Reading disorders in stuttering children. *Journal of Fluency Disorders,* 15, 175–189.

Nippold, M. A., Schwartz, I. E., & Jescheniak, J.-D. (1991). Narrative ability in school-age stuttering boys: A preliminary investigation. *Journal of Fluency Disorders,* 16, 289–308.

Nittrouer, S., & Cheney, C. (1984). Operant techniques used in stuttering therapy: A review. *Journal of Fluency Disorders,* 9, 169–190.

Nowack, W. J., & Stone, R. E. (1987). Acquired stuttering and bilateral cerebral disease. *Journal of Fluency Disorders,* 12, 141–146.

Nudelman, H. B., Herbrich, K. E., Hess, K. R., Hoyt, B. D., & Rosenfield, D. B. (1992). A model of the phonatory response time of stutterers and fluent speakers to frequency modulated tones. *Journal of the Acoustical Society of America,* 92 (4, pt. 1), 1882–1888.

Nudelman, H. B., Herbrich, K. E., Hoyt, B. D., & Rosenfield, D. B. (1989). A neuroscience model of stuttering. *Journal of Fluency Disorders,* 14, 399–427.

Nwokah, E. E. (1988). The imbalance of stuttering behavior in bilingual speakers. *Journal of Fluency Disorders,* 13, 357–373.

Oates, D. W. (1929). Left-handedness in relation to speech defects, intelligence, and achievement. *Forum of Education,* 7, 91–105.

Ojemann, R. H. (1931). Studies in sidedness: III. Relation of handedness to speech. *Journal of Educational Psychology,* 22, 120–126.

Okasha, A., Bishry, Z., Kamel, M., & Hassan, A. H. (1974). Psychosocial study of stammering in Egyptian children. *British Journal of Psychiatry,* 124, 531–533.

Onslow, M. (1992a). Choosing a treatment procedure for early stuttering: Issues and future directions. *Journal of Speech and Hearing Research,* 35, 983–993.

Onslow, M. (1992b). Identification of early stuttering: Issues and suggested strategies. *American Journal of Speech-Language Pathology,* 1(4), 21–27.

Onslow, M., Andrews, G., & Lincoln, M. (1994). A control/experimental trial of an operant treatment for early stuttering. *Journal of Speech and Hearing Research,* 37, 1244–1259.

Onslow, M., Hayes, B., Hutchins, L., & Newman, D. (1992). Speech naturalness and prolonged-speech treatments for stuttering: Further variables and data. *Journal of Speech and Hearing Research,* 35, 274–282.

Onslow, M., & Ingham, R. J. (1987). Speech quality measurement and the management of stuttering. *Journal of Speech and Hearing Disorders,* 52, 2–17.

Otsuki, H. (1958). Study on stuttering: Statistical observations. *Otorhinolaryngology Clinic,* 5, 1150–1151.

Paden, E. P. (1970). *A History of the American Speech and Hearing Association 1925–1958.* Washington, DC: American Speech and Hearing Association.

Palmer, M. F., & Gillette, A. M. (1938). Sex differences in the cardiac rhythms of stutterers. *Journal of Speech Disorders,* 3, 3–12.

Palmer, M. F., & Gillette, A. M. (1939). Respiratory cardiac arrhythmia in stuttering. *Journal of Speech Disorders,* 4, 133–140.

Paul-Brown, D. (1990). National Stuttering Project. *ASHA Reports,* 32 (1), 35.

Pauls, D. L. (1990). A review of the evidence for genetic factors in stuttering. *ASHA Reports,* 18, 34–38.

Peleman-Cappaert, V. (1994). The education and growth of a speech pathologist who treats stutterers. *Journal of Fluency Disorders,* 19, 199.

Penfield, W., & Roberts, L. (1959). *Speech and Brain Mechanisms.* Princeton, NJ: Princeton University Press.

Perkins, D. (1947). An item by item compilation and comparison of the scores of 75 young adult stutterers on the California Test of Personality. *Speech Monographs,* 14, 211.

Perkins, W. H. (1973). Replacement of stuttering with normal speech: II. Clinical procedures. *Journal of Speech and Hearing Disorders,* 38, 295–303.

Perkins, W. H. (1979). From psychoanalysis to discoordination. In H. H. Gregory (Ed.), *Controversies About Stuttering Therapy.* Baltimore, MD: University Park Press, pp. 97–127.

Perkins, W. H. (1981). Measurement and maintenance of fluency. In E. Boberg (Ed.), *Maintenance of Fluency.* New York: Elsevier North-Holland.

Perkins, W. H. (1983a). The problem of definition: Commentary on stuttering. *Journal of Speech and Hearing Disorders,* 48, 246–249.

Perkins, W. H. (1983b). Learning from negative outcomes in stuttering therapy: II. An epiphany of failures. *Journal of Fluency Disorders, 8,* 155–160.

Perkins, W. H. (1990a). What is stuttering? *Journal of Speech and Hearing Disorders, 55,* 370–382.

Perkins, W. H. (1990b). Gratitude, good intentions, and red herrings: A response to commentaries. *Journal of Speech and Hearing Disorders, 55,* 402–404.

Perkins, W. H. (1991). So near and yet so far: A response to Siegel. *Journal of Speech and Hearing Research, 34,* 1083–1086.

Perkins, W. H. (1992a). How can agreement be disagreement? A reply to Christensen. *Journal of Speech and Hearing Research, 35,* 1033.

Perkins, W. H. (1992b). Marching to different drummers: A reply to Smith. *Journal of Speech and Hearing Research, 35,* 1033–1039.

Perkins, W. H. (1993). The early history of behavior modification of stuttering: A view from the trenches. *Journal of Fluency Disorders, 18,* 1–11.

Perkins, W. H. (1994). Solving unsolvable stuttering. *American Journal of Speech-Language Pathology, 3*(3), 32–33

Perkins, W. H., & Curlee, R. F. (1969). Clinical impressions of portable masking unit effects in stuttering. *Journal of Speech and Hearing Disorders, 34,* 360–362.

Perkins, W. H., Kent, R., & Curlee, R. (1991). A theory of neuropsycholinguistic function in stuttering. *Journal of Speech and Hearing Research, 34,* 734–735.

Perkins, W. H., Rudas, J., Johnson, L., & Bell, J. (1976). Stuttering: Discoordination of phonation with articulation and respiration. *Journal of Speech and Hearing Research, 19,* 509–522.

Peters, H. F. M., & Hulstijn, W. (1984). Stuttering and anxiety: The difference between stutterers and nonstutterers in verbal apprehension and physiologic arousal during the anticipation of speech and non-speech tasks. *Journal of Fluency Disorders, 9,* 67–84.

Peters, H. F. M., & Starkweather, C. W. (1989). Development of stuttering throughout life. *Journal of Fluency Disorders, 14,* 303–321.

Peters, T. J., & Guitar, B. (1990). *Stuttering: An Integrated Approach to Its Nature and Treatment.* Baltimore, MD: Williams & Wilkins.

Pill, J. (1988). A comparison between two treatment programs for stuttering: A personal account. *Journal of Fluency Disorders, 13,* 385–398.

Pill, J. (1994). Report on support groups and Consumers Affairs Committee. *Journal of Fluency Disorders, 19,* 201.

Pill, J., & St. Louis, K. (1994). Self-help and speech professionals. *Journal of Fluency Disorders, 19,* 200–201.

Platt, L. J., & Basili, J. (1973). Jaw tremor during stuttering block: An electromyographic study. *Journal of Communication Disorders, 6,* 102–109.

Podolskaya, O. V., & Shklovsky, V. M. (1973). Ob osobennostyakh nefermentativnoi fibrinolitichkoi aktivnosti i obrazovania kompleksov adrenalin-geparin i noradrenalin-geparin v krovi bolnikh logonervozon. *Zh. Nevropatol.Psikhiat.*, 73, 711–715.

Polanyi, M. (1967). *The Tacit Dimension*. New York: Doubleday Anchor Books.

Porfert, A. R., & Rosenfield, D. B. (1978). Prevalence of stuttering. *Journal of Neurology, Neurosurgery, and Psychiatry*, 41, 954–956.

Porret, J. M. (1993). Psychoanalytical aspects of stammering. *ACTA Paedopsychiatrica*, 56(1), 57–61.

Porter, H. K. (1939). Studies in the psychology of stuttering: XIV. Stuttering phenomena in relation to size and personnel of audience. *Journal of Speech Disorders*, 4, 323–333.

Porterfield, C. L. (1969). Adaptative mechanisms of young disadvantaged stutterers and nonstutterers. *Journal of Projective Techniques for Personal Assessment*, 33, 371–375.

Postma, A., & Kolk, H. (1992). Error monitoring in people who stutter: Evidence against auditory feedback deficit theories. *Journal of Speech and Hearing Research*, 35, 1024–1032.

Postma, A., & Kolk, H. (1993). The covert repair hypothesis: Prearticulatory repair processes in normal and stuttered disfluencies. *Journal of Speech and Hearing Research*, 36, 472–487.

Poulos, M. G., & Webster, W. G. (1991). Family history as a basis for subgrouping people who stutter. *Journal of Speech and Hearing Research*, 34, 5–10.

Preacher, W. G., & Harris, W. E. (1946). Speech disorders in World War II: VIII. Stuttering. *Journal of Speech Disorders*, 11, 303–308.

Preus, A. (1972). Stuttering in Down's syndrome. *Scandanavian Journal of Educational Research*, 16, 89–104.

Preus, A. (1981). *Attempts at Identifying Subgroups of Stutterers*. Oslo, Norway: University of Oslo Press.

Preus, A. (1987). The cluttering type of stutterer. *Nordisk Tidsskrift for Logopedi og Foniatri*, 12, 3–19.

Preus, A. (1992). Cluttering and stuttering: Related, different, or antagonistic disorders? In F. Myers & K. O. St. Louis (Eds.), *Cluttering: A Clinical Perspective*. Leicester, England: Far Communications, 55–70.

Prins, D. (1972). Personality, stuttering severity, and age. *Journal of Speech and Hearing Research*, 15, 148–154.

Prins, D. (1993). Models for treatment efficacy studies of adult stutterers. *Journal of Fluency Disorders*, 18, 333–349.

Prins, D., & Hubbard, C. P. (1988). Response contingent stimuli and stuttering: Issues and implications. *Journal of Speech and Hearing Research*, 31, 696–709.

Prins, D., & Hubbard, C. P. (1992). Consistency of interstress intervals in the fluent speech of people who stutter during adaptation trials. *Journal of Speech and Hearing Research*, 35, 799–804.

Prins, D., Hubbard, C. P., & Krause, M. (1991). Syllabic stress and the occurrence of stuttering. *Journal of Speech and Hearing Research, 34*, 1011–1016.

Prins, D., & Lohr, F. (1972). Behavioral dimensions of stuttered speech. *Journal of Speech and Hearing Research, 15*, 61–71.

Prosek, R. A., Montgomery, A. A., & Walden, B. E. (1988). Constancy of relative timing for stutterers and nonstutterers. *Journal of Speech and Hearing Research, 31*, 654–658.

Prosek, R. A., Montgomery, A. A., Walden, B. E., & Hawkins, D. B. (1987). Formant frequencies of stuttered and fluent vowels. *Journal of Speech and Hearing Research, 30*, 301–305.

Quarrington, B. (1953). The performance of stutterers on the Rosenzweig Picture-Frustration Test. *Journal of Clinical Psychology, 9*, 189–192.

Quesal, R. W. (1989). Stuttering research: Have we forgotten the stutterer? *Journal of Fluency Disorders, 14*, 153–164.

Quinn, P. T. (1971). Stuttering: Some observations on speaking when alone. *Journal of the Australian College of Speech Therapists, 21*, 92–94.

Quinn, P. T. (1972). Stuttering, cerebral dominance, and dichotic word test. *The Medical Journal of Australia, 2*, 639–643.

Quinn, P. T., & Andrews, G. (1977). Neurological stuttering—A clinical entity? *Journal of Neurology, Neurosurgery, and Psychiatry, 40*, 699–701.

Quinn, P. T., & Peachey, E. (1975). Haloperidol in the treatment of stuttering. *British Journal of Psychiatry, 123*, 247–248.

Ramig, P. R. (1984). Rate changes in the speech of stutterers after therapy. *Journal of Fluency Disorders, 9*, 285–294.

Ramig, P. R. (1993). The impact of self-help groups on persons who stutter: A call for research. *Journal of Fluency Disorders, 18*, 351–361.

Ramig, P. R., Krieger, S., & Adams, M. (1982). Vocal changes in stutterers and nonstutterers when speaking to children. *Journal of Fluency Disorders, 6*, 15–33.

Ramig, P. R., & Wallace, M. L. (1987). Indirect and combined direct-indirect therapy in a dysfluent child. *Journal of Fluency Disorders, 12*, 41–49.

Rao, P. R. (1991). Neurogenic stuttering as a manifestation of stroke and a mask of dysphonia. *Clinics in Communication Disorders, 1*(1), 31–37.

Rastatter, M. P., & Dell, C. W. (1987a). Simple visual versus lexical decision vocal reaction times of stuttering and normal subjects. *Journal of Fluency Disorders, 12*, 63–69.

Rastatter, M. P., & Dell, C. W. (1987b). Vocal reaction times of stuttering subjects to tachistoscopically presented concrete and abstract words: A closer look at cerebral dominance and language processing. *Journal of Speech and Hearing Research, 30*, 306–310.

Rastatter, M. P., & Dell, C. W. (1988). Reading reaction times of stuttering and nonstuttering subjects to unilaterally presented concrete and abstract words. *Journal of Fluency Disorders, 13*, 319–329.

Rastatter, M. P., & Harr, R. (1988). Measurements of plasma levels of adrenergic neurotransmitters and primary amino acids in five stuttering subjects: A preliminary report (biochemical aspects of stuttering). *Journal of Fluency Disorders,* 13, 127–139.

Rastatter, M. P., & Loren, C. A. (1988). Visual coding dominance in stuttering: Some evidence from central tachistoscopic stimulation (tachistoscopic viewing and stuttering). *Journal of Fluency Disorders,* 13, 89–95.

Rastatter, M. P., Loren, C. A., & Colcord, R. (1987). Visual coding strategies and hemisphere dominance characteristics of stutterers. *Journal of Fluency Disorders,* 12, 305–315.

Rastatter, M. P., McGuire, R. A., & Loren, C. A. (1988). Linguistic encoding dominance in stuttering: Some evidence for temporal and qualitative hemispheric processing differences. *Journal of Fluency Disorders,* 13, 215–224.

Reed, C. G., & Godden, A. L. (1977). An experimental treatment using verbal punishment with two preschool stutterers. *Journal of Fluency Disorders,* 2, 225–233.

Reed, C. G., & Lingwall, J. B. (1976). Some relationships between punishment, stuttering, and galvanic skin responses. *Journal of Speech and Hearing Research,* 19, 197–205.

Reich, A., Till, J., & Goldsmith, H. (1981). Laryngeal and manual reaction times of stuttering and nonstuttering adults. *Journal of Speech and Hearing Research,* 24, 192–196.

Rice, M., & Kroll, R. (1994). A survey of stutterers' perceptions of challenges and discrimination in the workplace. *Journal of Fluency Disorders,* 19, 203.

Richardson, L. H. (1944). A personality study of stutterers and nonstutterers. *Journal of Speech Disorders,* 9, 152–160.

Richter, E. (1982). Ein Beitrag zur Ätiologie des Stotterns. *Sprachheilarb.,* 27, 239–245.

Rieber, R. W. (Ed.) (1977). *The Problem of Stuttering: Theory and Therapy.* New York: Elsevier North-Holland.

Riley, G. D. (1972). A stuttering severity instrument for children and adults. *Journal of Speech and Hearing Disorders,* 37, 314–321.

Riley, G. D. (1984). *Stuttering Prediction Instrument for Young Children.* Austin, TX: PRO-ED.

Riley, G. D., & Riley, J. (1979). A component model for diagnosing and treating children who stutter. *Journal of Fluency Disorders,* 4, 279–293.

Riley, G. D., & Riley, J. (1986). Oral motor discoordination among children who stutter. *Journal of Fluency Disorders,* 11, 335–344.

Riley, G. D., & Riley, J. (1989). Physician's screening procedure for children who may stutter. *Journal of Fluency Disorders,* 14, 57–67.

Ritzman, C. H. (1943). A cardiovascular and metabolic study of stutterers and nonstutterers. *Journal of Speech Disorders,* 8, 161–182.

Robb, M. P., Lybolt, J. T., & Price, H. A. (1985). Acoustic measures of stutterers' speech following an intensive therapy program. *Journal of Fluency Disorders,* 10, 269–279.

Robe, E., Brumlik, J., & Moore, P. (1960). A study of spastic dysphonia: Neurologic and electroencephalographic abnormalities. *Laryngoscope,* 70, 219–245.

Rosenbek, J., Messert, B., Collins, M., & Wertz, R. (1978). Stuttering following brain damage. *Brain and Language,* 6, 82–86.

Rosenberger, P. B. (1980). Dopaminergic systems and speech fluency. *Journal of Fluency Disorders,* 5, 255–267.

Rosenberger, P. B., Wheelden, J. A., & Kalotkin, M. (1976). The effect of haloperidol on stuttering. *American Journal of Psychiatry,* 133, 331–337.

Rosenfield, D. B., & Freeman, F. J. (1983). Stuttering onset after laryngectomy. *Journal of Fluency Disorders,* 8, 265–268.

Rosenfield, D. B., Jones, B. P., & Liljestrand, J. S. (1981). Effects of right hemisphere damage in an adult stutterer. *Journal of Fluency Disorders,* 6, 175–179.

Roth, C. R., Aronson, A. E., & Davis, L. J., Jr. (1989). Clinical studies in psychogenic stuttering of adult onset. *Journal of Speech and Hearing Disorders,* 54, 634–646.

Rotter, J. B. (1966). Generalized expectancies for internal versus external control of reinforcement. *Psychological Monographs,* 80 [Whole of No. 609].

Rousey, C. G., Arjunan, K. N., & Rousey, C. L. (1986). Successful treatment of stuttering following closed head injury. *Journal of Fluency Disorders,* 11, 257–261.

Rubin, T. I. (1969). *The Angry Book.* New York: Macmillan.

Runyan, C. M., & Adams, M. R. (1978). Perceptual study of the speech of "successfully therapeutized" stutterers. *Journal of Fluency Disorders,* 3, 25–29.

Runyan, C. M., & Adams, M. R. (1979). Unsophisticated judges' perceptual evaluations of the speech of "successfully therapeutized" stutterers. *Journal of Fluency Disorders,* 4, 29–38.

Ruscello, D. M., Lass, N. J., Schmitt, J. F., & Pannbacker, M. D. (1994). Special educators' perceptions of stutterers. *Journal of Fluency Disorders,* 19, 125–132.

Rutherford, B. R. (1938). Speech reeducation for the birth injured. *Journal of Speech Disorders,* 3, 199–206.

Ryan, B. P. (1971). Operant procedures applied to stuttering therapy for children. *Journal of Speech and Hearing Disorders,* 36, 264–280.

Ryan, B. P. (1974). *Programmed Therapy for Stuttering in Children and Adults.* Springfield, IL: Charles C. Thomas.

Ryan, B. P. (1992). Articulation, language, rate, and fluency characteristics of stuttering and nonstuttering preschool children. *Journal of Speech and Hearing Research,* 35, 333–342.

Ryan, B. P., & Ryan, B. V. K. (1995). Programmed stuttering treatment: Comparison of two establishment programs through transfer, maintenance, and follow-up. *Journal of Speech and Hearing Research,* 38, 61–75

Ryan, B. P., & Van Kirk, B. (1974). The establishment, transfer, and maintenance of fluent speech in 50 stutterers using delayed auditory feedback and operant procedures. *Journal of Speech and Hearing Disorders,* 39, 3–10.

Sakai, T., Miyamura, M., & Kuzuhara, S. (1992). Palilalia and acquired stuttering in a case of Parkinson's disease [Japanese]. *Rinsho Shinkeigaku,* 32(8), 859–863.

Salamy, J. N., & Sessions, R. B. (1980). Spastic dysphonia. *Journal of Fluency Disorders,* 5, 281–290.

Schaefer, S. D., Gerling, I. J., Finitzo-Hieber, T., & Freeman, F. J. (in press). Brainstem conduction abnormalities in spasmodic dysphonia. *Annals of Otology, Rhinology, and Laryngology.*

Schindler, M. D. (1955). A study of educational adjustment of stuttering and nonstuttering children. In W. Johnson & R. R. Leutenegger (Eds.), *Stuttering in Children and Adults.* Minneapolis: University of Minnesota Press.

Schlanger, B. B., & Gottsleben, R. H. (1957). Analysis of speech defects among the institutionalized mentally retarded. *Journal of Speech and Hearing Disorders,* 22, 98–103.

Schleier, E., Schelhorn, P., & Groh, F. (1991). Biochemical studies in stuttering in children [Polish]. *Otolaryngologia Polska,* 45(2), 141–144.

Schloss, P. J., Espin, C. A., Smith, M. A., & Suffolk, D. R. (1987). Developing assertiveness during employment interviews with young adults who stutter. *Journal of Speech and Hearing Disorders,* 52, 30–36.

Schloss, P. J., Freeman, C. A., Smith, M. A., & Espin, C. A. (1987). Influence of assertiveness training on the stuttering rates exhibited by three young adults. *Journal of Fluency Disorders,* 12, 333–353.

Schmidt, B. (1994). Perceptions in stuttering adults during speech disfluency. *Journal of Fluency Disorders,* 19, 206.

Schuell, H. (1946). Sex differences in relation to stuttering. Part I. *Journal of Speech Disorders,* 11, 277–298.

Schwartz, H. D. (1993). Adolescents who stutter. *Journal of Fluency Disorders,* 18, 289–302.

Schwartz, H. D. (1994). Transferring fluency: Older children and adolescents. *Journal of Fluency Disorders,* 19, 207.

Schwartz, H. D., Zebrowski, P. M., & Conture, E. G. (1990). Behaviors at the onset of stuttering. *Journal of Fluency Disorders,* 15, 77–86.

Schwartz, M. F. (1976). *Stuttering Solved.* New York: McGraw-Hill.

Schwartz, M. F., & Carter, G. L. (1986). *Stop Stuttering.* New York: Harper & Row.

Scripture, E. W. (1931). *Stuttering, Lisping, and Correction of the Speech of the Deaf.* New York: Macmillian.

Sedlacek, C. (1947–48). Reactions of the autonomic nervous system in attacks of stuttering. *Folia Phoniatrica,* 1, 97–103.

Seeman, M. (1934). Uber somatische befunde bei stottern. *Monatschrift für Ohren-heilkunde,* 68, 895–912.

Seider, R. A., Gladstein, K. L., & Kidd, K. K. (1982). Language onset and concomitant speech and language problems in subgroups of stutterers and their siblings. *Journal of Speech and Hearing Research, 25,* 482–486.

Seider, R. A., Gladstein, K. L., & Kidd, K. K. (1983). Recovery and persistence of stuttering among relatives of stutterers. *Journal of Speech and Hearing Disorders, 48,* 402–409.

Seligman, M. (1975). *Helplessness: On Depression, Development, and Death.* San Francisco: W. H. Freeman.

Sermas, C. E., & Cox, M. D. (1982). The stutterer and stuttering: Personality correlates. *Journal of Fluency Disorders, 7,* 141–158.

Shames, G. H. (1951). The relationship between the attitude toward stuttering of secondary stutterers and several of their personality characteristics. *Speech Monographs, 18,* 241.

Shames, G. H. (1975). Operant conditioning and stuttering. In J. Eisenson (Ed.), *Stuttering: A Second Symposium.* New York: Harper & Row, 263–332.

Shames, G. H. (1989). Stuttering: An RFP for a cultural perspective. *Journal of Fluency Disorders, 14,* 67–77.

Shames, G. H., & Egolf, D. B. (1976). *Operant Conditioning and the Management of Stuttering: A Book for Clinicians.* Englewood Cliffs, NJ: Prentice-Hall.

Shames, G. H., & Florance, C. L. (1980). *Stutter-free Speech: A Goal for Therapy.* Columbus, OH: Charles E. Merrill.

Shames, G. H., & Rubin, H. (Eds.) (1986). *Stuttering Then and Now.* Columbus, OH: Charles E. Merrill.

Shames, G. H., & Sherrick, C. E., Jr. (1963). A discussion of nonfluency and stuttering as operant behavior. *Journal of Speech and Hearing Disorders, 28,* 3–18.

Shapiro, A. I. (1980). An electromyographic analysis of the fluent and disfluent utterances of several types of stutterers. *Journal of Fluency Disorders, 5,* 203–231.

Shapiro, A. K. (1964). Factors contributing to the placebo effect: Implications for psychotherapy. *American Journal of Psychotherapy, 18* (Suppl. 1), 73–88.

Shearer, W. M., & Baud, H. E. (1970). Adaptation in mentally retarded stutterers and nonstutterers. *Journal of Communication Disorders, 3,* 118–122.

Sheehan, J. G. (1968). Stuttering as a self-role conflict. In H. H. Gregory (Ed.), *Learning Theory and Stuttering Therapy.* Evanston, IL: Northwestern University Press, 72–83.

Sheehan, J. G. (1970). *Stuttering: Research and Therapy.* New York: Harper & Row.

Sheehan, J. G. (1974). Stuttering behavior: A phonetic analysis. *Journal of Communication Disorders, 7,* 193–212.

Sheehan, J. G. (1979a). Current issues on stuttering and recovery. In H. H. Gregory (Ed.), *Controversies About Stuttering Therapy.* Baltimore, MD: University Park Press, 175–207.

Sheehan, J. G. (1979b). Level of aspiration of female stutterers: Changing times? *Journal of Speech and Hearing Disorders, 44,* 479–486.

Sheehan, J. G. (1984). Problems in the evaluation of progress and outcome. In W. Perkins (Ed.), *Current Therapy of Communication Disorders: Stuttering Disorders.* New York: Thieme-Stratton, 223–239.

Sheehan, J. G., & Costley, M. (1977). A re-examination of the role of heredity in stuttering. *Journal of Speech and Hearing Disorders, 42,* 47–49.

Sheehan, J. G., & Martyn, M. M. (1970). Spontaneous recovery from stuttering. *Journal of Speech and Hearing Research, 13,* 279–289.

Sheehan, J. G., & Voas, R. B. (1954). Tension patterns during stuttering in relation to conflict, anxiety-binding, and reinforcement. *Speech Monographs, 21,* 272–279.

Sheehan, J. G., & Zussman, C. (1951). Rorschachs of stutterers compared with a clinical control. *American Psychologist, 6,* 500.

Sheehy, G. (1976). *Passages: Predictable Crises of Adult Life.* New York: E. P. Dutton.

Shenker, R. C., & Finn, P. (1985). An evaluation of the effects of supplemental "fluency" training during maintenance. *Journal of Fluency Disorders, 10,* 257–267.

Shenker, R. C., Mayberry, M., Scobble, M., Grothe, M., & White, K. (1994). The gesture-speech relationship in stuttering. *Journal of Fluency Disorders, 19,* 207.

Sherman, D. (1952). Clinical and experimental use of the Iowa Scale of Severity of Stuttering. *Journal of Speech and Hearing Disorders, 17,* 316–320.

Shine, R. (1984). Assessment and fluency training with the young stutterer. In M. Peins (Ed.), *Contemporary Approaches in Stuttering Therapy.* Boston: Little, Brown.

Shirkey, E. A. (1987). Forensic verification of stuttering. *Journal of Fluency Disorders, 12,* 197–203.

Shklovskii, V. M., Krol, L. M., & Mikhailova, E. L. (1988). The psychotherapy of stuttering: On the model of stuttering patients' psychotherapy group. *Soviet Journal of Psychiatry and Psychology Today, 1,* 130–141.

Shopwin, C. D. (1959). An experimental investigation of the passive-dependency component in adult male stutterers. *Speech Monographs, 26,* 143.

Shumak, I. C. (1955). A speech situation rating sheet for stutterers. In W. Johnson (Ed.), *Stuttering in Children and Adults: Thirty Years of Research at the University of Iowa.* Minneapolis: University of Minnesota Press, 341–347.

Siegel, G. M. (1970). Punishment, stuttering, and disfluency. *Journal of Speech and Hearing Research, 13,* 677–714.

Siegel, G. M. (1991). Response to Perkins, "What is stuttering?" *Journal of Speech and Hearing Research, 34,* 1081–1083.

Siegel, G. M. (1993). Stuttering and behavior modification: Commentary. *Journal of Fluency Disorders, 18,* 109–114.

Siegel, G. M., & Haugen, D. (1964). Audience size and variations in stuttering behavior. *Journal of Speech and Hearing Research, 7,* 381–388.

Silverman, E.-M. (1972a). Generality of disfluency data collected from preschoolers. *Journal of Speech and Hearing Research, 14,* 84–92.

Silverman, E.-M. (1972b). Preschoolers' speech disfluency: Single syllable word repetition. *Perceptual and Motor Skills, 35,* 1002.

Silverman, F. H. (1960). Forensic therapy. *Quarterly Journal of Speech,* 46, 305–306.

Silverman, F. H. (1970a). Course of nonstutterers disfluency adaptation during 15 consecutive oral readings of the same material. *Journal of Speech and Hearing Research,* 13, 382–386.

Silverman, F. H. (1970b). Concern of elementary-school stutterers about their stuttering. *Journal of Speech and Hearing Disorders,* 35, 361–363.

Silverman, F. H. (1970c). Distribution of instances of disfluency in consecutive readings of different passages by nonstutterers. *Journal of Speech and Hearing Research,* 13, 874–882.

Silverman, F. H. (1970d). A note on the degree of adaptation by stutterers and nonstutterers during oral reading. *Journal of Speech and Hearing Research,* 13, 173–177.

Silverman, F. H. (1971a). The effect of rhythmic auditory stimulation on the disfluency of nonstutterers. *Journal of Speech and Hearing Research,* 14, 350–355.

Silverman, F. H. (1971b). A rationale for the use of the hearing-aid metronome in a program of therapy for stuttering. *Perceptual and Motor Skills,* 32, 34.

Silverman, F. H. (1974). Disfluency behavior of elementary-school stutterers and nonstutterers. *Language, Speech, and Hearing Services in Schools,* 5, 32–37.

Silverman, F. H. (1975). How "typical" is a stutterer's stuttering in a clinical environment! *Perceptual and Motor Skills,* 40, 458.

Silverman, F. H. (1976a). Communicative success: A reinforcer of stuttering. *Perceptual and Motor Skills,* 43, 398.

Silverman, F. H. (1976b). Long-term impact of a miniature metronome on stuttering: An interim report. *Perceptual and Motor Skills,* 42, 1322.

Silverman, F. H. (1980a). Dimensions of improvement in stuttering. *Journal of Speech and Hearing Research,* 23, 137–151.

Silverman, F. H. (1980b). The Stuttering Problem Profile: A task that assists both client and clinician in defining therapy goals. *Journal of Speech and Hearing Disorders,* 45, 119–123.

Silverman, F. H. (1981). Relapse following stuttering therapy. In N. J. Lass (Ed.), *Speech and Language: Advances in Basic Research and Practice (Volume 5).* New York: Academic Press.

Silverman, F. H. (1987). *Microcomputers in Speech-Language Pathology and Audiology: A Primer.* Englewood Cliffs, NJ: Prentice-Hall.

Silverman, F. H. (1988a). Impact of a T-shirt message on stutterer stereotypes. *Journal of Fluency Disorders,* 13, 279–281.

Silverman, F. H. (1988b). The monster study. *Journal of Fluency Disorders,* 13, 225–231.

Silverman, F. H. (1990). Are professors likely to have "beliefs" about the intelligence and competence of students who stutter? *Journal of Fluency Disorders,* 15, 319–321.

Silverman, F. H. (1992). *Legal-Ethical Considerations, Restrictions, and Obligations for Clinicians Who Treat Communicative Disorders.* Springfield, IL: Charles C. Thomas.

Silverman, F. H. (1993). *Research Design and Evaluation in Speech-Language Pathology and Audiology* (3rd Ed.). Englewood Cliffs, NJ: Prentice-Hall.

Silverman, F. H. (1995). *Speech, Language, and Hearing Disorders.* Needham Heights, MA: Allyn & Bacon.

Silverman, F. H., & Bloom, C. M. (1973). Spontaneous recovery of nonstutterers' disfluency following adaptation. *Journal of Speech and Hearing Research,* 16, 452–455.

Silverman, F. H., & Bohlman, P. (1988). Flute stuttering. *Journal of Fluency Disorders,* 13, 427–428.

Silverman, F. H., Gazzolo, M., & Peterson, Y. (1989). Impact of a T-shirt message on stutterer stereotypes: A systematic replication. *Journal of Fluency Disorders.*

Silverman, F. H., & Goodban, M. K. (1972). The effect of auditory masking on the fluency of normal speakers. *Journal of Speech and Hearing Research,* 15, 543–546.

Silverman, F. H., & Hummer, K. (1989). Spastic dysphonia: A fluency disorder? *Journal of Fluency Disorders,* 14, 285–293.

Silverman, F. H., & Paynter, K. K. (1990). Impact of stuttering on perception of occupational competence. *Journal of Fluency Disorders,* 15, 87–91.

Silverman, F. H., & Silverman, E.-M. (1971). Stutter-like behavior in manual communication of the deaf. *Perceptual and Motor Skills,* 33, 45–46.

Silverman, F. H., & Trotter, W. D. (1973a). Bibliography: Literature related to the use of instrumental aids in stuttering therapy. *Perceptual and Motor Skills,* 36, 247–251.

Silverman, F. H., & Trotter, W. D. (1973b). Bibliography related to the use of instrumental aids in stuttering therapy: Supplement 1. *Perceptual and Motor Skills,* 37, 552.

Silverman, F. H., & Trotter, W. D. (1973c). Impact of pacing speech with a miniature electronic metronome on the manner in which a stutterer is perceived. *Behavior Therapy,* 4, 414–419.

Silverman, F. H., & Trotter, W. D. (1974). Bibliography related to the use of instrumental aids in stuttering therapy: Supplement 2. *Perceptual and Motor Skills,* 38, 1329–1330.

Silverman, F. H., & Trotter, W. D. (1975). Bibliography related to the use of instrumental aids in stuttering therapy: Supplement 3. *Perceptual and Motor Skills,* 40, 240.

Silverman, F. H., & Williams, D. E. (1967). Loci of disfluencies in the speech of nonstutterers during oral reading. *Journal of Speech and Hearing Research,* 10, 790–794.

Silverman, F. H., & Williams, D. E. (1972a). Prediction of stuttering by school-age stutterers. *Journal of Speech and Hearing Research,* 15, 189–193.

Silverman, F. H., & Williams, D. E. (1972b). Performance of stutterers on a single-word adaptation task. *Perceptual and Motor Skills,* 34, 565–566.

Silverman, F. H., & Williams, D. E. (1973). Use of revision by elementary-school stutterers and nonstutterers during oral reading. *Journal of Speech and Hearing Research,* 16, 584–585.

Smith, A. (1990a). Factors in the etiology of stuttering. *ASHA Reports* (Number 18), 39–47.

Smith, A. (1990b). Toward a comprehensive theory of stuttering: A commentary. *Journal of Speech and Hearing Disorders,* 55, 398–401.

Smith, A. (1992). Commentary on "A theory of neuropsycholinguistic function in stuttering." *Journal of Speech and Hearing Research,* 35, 805–809.

Smith, A., & Luschei, E. S. (1983). Assessment of oral-motor reflexes in stutterers and normal speakers: Preliminary observations. *Journal of Speech and Hearing Research,* 26, 322–328.

Snidecor, J. C. (1947). Why the Indian does not stutter. *Quarterly Journal of Speech,* 33, 493–495.

Snidecor, J. C. (1955). Tension and facial appearance in stuttering. In W. Johnson & R. R. Leutenegger (Editors), *Stuttering in Children and Adults*. Minneapolis: University of Minnesota Press.

Spadino, E. J. (1941). *Writing and Laterality Characteristics of Stuttering Children*. New York: Columbia University Teachers College.

St. Louis, K. O. (Ed.) (1986). *The Atypical Stutterer: Principles and Practices of Rehabilitation*. Orlando, FL: Academic Press.

St. Louis, K. O. (1992). On defining cluttering. In F. Myers & K. O. St. Louis (Eds.), *Cluttering: A Clinical Perspective*. Leicester, England: Far Communications, 37–53.

St. Louis, K. O., & Hinzman, A. R. (1986). Studies of cluttering: Perceptions of cluttering by speech-language pathologists and educators. *Journal of Fluency Disorders,* 11, 131–149.

St. Louis, K. O., & Hinzman, A. R. (1988). A descriptive study of speech, language, and hearing characteristics of school-age stutterers. *Journal of Fluency Disorders,* 13, 331–355.

St. Louis, K. O., Hinzman, A. R., & Hull, F. M. (1985). Studies of cluttering: Disfluency and language measures in young possible clutterers and stutterers. *Journal of Fluency Disorders,* 10, 151–172.

St. Louis, K. O., & Rustin, L. (1992). Professional awareness of cluttering. In F. Myers & K. O. St. Louis (Eds.), *Cluttering: A Clinical Perspective*. Leicester, England: Far Communications, 23–35.

St. Onge, K. (1963). The stuttering syndrome. *Journal of Speech and Hearing Research,* 6, 195–197.

St. Onge, K., & Calvert, J. J. (1964). Stuttering research. *Quarterly Journal of Speech,* 50, 159–165.

Stager, S. V. (1990). Heterogeneity in stuttering: Results from auditory brainstem response testing. *Journal of Fluency Disorders,* 15, 9–19.

Stager, S. V., Ludlow, C., Gordon, C., Cotelingham, M., & Rapoport, J. (1994). Maintenance of fluency following long-term clomipramine treatment. *Journal of Fluency Disorders,* 19, 212.

Stampfl, T., & Levis, D. (1967). Essentials of implosive therapy. *Journal of Abnormal Psychology*, 72, 496–503.

Stansfield, J. (1995). Word-final disfluencies in adults with learning difficulties. *Journal of Fluency Disorders*, 20, 1–10.

Starbuck, H. B., & Steer, M. D. (1954). The adaptation effect in stuttering and its relation to thoracic and abdominal breathing. *Journal of Speech and Hearing Disorders*, 19, 440–449.

Stark, R. E., & Pierce, B. R. (1970). The effect of delayed auditory feedback on a speech-related task in stutterers. *Journal of Speech and Hearing Research*, 13, 245–253.

Starke, A. (1994). Why do stutterers reject artificial speech? The message incompatibility conflict. *Journal of Fluency Disorders*, 19, 213.

Starkweather, C. W. (1982). *Stuttering and Laryngeal Behavior: A Review* (ASHA Monographs Number 21). Rockville, MD: American Speech-Language-Hearing Association.

Starkweather, C. W. (1987). *Fluency and Stuttering*. Englewood Cliffs, NJ: Prentice-Hall.

Starkweather, C. W. (1990). Current trends in therapy for stuttering children and suggestions for future research. *ASHA Reports*, 18, 82–90.

Starkweather, C. W. (1993). Issues in the efficacy of treatment for fluency disorders. *Journal of Fluency Disorders*, 18, 151–168.

Starkweather, C. W. (1994). The electronic self-help group. *Journal of Fluency Disorders*, 19, 213.

Starkweather, C. W., Franklin, S., & Smigo, T. M. (1984). Vocal and finger reaction times in stutterers and nonstutterers: Differences and correlations. *Journal of Speech and Hearing Research*, 27, 193–196.

Starkweather, C. W., & Gottwald, S. R. (1990). The demands and capacities model II: Clinical implications. *Journal of Fluency Disorders*, 15, 143–157.

Starkweather, C. W., & Gottwald, S. R. (1993). A pilot of study of relations among specific measures obtained at intake and discharge in a program of prevention and early intervention for stuttering. *American Journal of Speech-Language Pathology*, 2(1), 51–58.

Starkweather, C. W., Gottwald, S. R., & Halfond, M. M. (1990). *Stuttering Prevention: A Clinical Method*. Englewood Cliffs, NJ: Prentice-Hall.

Starkweather, C. W., Hirshman, P., & Tannenbaum, R. S. (1976). Latency of vocalization onset: Stutterers versus nonstutterers. *Journal of Speech & Hearing Research*, 19, 481–492.

Starr, H. E. (1928). Psychological concomitants of high alveolar carbon dioxide: A psychobiochemical study of the etiology of stammering. *Psychological Clinics*, 17, 1–12.

Stern, E. (1948). A preliminary of bilingualism and stuttering in four Johannesburg schools. *Journal of Logopedics*, 1, 15–25.

Stewart, C., Evans, W. B., & Finch, J. L. (1985). Oral form perception skills of stuttering and nonstuttering children measured by stereognosis. *Journal of Fluency Disorders,* 10, 311–316.

Stewart, J. L. (1960). The problem of stuttering in certain North American Indian societies. *Journal of Speech and Hearing Disorders, Monograph 6* (Supplement).

Stewart, J. L. (1985). Stuttering Indians: A reply to Zimmermann et al. *Journal of Speech and Hearing Research,* 28, 313–315.

Stewart, T., & Grantham, C. (1993). A case of acquired stammering: The pattern of recovery. *European Journal of Disorders of Communication,* 28, 395–403.

Stigora, J. A., & DiSimoni, F. G. (1989). Resolution of opposing forces: An approach to the understanding and clinical management of stuttering. *Journal of Fluency Disorders,* 14, 293–302.

Still, A., & Griggs, S. (1979). Changes in the probability of stuttering following a stutter: A test of some recent models. *Journal of Speech and Hearing Research,* 22, 565–571.

Stocker, B. (1980). *The Stocker Probe Technique.* Tulsa, OK: Modern Education Corporation.

Stocker, B., & Gerstman, L. J. (1983). A comparison of the probe technique and conventional therapy for young stutterers. *Journal of Fluency Disorders,* 8, 331–339.

Stromsta, C. (1957). A methodology related to the determination of the phase angle of bone-conducted speech sound energy of stutterers and nonstutterers. *Speech Monographs,* 24, 147–148.

Stromsta, C. (1972). Interaural phase disparity of stutterers and nonstutterers. *Journal of Speech and Hearing Disorders,* 15, 771–787.

Studies in Tachyphemia (no date). New York: Speech Rehabilitation Institute.

Sugarman, M. (1980). It's O.K. to stutter: A personal account. *Journal of Fluency Disorders,* 5, 149–157.

Sussman, H. M., & MacNeilage, P. F. (1975). Hemispheric specialization for speech production and perception in stutterers. *Neuropsychologia,* 13, 19–26.

Szelag, E., Garwarska-Kolek, D., Herman, A., & Stasiek, J. (1993). Brain lateralization and severity of stuttering in children. *Acta Neurobiologiae Experimentalis,* 53(1), 263–267.

Tanner, D. C. (1980). Loss and grief: Implications for speech-language pathologists and audiologists. *Asha,* 22, 916–928.

Tatchell, R. H., Van Den Berg, S., & Lerman, J. W. (1983). Fluency and eye contact as factors influencing observers' perceptions of stutterers. *Journal of Fluency Disorders,* 8, 221–231.

Taylor, G. L. (1937). *An Observational Study of the Nature of Stuttering at Its Onset.* Unpublished masters thesis, University of Iowa.

Throneburg, R. N., Yairi, E., & Paden, E. P. (1994). Relation between phonologic difficulty and the occurrence of disfluencies in the early stage of stuttering. *Journal of Speech and Hearing Research, 37,* 504–509.

Thürmer, S., Thumfart, W., & Kittel, G. (1983). Elektromyographische Untersuchungsbefunde bei Stotterern. *Sprache-Stimme-Gehor, 7,* 125–127.

Tiger, R. J., Irvine, T. L., & Reis, R. P. (1980). Cluttering as a complex of learning disabilities. *Language, Speech, and Hearing Services in Schools, 11,* 3–14.

Till, J. A., Reich, A., Dickey, S., & Seiber, J. (1983). Phonatory and manual reaction times of stuttering and nonstuttering children. *Journal of Speech and Hearing Research, 26,* 171–180.

Tillis, M., & Wager, W. (1984). *Stutterin' Boy.* New York: Rawson Associates.

Tonev, P. (1994). Speech control, correction, and overcoming stuttering: A solution by Perfectly Mastered Breathing (PMB). *Journal of Fluency Disorders, 19,* 216.

Toscher, M. M., & Rupp, R. R. (1978). A study of the central auditory processes in stutterers using the Synthetic Sentence Identification (SSI) Test Battery. *Journal of Speech and Hearing Research, 21,* 779–792.

Travis, L. E. (1931). *Speech Pathology.* New York: Appleton-Century.

Travis, L. E. (1934a). Dissociation of the homologous muscle functioning in stuttering. *Archives of Neurology & Psychiatry, 31,* 127–133.

Travis, L. E. (1934b). Studies in stuttering. I. Dysintegration of breathing movements during stuttering. *Archives of Neurology and Psychiatry, 18,* 672–690.

Travis, L. E., Johnson, W., & Shover, J. (1937). The relation of bilingualism to stuttering. *Journal of Speech Disorders, 2,* 185–189.

Trotter, W. D., & Kools, J. (1955). Listener adaptation to the severity of stuttering. *Journal of Speech and Hearing Disorders, 20,* 385–387.

Trotter, W. D., & Lesch, M. M. (1967). Personal experiences with a stutter-aid. *Journal of Speech and Hearing Disorders, 32,* 270–272.

Trotter, W. D., & Silverman, F. H. (1973). Experiments with the stutter-aid. *Perceptual and Motor Skills, 36,* 1129–1130.

Trotter, W. D., & Silverman, F. H. (1974). Does the impact of pacing speech with a miniature metronome on stuttering wear off? *Perceptual and Motor Skills, 36,* 1129–1130.

Trotter, W. D., & Silverman, F. H. (1976). The stutterer as a character in contemporary literature: A bibliography. *Journal of Speech and Hearing Disorders, 41,* 553–554.

Tuck, A. E. (1979). An alaryngeal stutterer: A case history. *Journal of Fluency Disorders, 4,* 239–243.

Tudor, M. (1939). *An Experimental Study of the Effect of Evaluative Labeling on Speech Fluency.* Unpublished master's thesis, University of Iowa.

Turnbaugh, K., Guitar, B., & Hoffman, P. (1981). The attribution of personality traits. *Journal of Speech and Hearing Research, 24,* 288–291.

Tuthill, C. (1940). A quantitative study of extensional meaning with special reference to stuttering. *Journal of Speech Disorders,* 5, 189–191.

Van Lieshout, P. H. H. M., Peters, H. F. M., Starkweather, C. W., & Hulstijn, W. (1993). Physiological differences between stutterers and nonstutterers in perceptually fluent speech: EMG amplitude and duration. *Journal of Speech and Hearing Research,* 36, 55–63.

Van Riper, C. (1935). The quantitative measurements of laterality. *Journal of Experimental Psychology,* 18, 372–382.

Van Riper, C. (1936). Study of thoracic breathing of stutterers during expectancy and occurrence of stuttering spasm. *Journal of Speech Disorders,* 1, 61–72.

Van Riper, C. (1958). Experiments in stuttering therapy. In J. Eisenson (Ed.), *Stuttering: A Symposium.* New York: Harper & Brothers, 273–390.

Van Riper, C. (1970). *Historical approaches.* In J. Sheehan (Ed.), *Stuttering: Research and Therapy.* New York: Harper & Row.

Van Riper, C. (1973). *The Treatment of Stuttering.* Englewood Cliffs, NJ: Prentice-Hall.

Van Riper, C. (1975). The stutterer's clinician. In J. Eisenson (Ed.), *Stuttering: A Second Symposium.* New York: Harper & Row, 453–492.

Van Riper, C. (1979). *A Career in Speech Pathology.* Englewood Cliffs, NJ: Prentice-Hall.

Van Riper, C. (1982). *The Nature of Stuttering* (2nd ed.). Englewood Cliffs, NJ: Prentice-Hall.

Van Riper, C. (1984). Henry Freund: 1896–1982. *Journal of Fluency Disorders,* 9, 93–102.

Van Riper, C. (1992). Foreword. In F. Myers & K. O. St. Louis (Eds.), *Cluttering: A Clinical Perspective.* Leicester, England: Far Communications, vii–ix.

Vanryckeghem, M., & Brutten, G. J. (1992). The Communication Attitude Test: A test-retest reliability investigation. *Journal of Fluency Disorders,* 17, 177–190.

Wagaman, J. R., Miltenberger, R. G., & Arndorfer, R. E. (1993). Analysis of a simplified treatment for stuttering in children. *Journal of Applied Behavior Analysis,* 26(1), 53–61.

Wakaba, Y. Y. (1983). Group play therapy for Japanese children who stutter. *Journal of Fluency Disorders,* 8, 93–118.

Walker, S. T., & Walker, J. M. (1973). Differences in heart-rate variability between stutterers and nonstutterers following arousal. *Perceptual and Motor Skills,* 36, 926.

Wall, M. J. (1980). A comparison of syntax in young stutterers and nonstutterers. *Journal of Fluency Disorders,* 5, 345–352.

Walle, E. L. (1980). Masking devices and the Edinburgh Masker—Clinical applications within a prison setting. *Journal of Fluency Disorders,* 5, 69–74.

Wallen, V. (1961). Primary stuttering in a 28-year-old adult. *Journal of Speech and Hearing Disorders,* 26, 393–395.

Walton, D., & Mather, M. D. (1963). The relevance of generalization techniques to the treatment of stammering and phobic symptoms. *Behavior Research and Therapy,* 1, 121–125.

Ward, D. (1992). Outlining semi-intensive fluency therapy. *Journal of Fluency Disorders,* 17, 243–255.

Waterloo, K. K., & Gotestam, K. G. (1988). The regulated-breathing method for stuttering: An experimental evaluation. *Journal of Behavior Therapy and Experimental Psychiatry,* 19, 11–19.

Watson, B. C., Freeman, F. J., Chapman, S. B., Miller, S., Finitzo, T., Pool, K. D., & Devous, M. D. (1991). Linguistic performance deficits in stutterers: Relation to Laryngeal Reaction Time profiles. *Journal of Fluency Disorders,* 16, 85–100.

Watson, B. C., Freeman, F. J., Devous, M. D., Chapman, T. F., Finitzo, T., & Pool, K. D. (1994). Linguistic performance and regional cerebral blood flow in persons who stutter. *Journal of Speech and Hearing Research,* 37, 1221–1228.

Watson, J. B. (1987). Profiles of stutterers' and nonstutterers' affective, cognitive, and behavioral communication attitudes. *Journal of Fluency Disorders,* 12, 389–405.

Watson, J. B. (1988). A comparison of stutterers' and nonstutterers' affective, cognitive, and behavioral self-reports. *Journal of Speech and Hearing Research,* 31, 377–385.

Watson, J. B., Gregory, H. H., & Kistler, D. J. (1987). Development and evaluation of an inventory to assess adult stutterers' communication attitudes. *Journal of Fluency Disorders,* 12, 429–450.

Watson, P., & Guitar, B. (1986). Respiratory stuttering? A case history. *Journal of Fluency Disorders,* 11, 165–173.

Watts, F. (1971). The treatment of stammering by the intensive practice of fluent speech. *British Journal of Disorders of Communication,* 6, 144–147.

Webster, L. M. (1977). A clinical note on psychotherapy for stuttering. *Journal of Fluency Disorders,* 2, 253–255.

Webster, R. L. (1974). A behavioral analysis of stuttering: Treatment and theory. In K. S. Calhoun, H. E. Adams, & K. M. Mitchell (Eds.), *Innovative Treatment Methods in Psychopathology.* New York: Wiley.

Webster, R. L. (1979). Empirical considerations regarding stuttering therapy. In H. H. Gregory (Ed.), *Controversies About Stuttering Therapy.* Baltimore: University Park Press, 209–239.

Webster, R. L. (1980). Evolution of a target-based behavioral therapy for stuttering. *Journal of Fluency Disorders,* 5, 303–320.

Webster, R. L. (1986). Stuttering therapy from a technological point of view. In D. H. Shames & H. Rubin (Eds.), *Stuttering Then and Now.* Columbus, OH: Charles E. Merrill, pp. 407–414.

Webster, W. G. (1985). Neuropsychological models of stuttering—I. Representation of sequential response mechanisms. *Neuropsychologia,* 23, 263–267.

Webster, W. G., (1986). Response sequence organization and reproduction by stutterers. *Neuropsychologia,* 24, 813–821.

Webster, W. G. (1989). Sequence reproduction deficits in stutterers tested under nonspeeded response conditions. *Journal of Fluency Disorders,* 14, 79–86.

Wedberg, C. F. (1956). *The Stutterer Speaks.* Magnolia, MA: The Expression Company.

Weinberg, B. (1964). Stuttering among blind and partially sighted children. *Journal of Speech and Hearing Disorders,* 29, 322–326.

Weiner, A. (1981). A case of adult onset of stuttering. *Journal of Fluency Disorders,* 6, 181–185.

Weiss, A. L., & Zebrowski, P. M. (1992). Disfluencies in the conversations of young children who stutter: Some answers about questions. *Journal of Speech and Hearing Research,* 35, 1230–1238.

Weiss, A. L., & Zebrowski, P. M. (1994). The narrative production of children who stutter: A preliminary view. *Journal of Fluency Disorders,* 19, 39–63.

Weiss, D. A. (1964). *Cluttering.* Englewood Cliffs, NJ: Prentice-Hall.

Weiss, D. A. (1967). Similarities and differences between cluttering and stuttering. *Folia Phoniatrica,* 19, 98–104.

Wells, G. B. (1983). A feature analysis of stuttered phonemes. *Journal of Fluency Disorders,* 8, 119–124.

West, R. (1958). An agnostic's speculations about stuttering. In J. Eisenson (Ed.), *Stuttering: A Symposium.* New York: Harper & Brothers, 167–222.

West, R., & Ansberry, M. (1968). *The Rehabilitation of Speech* (4th ed.). New York: Harper & Row.

West, R., Kennedy, L., & Carr, A. (1947). *The Rehabilitation of Speech* (Rev. ed.). New York: Harper & Brothers.

West, R., Nelson, S., & Berry, M. (1939). The heredity of stuttering. *Quarterly Journal of Speech,* 25, 23–30.

Westby, C. E. (1979). Language performance of stuttering and nonstuttering children. *Journal of Communication Disorders,* 12, 133–145.

Wexler, K. B. (1982). Developmental disfluency in 2-, 4-, and 6-year-old boys in neutral and stress situations. *Journal of Speech and Hearing Research,* 25, 229–234.

Whitney, J. L., and Goldstein, H. (1989). Using self-monitoring to reduce disfluencies in speakers with mild aphasia. *Journal of Speech and Hearing Disorders,* 54, 576–586.

Williams, D. E. (1955). Masseter muscle action potentials in stuttered and nonstuttered speech. *Journal of Speech and Hearing Disorders,* 20, 242–261.

Williams, D. E. (1957). A point of view about "stuttering." *Journal of Speech and Hearing Disorders,* 22, 390–397.

Williams, D. E. (1968). Stuttering therapy: An overview. In H. H. Gregory (Ed.), *Learning Theory and Stuttering Therapy.* Evanston, IL: Northwestern University Press, 52–66.

Williams, D. E. (1978). The stuttering problem. In F. L. Darley & D. C. Spriesters-bach (Eds.), *Diagnostic Methods in Speech Pathology.* New York: Harper & Row, 65–72.

Williams, D. E. (1979). A perspective on approaches to stuttering therapy. In H. H. Gregory (Ed.), *Controversies About Stuttering Therapy.* Baltimore: University Park Press, pp. 241–268.

Williams, D. E. (1982). Stuttering therapy: Where are we going—and why? *Journal of Fluency Disorders, 7,* 159–170.

Williams, D. E., & Kent, L. R. (1958). Listener evaluations of speech interruptions. *Journal of Speech and Hearing Research, 1,* 124–131.

Williams, D. E., Melrose, B. M., & Woods, C. L. (1969). The relationship between stuttering and academic achievement in children. *Journal of Communication Disorders, 2,* 87–98.

Williams, D. E., & Silverman, F. H. (1968). Note concerning articulation of school-age stutterers. *Perceptual and Motor Skills, 27,* 713–714.

Williams, D. E., Silverman, F. H., & Kools, J. A. (1968). Disfluency behavior of elementary school stutterers and nonstutterers: The adaptation effect. *Journal of Speech and Hearing Research, 11,* 622–630.

Williams, D. E., Silverman, F. H., & Kools, J. A. (1969a). Disfluency behavior of elementary school stutterers and nonstutterers: The Consistency Effect. *Journal of Speech and Hearing Research, 12,* 301–307.

Williams, D. E., Silverman, F. H., & Kools, J. A. (1969b). Disfluency behavior of elementary school stutterers and nonstutterers: Loci of instances of disfluency. *Journal of Speech and Hearing Research, 12,* 308–318.

Williams, D. F., & Brutten, G. J. (1994). Physiologic and aerodynamic events prior to the speech of stutterers and nonstutterers. *Journal of Fluency Disorders, 19,* 83–111.

Wingate, M. E. (1964). A standard definition of stuttering. *Journal of Speech and Hearing Disorders, 29,* 484–489.

Wingate, M. E. (1976). *Stuttering: Theory and Treatment.* New York: Irvington Publishers.

Wingate, M. E. (1981a). Knowing what to look for: Comments on stuttering identification—standard definition and moments of stuttering. *Journal of Speech and Hearing Research, 24,* 622–623.

Wingate, M. E. (1981b). Questionnaire study of laryngectomee stutterers. *Journal of Fluency Disorders, 6,* 273–281.

Wingate, M. E. (1981c). Sound and pattern in artificial fluency: Spectographic evidence. *Journal of Fluency Disorders, 6,* 95–118.

Wingate, M. E. (1982). Early position and stuttering occurrence. *Journal of Fluency Disorders, 7,* 243–258.

Wingate, M. E. (1984a). Fluency, disfluency, dysfluency, and stuttering. *Journal of Fluency Disorders, 9,* 163–168.

Wingate, M. E. (1984b). Pause loci in stuttered and normal speech. *Journal of Fluency Disorders*, 9, 227–235.

Wingate, M. E. (1984c). A rational management of stuttering. In M. Peins (Ed.), *Contemporary Approaches to Stuttering Therapy*. Boston: Little, Brown.

Wingate, M. E. (1986a). Adaptation, consistency and beyond: I. Limitations and contradictions. *Journal of Fluency Disorders*, 11, 1–36.

Wingate, M. E. (1986b). Adaptation, consistency and beyond: II. An integral account. *Journal of Fluency Disorders*, 11, 37–53.

Wingate, M. E. (1987). Fluency and disfluency: Illusion and identification. *Journal of Fluency Disorders*, 12, 79–101.

Wingate, M. E. (1988). *The Structure of Stuttering: A Psycholinguistic Analysis*. New York: Springer-Verlag.

Winkelman, C. (1994). Treatment of the cluttering component in stuttering behavior. *Journal of Fluency Disorders*, 19, 220.

Winkler, L. E., & Ramig, P. (1986). Temporal characteristics in the fluent speech of child stutterers and nonstutterers. *Journal of Fluency Disorders*, 11, 217–229.

Witt, H. M. (1925). Statistische Erhebungen über den Einfluss des Singens und Flusterns auf das stottern. *Vox*, 11, 41–43.

Wolk, L., Edwards, M. L., & Conture, E. G. (1993). Coexistence of stuttering and disordered phonology in young children. *Journal of Speech and Hearing Research*, 36, 906–917.

Wolpe, J. (1958). *Psychotherapy by Reciprocal Inhibition*. Stanford, CA: Stanford University Press.

Wolpe, J. (1969). Behavior therapy in stuttering: Deconditioning the emotional factor. In B. Gray and G. England (Eds.), *Stuttering and the Conditioning Therapies*. Monterey, CA: The Monterey Institute for Speech and Hearing, 15–27.

Wolpe, J., & Lazarus, A. A. (1966). *Behavior Therapy Techniques: A Guide to the Treatment of Neurosis*. New York: Pergamon Press.

Woods, C. L., & Williams, D. E. (1976). Traits attributed to stuttering and normally fluent males. *Journal of Speech and Hearing Research*, 19, 267–278.

World Health Organization (1977). *Manual of the International Statistical Classification of Diseases, Injuries, and Causes of Death* (Vol. 1). Geneva: World Health Organization.

Wyatt, G. L. (1969). *Language Learning and Communication Disorders in Children*. New York: Free Press.

Yairi, E. (1981). Disfluencies of normally speaking two-year-old children. *Journal of Speech and Hearing Research*, 24, 490–495.

Yairi, E. (1982). Longitudinal studies of disfluencies in two-year-old children. *Journal of Speech and Hearing Research*, 25, 155–160.

Yairi, E. (1990). Subtyping child stutterers for research purposes. *ASHA Reports* (Number 18), 50–57.

Yairi, E. (1993). Epidemiologic and other considerations in treatment efficacy research with preschool age children who stutter. *Journal of Fluency Disorders*, 18, 197–219.

Yairi, E., & Ambrose, N. (1992a). Early childhood stuttering: Pediatricians' attitudes and practices. *American Journal of Speech-Language Pathology,* 1(3), 54–62.

Yairi, E., & Ambrose, N. (1992b). A longitudinal study of stuttering in children: A preliminary report. *Journal of Speech and Hearing Research,* 35, 755–760.

Yairi, E., & Ambrose, N. (1992c). Onset of stuttering in preschool children: Selected factors. *Journal of Speech and Hearing Research,* 35, 782–788.

Yairi, E., Ambrose, N., & Niermann, R. (1993). The early months of stuttering: A developmental study. *Journal of Speech and Hearing Research,* 36, 521–528.

Yairi, E., & Clifton, N. F., Jr. (1972). Disfluent speech behavior of preschool children, high school seniors, and geriatric persons. *Journal of Speech and Hearing Research,* 15, 714–719.

Yairi, E., & Lewis, B. (1984). Disfluencies at the onset of stuttering. *Journal of Speech and Hearing Research,* 27, 154–159.

Yaruss, J. S., & Conture, E. G. (1993). F2 transitions during sound/syllable repetitions of children who stutter and predictions of stuttering chronicity. *Journal of Speech and Hearing Research,* 36, 883–896.

Yoss, K. A., & Darley, F. L. (1974). Developmental apraxia of speech in children with defective articulation. *Journal of Speech and Hearing Research,* 17, 399–416.

Young, M. A. (1985). Increasing the frequency of stuttering. *Journal of Speech and Hearing Research,* 28, 282–293.

Yovetich, W. S. (1984). Message therapy: Language approach to stuttering therapy with children. *Journal of Fluency Disorders,* 9, 11–20.

Zebrowski, P. M. (1994). Duration of sound prolongation and sound/syllable repetition in children who stutter: Preliminary observations. *Journal of Speech and Hearing Research,* 37, 254–263.

Zebrowski, P. M., & Conture, E. (1989). Judgments of disfluency by mothers of stuttering and normally fluent children. *Journal of Speech and Hearing Research,* 32, 307–317.

Zebrowski, P. M., & Schum, R. L. (1993). Counseling parents of children who stutter. *American Journal of Speech-Language Pathology,* 2(2), 65–73.

Zimmermann, G. N. (1980). Stuttering: A disorder of movement. *Journal of Speech and Hearing Research,* 23, 122–136.

Zimmermann, G. N., & Hanley, J. M. (1983). A cinefluorographic investigation of repeated fluent productions of stutterers in an adaptation procedure. *Journal of Speech and Hearing Research,* 26, 35–42.

Zimmermann, G. N., Liljeblad, S., Frank, A., & Cleeland, C. (1983). The Indians have many terms for it: Stuttering among the Bannock-Shoshoni. *Journal of Speech and Hearing Research,* 26, 315–318.

Zimmermann, G. N., Smith, A., & Hanley, J. M. (1981). Stuttering: In need of a unifying conceptual framework. *Journal of Speech and Hearing Research,* 24, 25–31.

Author Index

Heilman, K. M., 219, 288
Helm, N. A., 219, 223, 293
Helm-Estabrooks, N. A., 219, 220, 222, 223, 293
Heltman, H. J., 57, 293
Henschen, T. L., 226, 293
Herbrich, K. E., 61, 127, 306
Herman, A., 320
Herodotus, 10, 11, 293
Herrick, L. C., 104, 293
Hertrich, I., 219, 293
Hess, K. R., 61, 306
Hicks, D. M., 48, 301
Hill, D., 181, 291
Hill, H., 54, 57, 293
Hillis, J. W., 203, 209, 293
Hilton, L. M., 48, 306
Hinzman, A. R., 62, 76, 212, 213, 214, 219, 163, 318
Hippocrates, 293
Hirshman, P., 61, 319
Hoddinott, S., 276
Hoepfner, T., 80, 293
Hoffman, P., 68, 321
Hood, S. B., 42, 59, 62, 275, 278, 299
Hoops, R., 150, 294
Horii, Y., 41, 294
Horlick, R. S., 67, 294
Horner, J., 219, 294
Horovitz, L. J., 62, 63, 294
Horsburgh, G., 37, 157, 295
Howe, S. W., 62, 286
Howie, P., 10, 35, 107, 202, 203, 276, 279, 294
Hoyt, B. D., 61, 127, 306
Hubbard, C. P., 33, 34, 39, 41, 129, 294, 309, 310
Hulit, L. M., 6, 25, 41, 294
Hull, F. M., 212, 213, 219, 318
Hull, H. C., 67, 281
Hulstijn, W., 28, 49, 308, 322
Hummer, K., 211, 225, 317
Hunt, H., 10, 12, 17, 294
Hurst, M., 28, 206, 284, 294
Hutchins, L., 203, 307
Hutchinson, J. M., 49, 294

Ingham, J. C., 187, 188, 295
Ingham, R. J., 2, 5, 18, 27, 28, 36, 37, 39, 101, 129, 157, 187, 170, 189, 190, 193, 202, 209, 276, 284, 288, 295, 307
Irvine, T. L., 212, 218, 219, 321
Irving, R. W., 227, 295
Irwin, J., 121, 296
Izedebski, K., 226, 275

Jacobson, E., 41, 186, 192, 296
James, J. E., 39, 296
Jäncke, L., 61, 296
Janssen, P., 55, 298
Jayaram, M., 32, 296
Jensen, P. H., 63, 296
Johannsen, H. S., 54, 60, 296
Jordahl, N., 48, 61, 292
Jerger, J., 62, 163, 291
Jescheniak, J.-D., 76, 306
Johnson, G. F., 170, 183, 202, 296
Johnson, L., 36, 38, 302, 303, 308
Johnson, S. B., 62, 63, 294
Johnson, W., 1, 2, 3, 18, 19, 21, 23, 24, 26, 27, 28, 29, 30, 34, 35, 36, 38, 41, 44, 47, 49, 57, 64, 65, 67, 69, 70, 73, 75, 78, 79, 80, 81, 82, 87, 88, 92, 94, 104, 105, 108, 111, 114, 116, 117, 122, 125, 139, 140, 151, 153, 159, 177, 178, 181, 182, 184, 196, 205, 209, 275, 296, 297, 298, 321
Johnston, S. J., 56, 297
Jones, B. P., 59, 312
Jones, R., 59, 223, 297
Juhl, P., 191, 302

Kalinowski, J., 38, 176, 188, 287, 297
Kalinowski, L. S., 72, 74, 162, 264, 297
Kalotkin, M., 193, 312
Kamel, M., 65, 307
Kamhi, A. G., 40, 202, 203, 297
Kampman, K., 193, 297
Karlin, I. W., 57, 297
Katsovskaia, I. I. K., 123, 297
Katz, J., 193, 287
Katz, L., 65, 67, 163, 297
Katz, M., 13, 297

Subject Index

Abstract thinking, capacity for, 65
Academic achievement (*see* Educational achievement)
Achievement drive, 65
Action potentials, 54
Acupuncture, 193
Adaptation effect, 41–42, 44–45, 221, 225
Adjacency effect, 34
Aesop, 7
Aggression, 65, 113, 145
Agoraphobia, 133
Alone, speaking while, 38
American Academy of Speech Correction (*see* American Speech-Language-Hearing Association)
American Indians, 106, 115
American Method (*see* Yates)
American Speech-Language-Hearing Association, 17, 164, 201
Amino acids, 57
Amman, 17
Anal eroticism, 65, 113
Anger, 69, 113, 142, 194
Animals, speaking to, 38
Anoxia, 220
"Answerable" questions, 139–140, 141
Anticipation of stuttering (*see* Expectancy phenomenon)
Anticipatory-struggle hypotheses (*see* Stuttering)
Anxiety, 6, 55, 60, 65, 71–72, 73, 111, 199–202
Aphasia, 221
Approach-avoidance conflict, 113 (*see also* Stuttering)

Apraxia, 107, 143
Arapesh tribe, 106
Aristotle, 7, 11
Arnott, 17
Art therapy, 182
Arthur the Young Rat, 154, 245
Articulation errors, 76, 213, 214
Articulatory musculature, 49
Aspiration, level of, 65
Assertiveness, 145, 149, 175, 201
Assessment (*see* Evaluation)
Assignments, 25–26, 51, 77, 96, 135, 168, 209–210, 232
Attitude toward disorder, 44
Audience size, 44
Auditory functioning (*see* Hearing)
Auditory perception (*see* Hearing)
Auditory system (*see* Hearing)
Auditory tracking, 60
Australian aborigines, 106
Authority figures, speaking to, 43
Autonomic nervous system functioning, 52, 45, 55, 61–62
Auto-suggestion, 41
Avocations, choice of, 6
Avoidance strategies (*see* Stuttering)

Barton, Clara, 7
Basal metabolic rate, 56
Bates, 13
Battus, 10
Bell Adjustment Inventory, 66
Bell, Alexander, Graham, 17
Bell, Alexander Melville, 17
Bernrueter Personality Inventory, 66